G.K. Krieglstein

Glaucoma Update VI

Springer-Verlag Berlin Heidelberg GmbH

G. K. Krieglstein

Glaucoma Update VI

With 41 Figures

Springer

Glaucoma Society of the International Congress of Ophthalmology
Edingburgh/Scotland, June 1998

Professor Dr. G.K. Krieglstein
Universitäts-Augenklinik
Josef-Stelzmann-Straße 9
50931 Köln

ISBN 978-3-642-62985-3 ISBN 978-3-642-57056-8 (eBook)
DOI 10.1007/978-3-642-57056-8

Die Deutsche Bibliothek - CIP-Einheitsaufnahme
Glaucoma update ... - Berlin ; Heidelberg ; New York ; Barcelona ; Hongkong ; London ; Mailand ; Paris ; Singapur ; Tokio : Springer
ISSN 1430-631X

Vol. 6. - (2000) -

Originally published by Springer-Verlag Berlin Heidelberg in 2000
Softcover reprint of the hardcover 1st edition 2000

Production: PRO EDIT GmbH, D-69126 Heidelberg, Germany
Cover design: d & p, D-69121 Heidelberg
Typesetting: Mitterweger Werksatz, 68723 Plankstadt, Germany
SPIN: 10665454 24/3135-5 4 3 2 1 0 - Printed on acid-free paper

Preface

On 14–18 June 1998, the closed meeting of the Glaucoma Society of the International Congress of Ophthalmology was held in Edinburgh, Scotland. Following tradition, the meeting preceded the International Congress of Ophthalmology and was attended by the members of the society and invited guests. The structure of the scientific program and the local organization was in the hands of Roger Hitchings, London. The aim of the meeting was to exchange information regarding the latest progress in worldwide glaucoma research - basic aspects as well as clinical applications - with ample discussion time between the individual scientific presentations. The number of attendees was limited to favor a maximum amount of discussion.

Glaucoma Update VI comprises the scientific presentations of this meeting now available for everyone interested in glaucoma research and its clinical use to improve the care of our patients.

The society is indebted to both Pharmacia and Upjohn, Germany, for supporting the printing expenses of this proceeding volume so generously, and Springer Verlag, Heidelberg, for printing in a timely fashion.

Günter K. Krieglstein, MD

Executive Committee of the Glaucoma Society of the International Congress of Ophthalmology

Contents

Visual Function

Normal Pressure Glaucoma

Surgery I

Surgery II

Surgery III

Contributors

H. ABE
Department of Ophthalmology Niigata University, School of Medicine, 1-757, Asahimachi-dori, Niigata, 951-8510, Japan

P. J. AIRAKSINEN
Department of Ophthalmology, University of Oulu, SF-90220 Oulu 22, Finland

H. I. ALANKO
Department of Ophthalomology, University of Oulu, SF-90220 Oulu, Finland

R. R. ALLINGHAM
Duke University Eye Center, Duke University Medical Center, Box 3802, Erwin Rd. Durham, NC 27710, USA

W. L. M. ALWARD
Department of Ophthalmology, College of Medicine, The University of Iowa, 200 Hawkins Drive, Iowa City, Iowa 52242, USA

M. ARAIE
Department of Ophthalmology, University of Tokyo School of Medicine, 7-3-1, Hongo, Bunkyo-ku, Tokyo, 113-8655, Japan

I. AZUMA
Department of Ophthalmology, Osaka Medical College, Takatsuki, Osaka, Japan

K.-U. BARTZ-SCHMIDT
Division of Vitreo-retinal Surgery, Department of Ophthalmology, University of Cologne, Germany

M. BATTERBURY
University Of Liverpool, St Pauls Eye Unit, Liverpool, UK

A. Béchetoille
Ophtalmologie, Centre Hospitalier Universitaire d'Angers,
F-49033 Angers cedex 01, France

B. Becker
Department of Ophthalmology and Visual Science,
Washington University Medical School, St. Louis, MO, USA

B. Bengtsson
Department of Ophthalmology, Malmö University Hospital,
Malmö, Sweden

M. Berkani
Glaucoma Institute, Saint-Joseph Hospital Foundation, Paris, France

C. F. Bosworth
Visual Function Laboratory and Glaucoma Center,
Department of Ophthalmology, University of California at San Diego

H. Bresson-Dumont
Ophtalmologie, Centre Hospitalier Universitaire d'Angers,
F-49033 Angers cedex 01, France

B. Broomer
Duke University Eye Center, Duke University Medical Center, Box 3802,
Erwin Rd. Durham, NC 27710, USA

W. M. Budde
Department of Ophthalmology and Eye Hospital,
University Erlangen-Nürnberg, Germany

N. Calixto
Glaucoma Service, São Geraldo Eye Hospital,
Federal University of Minas Gerais, Belo Horizonte, Brazil

C. B. Camras
Department of Ophthalmology, University of Nebraska Medical Center,
Omaha, NE, USA

Y. C. Chen
Department of Ophthalmology, National Taiwan University Hospital,
#7, Chung-Shan South Road, Taipei 100, Taiwan

P. T. K. Chew
Department of Ophthalmology, National University Hospital, Singapore

G. A. Cioffi
Devers Eye Institute, Portland, Oregon

S. Cronemberger
Glaucoma Service, São Geraldo Eye Hospital, Federal University of Minas Gerais, Belo Horizonte, Brazil

L. Daugeliene
Department of Ophthalmology, Gifu University School of Medicine, 40 Tsukasa-machi, Gifu-shi, Japan, 500-8705

M. A. de la Paz
Duke University Eye Center, Duke University Medical Center, Box 3802, Erwin Rd. Durham, NC 27710, USA

E. A. Del Bono
New England Medical Center, Boston, MA, USA

P. Demailly
Glaucoma Institute, Saint-Joseph Hospital Foundation, Paris, France

J. G. Devereux
Singapore National Eye Centre and Singapore Eye Research Institute, Singapore

C. A. Downs
Department of Ophthalmology, The University of Michigan, W. K. Kellogg Eye Center, 1000 Wall Street, Ann Arbor, Michigan, USA

J. H. Fingert
Department of Ophthalmology, College of Medicine, The University of Iowa, 200 Hawkins Drive, Iowa City, Iowa 52242, USA

A. Floyd
University Of Liverpool, St Pauls Eye Unit, Liverpool, UK

P. J Foster
Singapore National Eye Centre and Singapore Eye Research Institute, Singapore

B. T. Gabelt
Department of Ophthalmology and Visual Sciences, University of Wisconsin, Madison, WI 53792-3220, USA

D. D. Gaton
The Glaucoma Center, University of California San Diego, 9500 Cilman Drive, La Jolla, California 92093-0946, USA

S. J. GEDDE
Department of Ophthalmology, University of Miami School of Medicine, Miami, Florida, USA

B. GEIGER
Department of Molecular Cell Biology, Weizmann Institute of Science, Rehovot, Israel 76100

A. GEMPERLI
Department of Ophthalmology and Visual Sciences University of Illinois College of Medicine, Chicago, Illinois, USA

E. GRAMER
Universitäts-Augenklinik Würzburg, Josef-Schneider-Str. 11, D-97080 Würzburg, Germany

F. GREHN
Universitäts-Augenklinik Würzburg, Josef-Schneider-Str. 11, D-97080 Würzburg, Germany

I. GRIERSON
University Of Liverpool, St Pauls Eye Unit, Liverpool, UK

J. L. HAINES
Vanderbilt University, Nashville, TN, USA

S. HASEGAWA
Department of Ophthalmology Niigata University, School of Medicine, 1-757, Asahimachi-dori, Niigata, 951-8510, Japan

N. HAYASHI
Department of Ophthalmology, Gifu University School of Medicine, 40 Tsukasa-machi, Gifu-shi, Gifu, 500 Japan

S. S. HAYREH
Department of Ophthalmology and Visual Sciences, University Hospitals & Clinics, College of Medicine, University of Iowa, 200 Hawkins Drive, Iowa City, Iowa 52242-1091, USA

A. HEIJL
Department of Ophthalmology, Malmö University Hospital, Malmö, Sweden

K. HEIMANN
Division of Vitreo-retinal Surgery, Department of Ophthalmology, University of Cologne, Germany

D. K. Heuer
Department of Ophthalmology, Medical College of Wisconsin, Milwaukee, Wisconsin, USA

H. D. Hoskins
Clinical Professor of Ophthalmology,
University of California School of Medicine - San Francisco,
655 Beach Street, San Francisco CA 94109 USA

P. T. Hung
Department of Ophthalmology, National Taiwan University Hospital, #7, Chung-Shan South Road, Taipei 100, Taiwan

P. Hyytinen
Department of Ophthalomology, University of Oulu, SF-90220 Oulu, Finland

K. Ishida
Department of Ophthalmology, Gifu University School of Medicine, 40 Tsukasa-machi, Gifu-shi, Japan, 500-8705

H. Ishikawa
The Ocular Imaging Center, The New York Eye and Ear Infirmary, 310 East 14th Street, New York, NY 10003, USA

A. T. Johnson
Department of Ophthalmology, College of Medicine,
The University of Iowa, 200 Hawkins Drive, Iowa City, Iowa 52242, USA

J. Jonas
Universitäts-Augenklinik, Schwabachanlage 6, D-91054 Erlangen, Germany

K. H. Jones
Duke University Eye Center, Duke University Medical Center, Box 3802, Erwin Rd. Durham, NC 27710, USA

A. Juutinen
Department of Ophthalomology, University of Oulu, SF-90220 Oulu, Finland

K. Kashiwagi
The Glaucoma Center, University of California San Diego, 9500 Cilman Drive, La Jolla, California 92093-0946, USA

P. L. Kaufman
Department of Ophthalmology and Visual Sciences,
University of Wisconsin, Madison, WI 53792-3220, USA

J. Kern
New England Medical Center, Boston, MA, USA

P. T. Khaw
Institute of Ophthalmology and Moorfields Eye Hospital, London, England

B. Kirchhof
Department of Ophthalmology, University of Aachen (RWTH), Pauwelsstrasse 30, 52057 Aachen, Germany

Y. Kitazawa
Department of Ophthalmology, Gifu University School of Medicine, 40 Tsukasa-machi, Gifu-shi, Japan, 500–8705

G. K. Krieglstein
University of Cologne, Department of Ophthalmology, Division Glaucoma Service (Universitäts-Augenklinik), Joseph-Stelzmann-Straße 9, 50931 Köln, Germany

Y. H. Kwon
Department of Ophthalmology, College of Medicine, The University of Iowa, 200 Hawkins Drive, Iowa City, Iowa 52242, USA

Y. Lachkar
Glaucoma Institute, Saint-Joseph Hospital Foundation, Paris, France

P. J. Lang
Department of Ophthalmology and Eye Hospital, University Erlangen-Nürnberg, Germany

B. L. Lee
Visual Function Laboratory and Glaucoma Center, Department of Ophthalmology, University of California at San Diego

P.-Y. Lee
Department of Ophthalmology, Box 1183, Mount Sinai School of Medicine, One Gustave L. Levy Place, New York, NY 10029, USA

P. R. Lichter
Department of Ophthalmology, The University of Michigan, W. K. Kellogg Eye Center, 1000 Wall Street, Ann Arbor, Michigan, USA

J. M. Liebmann
The Ocular Imaging Center, The New York Eye and Ear Infirmary, 310 East 14th Street, New York, NY 10003, USA

J. D. Lindsey
The Glaucoma Center, University of California San Diego,
9500 Cilman Drive, La Jolla, California 92093–0946, USA

C. G. Machado
Department of Ophthalmology, University of São Paulo,
Av. São Gualter 99 05455–000, São Paulo, Brazil

A. Mandahl
Pharmacia and Upjohn Company, Uppsala, Sweden

T. Mittag
Department of Ophthalmology, Box 1183,
Mount Sinai School of Medicine, One Gustave L. Levy Place,
New York, NY 10029, USA

K. Muta
Department of Ophthalmology, University of Tokyo School of Medicine, 7–3–1, Hongo, Bunkyo-ku, Tokyo, 113–8655, Japan

S. Nagasubramanian
Glaucoma Unit, Moorfields Eye Hospital, London, United Kingdom

A. Nelson
University Of Liverpool, St Pauls Eye Unit, Liverpool, UK

G. Nelson
Department of Ophthalmology
and Visual Sciences University of Illinois College of Medicine,
Chicago, Illinois, USA

F. T. S. Oen
Singapore National Eye Centre and Singapore Eye Research Institute,
Singapore

A. Ohinmaa
Department of Economics, University of Oulu, Oulu, Finland

H. Oku
Department of Ophthalmology, Osaka Medical College, Takatsuki,
Osaka, Japan

A. Ooshima
Department of Ophthalmology Niigata University, School of Medicine,
1–757, Asahimachi-dori, Niigata, 951–8510, Japan

R. K. Parrish II
Department of Ophthalmology,
University of Miami School of Medicine, Miami, Florida, USA

K. Patterson
New England Medical Center, Boston, MA, USA

J. S. Perez
Visual Function Laboratory and Glaucoma Center,
Department of Ophthalmology, University of California at San Diego

M. A. Pericak-Vance
Duke University Eye Center, Duke University Medical Center,
Box 3802, Erwin Rd. Durham, NC 27710, USA

J. A. Peterson
Department of Ophthalmology and Visual Sciences,
University of Wisconsin, Madison, WI 53792-3220, USA

B. L. Petrig
Institut de Recherche en Ophtalmologie, Sion, Switzerland

B. L. Petrig
Scheie Eye Institute, University of Pennsylvania, Philadelphia

S. M. Podos
Department of Ophthalmology, Box 1183,
Mount Sinai School of Medicine, One Gustave L. Levy Place,
New York, NY 10029, USA

R. Polk
Glaucoma Service, Doheny Eye Institute,
University of Southern California School of Medicine,
1450 San Pablo Street, Los Angeles, CA 9003, USA

J. Rhodes
University Of Liverpool, St Pauls Eye Unit, Liverpool, UK

J. E. Richards
Department of Ophthalmology, The University of Michigan,
W. K. Kellogg Eye Center, 1000 Wall Street, Ann Arbor, Michigan, USA

R. Ritch
Glaucoma Service, Department of Ophthalmology,
The New York Eye and Ear Infirmary,
310 East 14th Street, New York, NY 10003, USA

C. E. Riva
Institut de Recherche en Ophtalmologie, Sion, Switzerland

C. E. Riva
Scheie Eye Institute, University of Pennsylvania, Philadelphia, USA

C. E. Riva
University of Lausanne, Switzerland

F. W. Rozsa
Department of Ophthalmology, The University of Michigan,
W. K. Kellogg Eye Center, 1000 Wall Street, Ann Arbor, Michigan, USA

T. Sagara
The Glaucoma Center, University of California San Diego,
9500 Cilman Drive, La Jolla, California 92093-0946, USA

J. R. Sampaolesi
University of Buenos Aires, Parana 1239-1A, 1018 Buenos Aires, Argentina

R. Sampaolesi
University of Buenos Aires, Parana 1239-1A, 1018 Buenos Aires, Argentina

P. A. Sample
Department of Ophthalmology, 9500 Gilman Dr., La Jolla, California, 92093-0946, USA

R. A. Schumer
Department of Ophthalmology, Mt. Sinai School of Medicine, New York, NY, USA

S. K. L. Seah
Singapore National Eye Centre and Singapore Eye Research Institute, Singapore

J. B. Serle
Department of Ophthalmology, Box 1183,
Mount Sinai School of Medicine, One Gustave L. Levy Place,
New York, NY 10029, USA

V. C. Sheffield
Department of Pediatrics, College of Medicine
and the Howard Hughes Medical Institute, The University of Iowa,
200 Hawkins Drive, Iowa City, Iowa 52242, USA

S. Shimizu
Department of Ophthalmology, The University of Michigan,
W. K. Kellogg Eye Center, 1000 Wall Street, Ann Arbor, Michigan, USA

S. Shirato
Department of Ophthalmology, Hachiohji Medical Center,
Tokyo Medical University, 1163 Tatemachi, Hachiohji,
Tokyo 193-8639, Japan

G. L. Spaeth
Glaucoma Service, Wills Eye Hospital, Jefferson Medical College,
900 Walnut St, Philadelphia, PA 19107 Pennsylvania

E. M. Stone
Department of Ophthalmology, College of Medicine,
The University of Iowa, 200 Hawkins Drive, Iowa City, Iowa 52242, USA

P. Sullivan
Devers Eye Institute, Portland, Oregon

R. Susanna Jr
Department of Ophthalmology, University of São Paulo,
Av. São Gualter 99 05455-000, São Paulo, Brazil

Y. Suzuki
Department of Ophthalmology,
University of Tokyo School of Medicine, Tokyo, Japan

R. Takada
Department of Ophthalmology Niigata University, School of Medicine,
1-757, Asahimachi-dori, Niigata, 951-8510, Japan

M. Takagi
Department of Ophthalmology Niigata University, School of Medicine,
1-757, Asahimachi-dori, Niigata, 951-8510, Japan

D. A. Tallett
Duke University Eye Center, Duke University Medical Center,
Box 3802, Erwin Rd. Durham, NC 27710, USA

F. Taniguchi
Department of Ophthalmology,
University of Tokyo School of Medicine,
Tokyo, Japan

A. Tawara
Department of Ophthalmology, Wakayama Medical College, Wakayama, Japan

C. Tebbs
University Of Liverpool, St Pauls Eye Unit, Liverpool, UK

P. Teesalu
Department of Ophthalmology, University of Tartu, Estonia

H. Thiele
Universitäts-Augenklinik Würzburg, Josef-Schneider-Str. 11, D-97080 Würzburg, Germany

B. Tian
Department of Ophthalmology and Visual Sciences, University of Wisconsin, Madison, WI 53792-3220, USA

G. Tomita
Department of Ophthalmology, Gifu University School of Medicine, 40 Tsukasa-machi, Gifu-shi, Gifu, 500 Japan

E. Toppinen
Ylivieska Health Care Center, Ylivieska, FIN-84100 Finland

A. Tuulonen
Department of Ophthalmology, University of Oulu, SF-90221 Oulu 22, Finland

T. Usui
Department of Ophthalmology Niigata University, School of Medicine, 1-757, Asahimachi-dori, Niigata, 951-8510, Japan

N. Urier
Ophtalmologie, Centre Hospitalier Universitaire d'Angers, F-49033 Angers cedex 01, France

E. M. Van Buskirk
Devers Eye Institute, Portland, Oregon

R. Varma
Glaucoma Service, Doheny Eye Institute,
University of Southern California School of Medicine,
1450 San Pablo Street, Los Angeles, CA 9003, USA

D. Vollrath
Department of Genetics, Stanford Medical School, Stanford, CA, USA

L. Wang
Devers Eye Institute, Portland, Oregon

R.-F. Wang
Department of Ophthalmology, Box 1183,
Mount Sinai School of Medicine, One Gustave L. Levy Place,
New York, NY 10029, USA

R. N. Weinreb
The Glaucoma Center, University of California San Diego,
9500 Cilman Drive, La Jolla, California 92093-0946, USA

R. N. Weinreb
Visual Function Laboratory and Glaucoma Center,
Department of Ophthalmology, University of California at San Diego, USA

J. L. Wiggs
New England Medical Center, Boston, MA, USA

J. T. Wilensky
Department of Ophthalmology and Visual Sciences University of
Illinois College of Medicine, Chicago, Illinois, USA

T. Yamamoto
Department of Ophthalmology, Gifu University School of Medicine,
40 Tsukasa-machi, Gifu-shi, Japan, 500-8705

General Aspects

CHAPTER 1

Definitions, Terminology, and a New Way of Staging Glaucoma

G. L. Spaeth

"In the beginning was the word." Humankind can manipulate the environment, largely due to its ability to think in symbols. Words are the major symbols involved in our thinking. Symbols, whether mathematical or verbal, allow communicating, perpetuating, and interpreting reality in a way not possible without such symbols. Augustine said, "A sign is the thing which, over and above the impression it makes on the senses, causes something else to come into mind as a consequence of itself." The word "glaucoma" is a symbol. When we say "glaucoma" something comes to mind of which the word is a sign.

Science requires symbols. Science is the process of defining reality in symbolic terms that have sufficient clarity of meaning that they can be manipulated in a systematic manner, resulting in new meanings not previously present. Essential to science, essential to clarity of thinking, is clarity of definition. To define, means to place limits. Symbols must have well-defined edges. They must occupy a specific space. There must be agreement that a specific symbol has a particular meaning that has some permanence to it. If it is agreed that the meaning is no longer correct, then the old symbol must be discarded and a new symbol with a defined meaning must take its place. If the number 1 could mean the number 1 or the number 2, science would be impossible. If "love" also could mean what most people think of as "hate," communication would be impossible. Living in such a world would be an extension of a world even more absurd and tragic than that portrayed in Kafka's *The Castle*. Perhaps one of the reasons why much contemporary music fails to communicate meaningfully, fails to move and enlighten or delight, as music did in past times, is that current musical signs have become so ill-defined that the listener cannot make sense of what is being said. Unless there is common agreement regarding the meaning of symbols there can be no meaningful communication, no memory, and no logical interpretation.

One of the principal problems in the field of glaucoma today is an imprecision of terminology. The current presentation will deal with a specific aspect of this imprecision: staging.

One thing is clear – the course of glaucoma is highly variable. However, there is one similarity that applies to all the many types and subtypes of glaucoma. Specifically, the glaucomas are entities that pass through various stages in the same order. Initially, there is some "precursor," some phase in which there is a likelihood that a subsequent stage will occur. Secondly, damage occurs. This damage may be to retinal ganglion cells, glial tissue, corneal endothelial cells, or other tissues. Perhaps it even involves cells in the lateral geniculate body, but wherever and however, the second stage is damage. The third and final stage is the development of functional loss caused by the damage: pain, loss of visual field, loss of central acuity, loss of color vision, etc. These symptoms may occur fulminantly, as in acute primary angle-closure glaucoma, or insidiously as in so-called primary, adult-onset, open-angle glaucoma. The functional loss can be trivial or incapacitating, the final phase of the third stage being functional incapacitation.

The potential deterioration of glaucoma through precursor, damage, and functional loss is a constant similarity applicable to all cases. "Symptoms," the awareness of some problem, are related to anxiety, side effects or medications, or the damage caused by the glaucomatous process. They are essential to assess, as prevention or alleviation of symptoms is the ultimate goal of therapy.

The deterioration of glaucoma through stages is clear. The present thinking regarding goals of treatment are less clear. Ophthalmologists, questioned about what they are trying to achieve in caring for patients with glaucoma, will answer "Control the intraocular pressure," or "Prevent visual field loss." But those are not appropriate ultimate end-points, outcomes, or results. The proper goal is the preservation or enhancement of the patient's health; the proper goal is assisting the patient to celebrate life fully. Controlling intraocular pressure or preventing visual field loss are sometimes necessary steps on the way to achieving the ultimate goal, but unless the desired destination of the journey is well remembered, it is easy to get lost on the way, and believe preventing visual field loss, for example, is what we ophthalmologists ultimately are trying to do in our efforts to help patients with glaucoma. Indeed, is this not where we are now? Is this not what we routinely hear?

While we are now bemused at those who had as a goal lowering intraocular pressure below 21 mmHg, are we similarly critical of those who have as a goal lowering intraocular pressure below 10 mmHg? We should be! Controlling intraocular pressure may be an appropriate step towards preserving visual field, and preserving visual field may be an appropriate step towards maintaining health, but it is easy to substitute the stops on the way for the ultimate destination. Lowering intraocular pressure is not the ultimate outcome in preventing or managing glaucoma. There may be reasons for lowering intraocular pressure in patients with "elevated" intraocular pressure (such as 30 mmHg) other than prevention or alleviation of glaucoma. For example, when the intraocular pressure is 60 mmHg it will cause an anterior ischemic optic neuropathy. The pressure needs to be lowered to prevent that. Also there may be a role of elevated intraocular pressure in causing vein occlusion. Other reasons for lowering intraocular pressure may also exist.

Thus, the similarity in the glaucomas is that they pass through stages: precursor, then damage and, in some cases, eventually loss of function. There are difficulties attendant to developing a system of staging on the basis of damage and function. In the first place, there is an uncertain correlation between function and symptoms, between function and findings, and between function and the results of questionnaires. It is impossible at present using currently available methodology to measure change in the stage of functional loss. It is also difficult to measure deterioration in the precursor stage. As a result, current methodologies of plotting change in glaucoma consider only one of the three phases, specifically the damage stage. We have little information about which precursors actually lead to incapacitation, or to significant symptoms and, in fact, that is what we really want to know.

The dissimilarities regarding the deterioration of glaucoma are the *rate*, the *pattern* of change, and the *duration* over which the change will take place. A simple analogy clarifies why these three factors are key. Consider the traveler embarking on a journey through the desert to a destination well known to him, say, 500 miles away. He needs, obviously, to take sufficient water to nourish him throughout the trip. In order to calculate the amount of water he needs to take with him, he needs to know how much water he will drink each day, and he must know the number of days that he will be traveling. He must know the rate at which he uses the water, the pattern with which he will be using the water, and the duration of his voyage. And so it is with glaucoma. We *must* know the rate and pattern of and duration over which the glaucoma will be causing damage. Without this knowledge we cannot make a meaningful assessment of the outcome.

I propose the following staging system. The elements that are known to be "precursors" will change as we learn more. The definition of "damage" will also change as we learn to identify earlier defects with greater specificity and sensitivity. Our ability to detect change will increase as technology improves. There is, as of yet, no method of assessing actual functional status. There has been almost no work done in this regard. However, in order to measure how precursors lead through damage to func-

Table 1. Definition and terminology

Glaucoma	Ocular tissue damage at least partially related to intraocular pressure
Glaucomatous disease	Functional loss caused by glaucoma
Ocular hypertension	Intraocular pressure above 21 mmHg (with or without damage or functional loss)
Precursor	A finding that suggests the subsequent development of glaucomatous damage

Table 2. Stages of glaucoma

0. Normal	
I. Glaucoma suspect	Positive family history of: 1. Angle-closure attack 2. Visual loss due to chronic glaucoma
	Bearer of gene for glaucoma Intraocular pressure 20–30 mmHg Elevation of intraocular pressure in response to topical steroids Exfoliation syndrome or pigment dispersion syndrome
	Disc appearance 1. Cup asymmetry 0.1–0.2 C/D 2. Rim width at inferior or superior pole 0.2 to 0.3 C/D 3. Cup 0.5 C/D or larger 4. Vertical cup 0.1 C/D larger than horizontal cup
	Visual field 1. Nasal hemifield loss, one spot 5–10 dB 2. Paracentral hemifield loss, one spot 5–10 dB 3. Generalized loss 1–5 dB
	Occludable anterior chamber angle 1. C10r or narrower angle 2. D10r or narrower angle

Table 2. (Continued)

	3. C15 s or narrower angle 4. D10 s or narrower angle 5. Shaffer 0 or 1
II. Damage without functional loss	Questionable damage 1. Intraocular pressure 31–40 mmHg 2. Disc appearance a. Asymmetry 0.2–0.3 C/D b. Rim width 0.1–0.2 C/D c. Questionable notch d. Questionable saucer e. Temporal/inferior rim ratio less than 1/2 f. Temporal/superior rim ratio less than 2/3 3. Visual field loss a. Nasal hemifield loss, 2 contiguous spots, 5–10 dB b. Nasal hemifield loss, 1 spot, 10–15 dB c. Paracentral hemifield loss, 2 contiguous spots, 5–10 dB d. Paracentral hemifield loss, 1 spot, 10–15 dB e. Generalized loss, mean defect 5 dB 4. Optically closed angle with questionable peripheral anterior synechiae
	Definite damage 1. Intraocular pressure 41–50 mmHg 2. Disc appearance a. Asymmetry 0.3 or greater b. Rim lost in no more than one quadrant c. Definite notch d. Definite acquired pit of optic nerve e. Disc hemorrhage crossing rim edge 3. Visual field loss a. Nasal hemifield loss, 3 contiguous spots, 5–15 dB b. Nasal hemifield loss, 2 contiguous spots, 10–20 dB c. Arcuate loss, 3 contiguous spots, 10–20 dB d. Arcuate loss, 4 contiguous spots, 10–15 dB e. Generalized loss, mean defect 5–10 dB 4. Peripheral anterior synechiae less than 50 % of angle
	Marked damage 1. Intraocular pressure above 51 mmHg 2. Disc appearance a. Rim lost in more than one quadrant b. Superior and inferior notch 3. Visual field loss a. Nasal hemifield loss, 4 contiguous spots, 5–15 dB b. Nasal hemifield loss, 3 contiguous spots, 15–20 dB c. Arcuate loss, 4 contiguous spots, 10–20 dB d. Arcuate loss, 3 contiguous spots, 20–30 dB 4. Peripheral anterior synechias more than 50 % of angle
III. Damage with functional loss	Questionable functional loss 1. No definite limitation of function, but sense that vision is not "right" and function is not perfect
	Early functional loss 1. Unable to do activities requiring good vision: loses place on page, sees poorly in dark, problems driving, difficulty reading
	Moderate functional loss Major change in lifestyle required because of loss of vision: can no longer drive, difficulty reading, limits work opportunities, etc Severe functional loss Incapacitated by visual loss and/or pain

tional difficulty we must, obviously, have a system of evaluating functional problems. A method of quantifying functional loss must be developed; the quantification of symptoms is evolving as various quality of life assessments are developed, evaluated, and modified.

"A journey of a thousand miles starts with one step." I propose here a first step, a series of definitions (Table 1) and stages (Table 2).

The Glaucoma Graph

The glaucoma graph is a way of determining and understanding the clinical course of glaucoma in an individual patient. On the *y* axis of the graph is the stage of the glaucoma, and on the *x* axis the life expectancy. The slope and the curve of each of the individual lines are determined and graphed in different ways:

- Dotted lines indicate that the slope and the curve have been determined by plotting the results of serial studies, such as repeated disc photographs taken yearly or repeated visual field examinations.
- Solid lines depict the clinical course as described in the patient's history.
- Dashed lines are extrapolations that are presumed to represent what will happen in the future. These hypothetical, extrapolated future courses are based on the nature of the previous courses and on knowledge of what has happened since a known point in time.

The glaucoma graph (Fig. 1) is a way of determining the courses of seven different patients with different manifestations of glaucoma:

- A patient at point "*A*" has minimal glaucoma, and about one-third of his or her life still to live.
- A patient at point "*B*" has advanced glaucoma and has about one-third of his or her life still to live.
- A patient at point "*C*" has very early glaucoma and only a few years to live.
- A patient at point "*D*" has advanced glaucoma and only a few years to live.
- Patient no. 1, considered at point "*A*" has one-third of his or her life to live and is in an early stage of glaucoma. About one-third of his or her life earlier, this patient was noted to have elevated pressure and was followed without treatment. The patient continued to be followed without treatment and no damage to the optic nerve or visual field was ever noted. It is reasonable to assume that, if the patient continues to have intraocular pressures around the same level as those noted initially, he or she will probably follow the course described by *line 1*, and will die without any evidence of glaucoma damage.
- Patient no. 2, also considered at point "*A*", i.e., has minimal damage with one-third of his or her life left to live. In this case, however, the patient's intraocular pressure rose continuously, and the patient was noted to develop early disc and field damage, which then continued at the rate depicted by the *dashed line 2*. This patient, if untreated, would develop definite asymptomatic damage. However, the patient would have no functional loss at the time of his or her death.
- Patients no. 3 and no. 4, at point "*B*"; both have advanced glaucoma and one-third of their lives left to live. However, patient no. 3 is deteriorating rapidly and will be

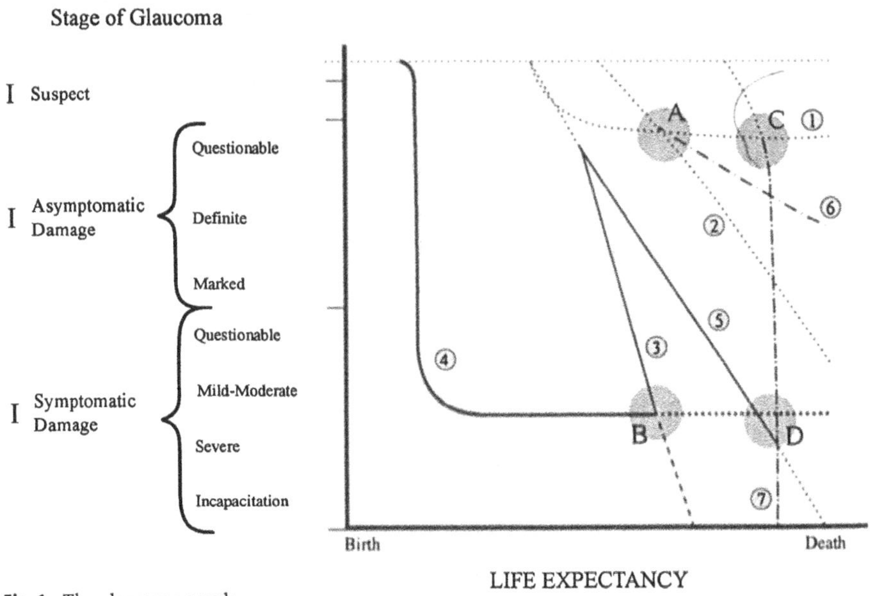

Fig. 1. The glaucoma graph

blind long before he or she dies, whereas patient no. 4, who had a blow to the eye as a child and lost vision to a steroid-induced glaucoma at that time, has had stable vision for most of his or her life. It is reasonable to expect that this will continue to be stable.

- Patients at points "*C*" and "*D*" have only a few years to live, but those at point "*C*" (like patients no. 1 and no. 2 at point "*A*") have minimal damage, and those at point "*D*" (like patient no. 4 at point "*B*") have marked damage.
- Patient no. 5 started with a clinical course similar to that of patient no. 3 (advanced glaucoma deteriorating rapidly), but around the midpoint of his or her life, the glaucoma became less severe. Nevertheless, this patient will be blind at the time of his or her death unless there is effective intervention. Compare patient no. 4, who at point "*D*" has the same life expectancy and the same amount of damage as patient no. 5 (only a few years to live and advanced glaucoma). Patient no. 4, however, has a stable clinical course and does not appear to need a change in therapy. In contrast, patient no. 5 needs lowering of intraocular pressure urgently.
- Patient no. 6, at around point "*C*" also has only a few years of life remaining, but has a glaucoma that is getting worse a little bit more slowly than that affecting patients no. 2 and 5. However, since patient no. 6 has so little damage to start with, no treatment is necessary, even though he or she is getting worse. Even without treatment, he or she will not have enough damage or visual loss due to glaucoma at the time of death that he or she will have any limitation in function.
- Patient no. 7 at point "*C*" has only a few years left to live, but has a type of glaucoma that is deteriorating so rapidly that, even though he or she has only a short period of time to live, he or she will be blind well before the time of death.

Using the glaucoma graph to define and characterize the nature of the clinical course helps the physician and patient to understand that:

- Patients no. 1, 4, and 6 do not need any treatment at all; patient no. 1 will never develop damage, patient no. 4 has marked damage but it is not getting worse, and patient no. 6 is getting worse so slowly that it will not interfere with his or her life.
- Patients no. 3, 5, and 7 can be seen to need treatment urgently in order to prevent them from becoming totally blind prior to the time of their deaths.
- For patient no. 2, the need for treatment is controversial. Since this patient would never develop glaucoma, perhaps he or she should not be treated at all. But since he or she would develop some damage, those who want to prevent any damage at all would advise therapy.

In patients with "elevated" intraocular pressure (such as 30 mmHg) there may be reasons for lowering it other than prevention or alleviation of glaucoma. For example, when the intraocular pressure is 60 mmHg, it will cause an anterior ischemic optic neuropathy. The pressure needs to be lowered to prevent that. Also there may be a role of elevated intraocular pressure in causing vein occlusion. Other reasons for lowering intraocular pressure also may exist.

CHAPTER 2

Remote Ophthalmology Care in Northern Finland

The Application of Teleophthalmology in Examining Patients with Glaucoma

A. Tuulonen · H. I. Alanko · P. Hyytinen · A. Juutinen · E. Toppinen · A. Ohinmaa

Abstract. *Purpose:* During the last decade the number of glaucoma patients has increased by 50 % in Finland. The tightened budget and the 1993 subsidy reform lead to growing community orientation and quality awareness, e.g. equal services regardless of residence. We introduce a pilot study in which teleophthalmology is applied in the care of glaucoma patients in a rural area, as well as for training purposes. *Methods:* A video slit-lamp, a perimeter and a non-mydriatic fundus camera and a videoconferencing system were installed in a health care center in a rural area. The camera was equipped with a video camera and a digital still recorder to obtain images from the optic disc and nerve fiber layer (RNFL). The images and visual fields were compared with the patients' previous digital images and visual fields stored in the database. ISDN connections and special application software were utilized to meet the transfer and data storage needs. An interactive video consultation was created to the university glaucoma clinic. Twenty-nine patients with glaucoma were examined in the rural health care center in stead of the university eye clinic. The control group consisted of 41 patients examined at the eye clinic one year earlier. *Results:* Both patient groups were equally satisfied with the ophthalmic service. Nearly all patients in the telemedicine group (96 %) wanted to have their next visit in their own health care center. The most important reasons were reduction of travelling (93 %), costs (91 %) and time (87 %). With the current technique the evaluation of the optic disc was possible in all cases while RNFL presented less satisfactorily. *Conclusion:* The study will report our first experiences in setting up and applying a teleophthalmology system between two health care units. Further research is needed for evaluation of methods, technology and economics of teleophthalmology.

Introduction

Telemedicine uses electronic signals to transfer medical data, i.e., images, patient records, sounds, and videoconferencing, from one site to another. The transfer of medical data may use the inter- and intranets, personal computers (PCs), satellites, videoconferencing equipment and telephones [1]. Ophthalmology is an ideal application for telemedicine since images and data from most peripherals used for diagnosis and follow-up can be transferred form one site to another – either in real-time or store-and-forward format – such as slit lamp and operating microscopes, fundus and other digital images, keratometers, ophthalmoscopes, scanning laser ophthalmoscopes, visual fields and other psyschophysical data, ultrasound, computed tomography (CT) and magnetic resonance imaging (MRI).

The cut down of financial resources in health care and the 1993 subsidy reform in Finland lead to growing community orientation and quality awareness of health care services, e.g., demand of equal services regardless of residence. Together with the rapid advances in information technology, they resulted in a need to create new innovations to promote collaboration between hospitals and primary health care. The applications of telemedicine support the goal of shared, seamless care between primary and specialized health care [2]. Instead of the patient transportation, the data is transferred which saves travel costs and offers specialized services in the home district.

During the last decade in Finland, the number of patients entitled to refunds of medical treatment for glaucoma has increased by 50 % [3]. In addition to the constantly increasing number of patients requiring follow-up, large remote areas in Northern Finland have suffered from a lack of ophthalmologists since the 1970s. The maldistribution of physician manpower is reflected also in the screening of diabetes, in which Finland has the highest incidence in the world (type I). In this pilot study, we report our first experiences of teleophthalmology in examining patients with glaucoma.

Material and Methods

The University Hospital of Oulu covers a large area up to 600 km (375 miles) away. The population of this area (733,000 inhabitants) is only 15 % of that of the whole country, while in area (168,000 km^2) it covers 50 % of Finland (equals in area half that of Germany, half of Japan, one-third of British Columbia, or one quarter of Texas). Three remote hospital districts have suffered from a chronic lack of ophthalmologists for more than three decades.

Our model for teleophthalmology applications is presented in Fig. 1. The present pilot study was undertaken using a block of the lowest costs. An Inami video slit lamp, a Humphrey HF II perimeter, a Canon CR5-45NM non-mydriatic fundus camera and a Videra viodeoconferencing system were installed in the Ylivieska health care center. The fundus camera was equipped with a Sony DXC-950P 3CCD color video camera and a Sony DKR-700P digital still recorder to obtain still images from the optic disc and the nerve-fiber layer. In the health care center, the new images and visual fields were compared with the patients' previous digital images and visual fields stored on the database. A real-time, interactive video consultation session was created with a glaucomatologist (AT) at the university clinic. Visual field data was transferred to the university clinic with the aid of a document camera. Integrated services digital network (ISDN) connections and a special application software were utilized to meet the image transfer and data storage needs between the two health care units.

Thirty consecutive patients scheduled for routine glaucoma check-up at the university eye clinic between February and May 1998 were invited to visit their local health care center instead of the eye clinic. As one patient refused, a total of 29 patients (telemedicine group) were examined in the rural health center.

An ophthalmic resident examined the patients and taught, at the same time, a local general practitioner how to both use the telemedicine equipment and examine eye patients, i.e., how to use slit lamp, goniolens, tonometer, and fundus examination. A video contact to the university clinic was created ten times for consultation.

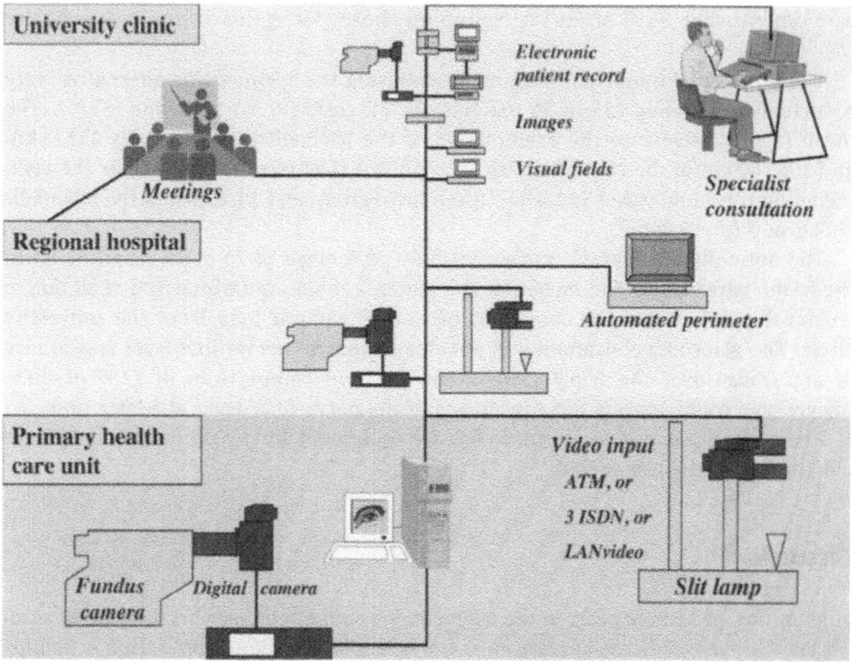

Fig. 1. Our model for teleophthalmology application offers different levels or blocks of technology in telemedicine consultation, depending on the client's resources and needs in the community. A fundus camera with a digital camera body is required for diabetic screening and, for consultation of acute cases, a slit lamp microscope with video input. At the level of regional hospitals other examination data, such as visual field, will be included. The university hospital represents the highest technical level including an electronic patient record. The regional hospitals participate in the university meeting and Continuous Medical Education (*CME*) program. For each block in the model and for each health care unit, we calculate the costs and the critical mass of population required to cover the costs and expenses of the application compared with conventional visits to the eye clinic

A control group consisted of 41 consecutive patients from the same geographic area who had visited the glaucoma clinic of the university hospital a year earlier, i.e., between January and May 1997. In order to analyze both direct and indirect costs, both groups filled in a questionnaire with 23 parameters altogether, including demographic data, housing conditions, distance to check-up at the health care unit, travel costs, escort, total time spent for the visit, waiting times, and satisfaction with care, among other things. In addition, the physicians analyzed the technical characteristics and the quality of images.

Results

The mean (±SD) age of the subjects partaking in this telemedicine study was 64±14 years and 64±15 years in the control group (NS). Both patient groups were equally satisfied with the ophthalmic and overall service. Nearly all patients (96 %) in the telemedicine group wanted to have their next follow-up visit in their own health care center, while 81 % of the control group chose that option in the questionnaire ($p = 0.062$).

The three most important reasons for choosing the telemedicine alternative were reduction of traveling (52 of 56 patients, 93 %), costs (91 %) and time (87 %). The mean (±SD) distance to the examination of the telemedicine group was 25±13 km and 196±60 km in the control group ($p = 0.0000$). The total time spent for the visit, including traveling, was 8.5±2.4 h in the control group and 2.0±1.0 h in the telemedicine group ($p = 0.0001$).

The optic disc evaluation was successfully performed in 24 of 29 cases (83 %) in the health care center. The images of five patients could not be analyzed at all due to technical problems, which could not be solved without help from the university clinic. The glaucoma consultant was not able to analyze nerve-fiber layer appearance of any image over the triple ISDN connection. In comparison, in 72 % of these images, she could analyze the appearance of the nerve-fiber layer at a later time.

The general practitioner learnt to use the equipment and learnt to examine an eye patient during the test period.

Discussion

High initial investment costs in the telemedicine equipment have been regarded as an obstacle for telemedicine applications. Our teleophthalmology application – Remote Ophthalmology Care in Northern Finland (ROC-NF) – forms a part of the RHC-NF (Remote Health Care in Northern Finland) project, which covers half of the country in area. Total investment costs in infrastructure in the whole RHC-NF project, including most specialties, have been estimated to be between Euros 25–33, or US $30–$40 million [4].

The greatest benefit in using telemedicine will be saving, traveling, time and costs, both for the patient and the community, since the traveling costs are also partly subsidized in Finland. Our analysis showed that the mean distance to follow-up visit and the time spent for the visit was reduced to one-fourth using telemedicine applications. The final cost analysis of the present model, which will also include acute cases and diabetic patients, will be reported separately. Since care facilities for diabetic patients are spread out throughout the community, it is most appropriate that their retinas should be examined there [5].

With telemedicine applications, the quality of care also improves since expert opinions are available immediately. In this study, we simulated a model in which the resident and his consultant were physically in different health care units, no matter how far apart. With this application, the ophthalmic residents could work for longer periods of time in remote, regional hospitals and thus help their chronic lack of physician manpower.

With telemedicine the total health care costs will be cut, e.g., when visits for expert consultation can be reduced and the need for transportation in acute cases can be determined by a specialist at the university clinic. Telemedicine also has great potential in education of health personnel. Although the general practitioner learnt about ophthalmology and telemedicine in this study, there is no doubt that the equipment set and software applications used in this pilot study were not user friendly enough to be marketed as a product, but should be regarded merely as a beginning. For the present, there is very little knowledge available on the effects and efficacy of telemedicine applications. Therefore, there is a need for evaluation for both methods and technology as well economics. Another field in need of development and resources is the security and safety issues.

At first being extremely expensive and used by only a few, in recent years, we have witnessed the rapid spread of using, for example, e-mail, telefax, and cellular phones. Nowadays almost every household in Finland has at least one of these modes of communication. Today we use clumsy ISDN lines, the next step of conferencing and telemedicine lies in high-speed wide-area network connections. The future technical development will have revolutionary possibilities in telemedicine. With improvement of safety, transfer speed, and image resolution, the physician can be reached anywhere in the world.

References

1. Telemedicine Research Center (http://tie.telemed.org)
2. The Cluster of Welfare in Oulu (http://www.intermin.fi/sm/laanit/olh/wllness)
3. National Agency for Medicines and Social Insurance Institution (1997) Finnish Statistics on Medicines 1996, Helsinki
4. Report of Application of Telemedicine in the Northern Ostrobothnian Hospital District, vol 1 (1997) Oulu
5. Williamson TH, Keating D (1998) Telemedicine and computers in diabetic retinopathy screening. Br J Ophthalmol 82:5–7

CHAPTER 3

Pigment Dispersion Syndrome

N. Calixto · S. Cronemberger

Introduction

The purpose of this study is to present some data not yet well established in the literature concerning pigment dispersion syndrome (PDS). It represents our experience dealing with this syndrome. Krukenberg (1899), who was probably the pioneer in the study of this syndrome, described without slit-lamp, three cases of "bilateral congenital corneal melanosis" (one of them with glaucoma). Sugar and Barbour (1949) characterized pigmentary glaucoma (PG) and Malbran (1957) showed congenital gonioscopic changes in PG. Scheie and Fleischhauer (1958) found that 21 (43 %) of 49 patients (97 eyes), who were followed up for 10 years, had PG and the other 28 patients (57 %) had PDS. Brachet and Chermet (1974) emphasized the association between PG and retinal detachment (RD). In the thesis of Calixto (1981), a review of PDS emphasizing the contributions of each author to the knowledge of this syndrome was presented.

Patients and Methods

In this paper, we present a study of 68 patients: 47 males (69 %) and 21 females (31 %), aged from 17 years to 64 years: 2 patients were less than 20 years; 17 patients 20–29 years; 17 patients 30–39 years; 13 patients 40–49 years; 16 patients 50–59 years; and 3 patients more than 59 years old.

Myopia and myopic astigmatism were present in 81 % of the patients; emmetropia in 9 % and hypermetropia and mixed astigmatism in 10 %. The patients were distributed into three groups:

Group I The ophthalmological examination was normal in relation to intraocular pressure (IOP), optic disc and visual fields – 20 patients (11 males and 9 females).

Group II The IOP values varied between 18 mmHg and 25 mmHg (applanation), but the visual fields were normal – 18 patients (12 males and 6 females).

Group III Showed typical pigmentary glaucoma [IOP > 25 mmHg, cup/disc (C/D) ratio > 0.7 and damaged visual fields] – 30 patients (24 males and 6 females).

Besides the routine ophthalmological examination, the patients were submitted to the following examinations:

1. Visual fields (first in the Goldmann perimeter and, starting in 1992, in the Octopus 1-2-3 automated perimeter)
2. Gonioscopy with a 3-mirror Goldmann lens (with dilated pupil and afterwards repeated with dynamic pupil)
3. Tonography ("crescent" tonometer coupled to a Honeywell Electronic model 193 printer), preceded by applanation and differential tonometry with standardized Schioetz-Sklar tonometer
4. Ophthalmodynamometry using Mueller's dynamometer
5. Diurnal curve of pressure
6. Permeability of the hemato-ocular barrier (Amsler–Huber test)
7. Keratometry (Bausch & Lomb and Zeiss instruments) and measurements (Pachometer I and II) in the Haag Streit Biomicroscope (Model 900) of:
   a. Cornea thickness
   b. Dynamic and static anterior chamber depth
   c. Lens thickness

Patients using miotics and other hypotensive drugs interrupted their use for 2–3 days in order to study the eyes without medication.

The diagnosis of PDS was established based on biomicroscopic and gonioscopic findings. For the study and the measurements of anterior ocular segment (keratometry, cornea thickness, anterior chamber depth and lens thickness), the initial three groups were abandoned and the patients were rearranged according to age.

Results and Discussion

Iris Transillumination

Iris transillumination was studied in dark-room conditions with dynamic pupil in 129 eyes. A comparison was made to the papers of Scheie and Fleischhauer (1958) and Lichter et al. (1969) regarding occurrence of positive iris transillumination:

1. Scheie et al.: 85 of 97 eyes (87 %)
2. Lichter et al.: 69 of 202 eyes (34 %)
3. This paper: 91 of 129 eyes (71 %)

This finding is important to characterize PDS; iris depigmentation is located in the ciliary portion of the iris.

Zonular Pigmentation and Detachment of the Zonular Hyaloid Membrane

Very wide mydriasis and the gonioscopic mirror of 3-mirror Goldmann lens are required to observe these findings. The zonular pigmentation (mainly in the posterior zonular fibers) was very frequently observed and was independent of the retrolental annular pigmentation. Besides the fluctuation of the anterior hyaloid mem-

Fig. 1. Detachment of zonular hyaloid membrane (*arrows*)

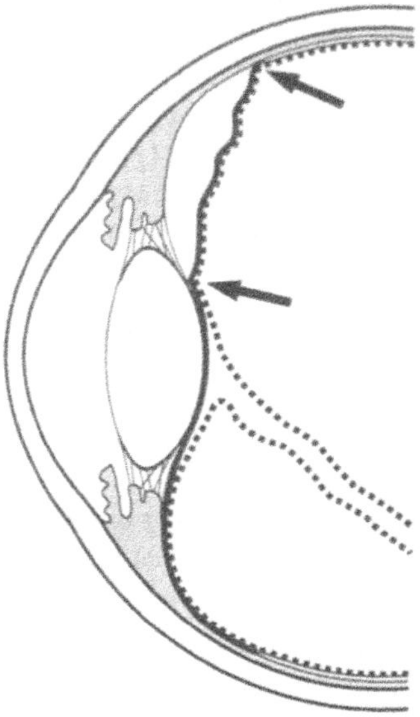

brane with pigments on its anterior face, a true detachment of this membrane was observed (Fig. 1). It was possible to follow the detachment to the vitreous' base around the ora serrata. In this study, detachment of the zonular hyaloid membrane was found in:

Group I 6 (23 %) of 26 eyes examined
Group II 0 (0 %) of 24 eyes examined
Group III 19 (43.2 %) of 44 eyes examined

Therefore, we found the detachment of the zonular hyaloid membrane in 25 (26.6 %) of 94 eyes. When Calixto published these findings in 1981, there was only one reference in the literature, a paper by Sampaolesi (1975), in which he mentioned, from 40 patients with PG, only one with "anterior and posterior detachment of the vitreous body". It may be possible that the detachment of the zonular hyaloid membrane has a role in the changes found in the periphery of the retina leading to retinal detachment.

PDS and Retinal Detachment

Since the first reference to RD in patients with Krukenberg spindle (Kraupa 1917), many papers have been published regarding the association between PG and RD, including that by Brachet and Chermet (1974), who found 19 cases of RD in 40 patients with PG. Our findings were as follows:

Group I No RD, but lattice degeneration and cystoid degeneration in some eyes (30 eyes examined)
Group II Peripheral retinoschisis in four eyes and retinal breaks in two eyes (20 eyes examined)

Group III From 50 eyes examined, 6 eyes with RD and 5 eyes with retinal breaks without RD

Cardoso (1985) found a higher incidence of RD in PG than in open-angle glaucoma and in myopic eyes (≥1.0 diopter) without PDS. It is probably important to emphasize the possible role of the detachment of the zonular hyaloid membrane in the genesis of RD in patients with PG.

Intraocular Pressure Parameters

In Tables 1–3 and Fig. 2, the PDS data of IOP obtained from group I (normal values of IOP), which were compared to values obtained from a normal sample from a previous paper by Calixto (1967). Not only the data relative to isolated measurements of IOP, but all the values of the diurnal curve of intraocular pressure (DCP_o) and tonographic coefficients (Figs. 3, 4) were statistically different, with one exception; the ocu-

Table 1. IOP and ocular rigidity

	No. of patients	Applanation (x±σ)	Differential tonometry (x±σ)	Ocular rigidity (differential tonometry) (x±σ)	Ocular rigidity (Applanation +7.5 weight Schioetz) (x±σ)
Normal sample	240	13.10±1.84	15.88±2.33	0.0192±0.0039	0.0216±0.0022
Group I	36	14.33±2.73	17.44±3.28	0.0198±0.0031	0.0226±0.0038
"*t*"		-3.52	-3.53	-0.9	-2.22
p<		0.001	0.001	-	0.05

Table 2. Tonographic coefficients

	No. of patients	C (x±σ)	F (x±σ)	C_{3-7} (x±σ)
Normal sample	240	0.34±0.09	2.26±1.19	0.19±0.03
Group I	34	0.27±0.09	1.40±0.78	0.14±0.05
"*t*"	–	4.25	3.90	8.25
p<	–	0.001	0.001	0.001

Table 3. Diurnal curve of pressure

	No. of patients	Mean pressure (*Pm*) (x±σ)	Standard-deviation of seven measurements (*V*) (x±σ)
Normal sample	86	12.87±2.22	1.51±0.45
Group I	32	13.31±2.56	1.99±0.69
"*t*"	–	-0.92	-4.42
p<	–	–	0.001

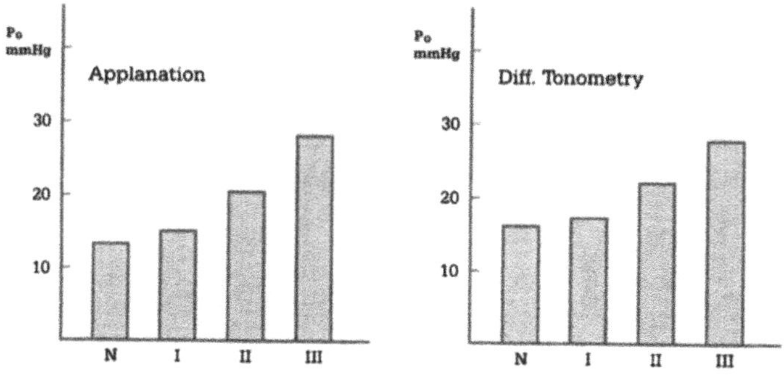

Fig. 2. Histogram of IOP measured by applanation and differential tonometry in normal patients (*N*) and the three PDS groups (*I–III*)

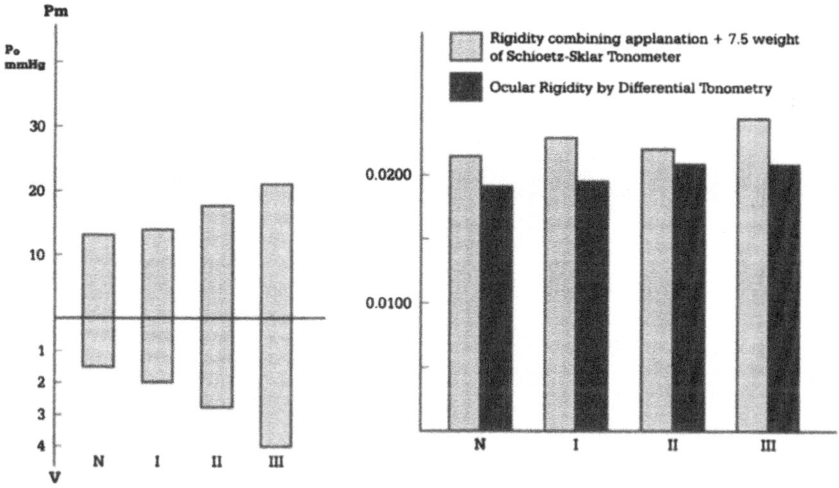

Fig. 3. Histogram of DCP_0 and ocular rigidity of PDS in comparison to normal patients

lar rigidity was similar in both groups (marginally higher in group I when it was measured combining applanation tonometry with the 7.5 weight of the Schioetz-Sklar tonometer). In relation to tonographic coefficients (all of them with significant statistical differences), it is important to comment on the aqueous humor flow. In PDS, the epithelial layer of the anterior uvea is damaged clinically and histologically (Hanssen, Kupfer, etc). We know that the aqueous humor is produced in the ciliary body and circulates in the posterior and anterior chambers with diffusional exchanges in the iris. The minute volume of aqueous humor in group I was reduced to almost half of the value of the normal sample; this tonographic parameter indeed expresses the anatomic and functional change in the anterior segment of the eye. The data are different from those of Brown and Brubaker (1989). In relation to DCP_0, the comparison also showed a statistically significant difference, but this difference occurred only in the

Fig. 4. Tonographic coefficients comparing normal patients (*N*) and the three PDS groups (*I–III*)

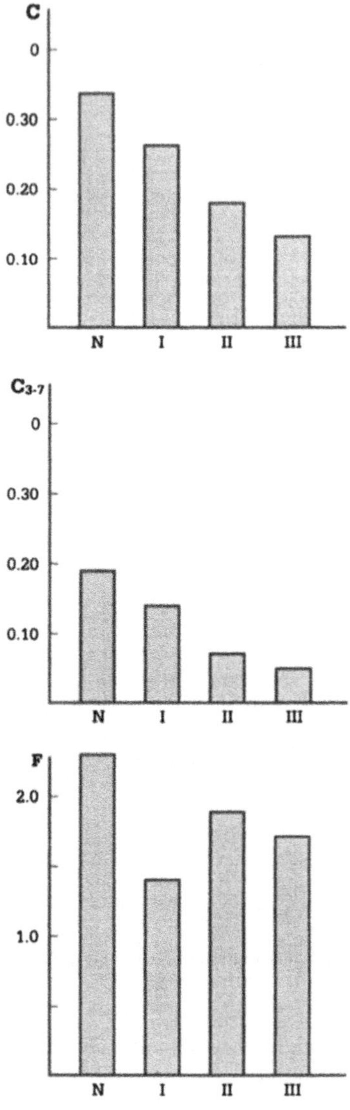

standard deviation of the seven measurements (*V*) because the mean values of IOP (*Pm*) were not statistically different. This finding seems to express the spreading out of the normal circadian variations of IOP. Therefore, group I of patients with PDS is different from the normal population with respect to the IOP parameters.

Cornea Thickness

As previously mentioned, groups I–III were rearranged according to age to study them comparatively relative to normal subjects of the same age groups. The cornea in PDS is thinner and slightly plainer than in the normal sample from the statistical point of view in all groups, with one exception; the keratometric values in both meridians (90° and 180°) were similar in the statistical comparison (Tables 4–6) (Fig. 5).

Anterior Chamber Depth and Lens Thickness

The measurements of the anterior chamber depth were made with dynamic pupil (unmedicated) and under cycloplegia (static measurement). Following this, the lens thickness was measured using the same pachometer II which was used to measure the anterior chamber depth. Some authors measured the anterior chamber depth in few cases of PG, emphasizing its increased depth. Here, a statistically significant difference was also found in all age groups, by dynamic or static measurements (Tables 7, 8) (Fig. 5).

In relation to the lens thickness (Table 9) (Fig. 5), the comparison showed a statistically significant difference between the normal sample and the PDS group, also with one exception; the 41-year to 50-year-old group did not show any difference. In this age group, there were only 13 eyes that had PDS and it was numerically the smallest group. By increasing the number of eyes in this age group, a difference may appear.

The Breakdown of the Hemato-Aqueous Barrier

Fifty eyes (group I = 14 eyes; group II = 10 eyes, group III = 26 eyes) were studied using the Amsler–Huber test to check the permeability of the hemato-aqueous barrier. In the three groups, the barrier was conspicuously and uniformly broken down, very similar to what is found in pseudo-exfoliation syndrome, independent of the presence of glaucoma or ocular hypertension (Fig. 6). These findings are different from those of Sampaolesi (1974), who found a slight increase in the permeability of the barrier in PG and simple glaucoma. This finding reflects a functional disturbance of the anterior segment of the eye, possibly secondary to the anatomic changes as previously mentioned in this paper.

Ophthalmodynamometry

Groups I and II of PDS had an IOP below or slightly higher than 20 mmHg. It was possible to compare mean blood pressure and mean ophthalmic artery pressure taking into account the initial value of IOP (the IOP limit in the table for comparison is 20 mmHg). The values are shown in Table 10. The values that we obtained individually were compared with tabular values obtained in normal eyes by Weigelin and Lobstein (1963) and, afterwards, the mean plus standard deviation was calculated and compared by means of paired-t tests. The differences were highly significant from a statistical point of view and the mean values in PDS were lower than those found by Weigelin and Lobstein (1963). If these values are confirmed by others, they will indi-

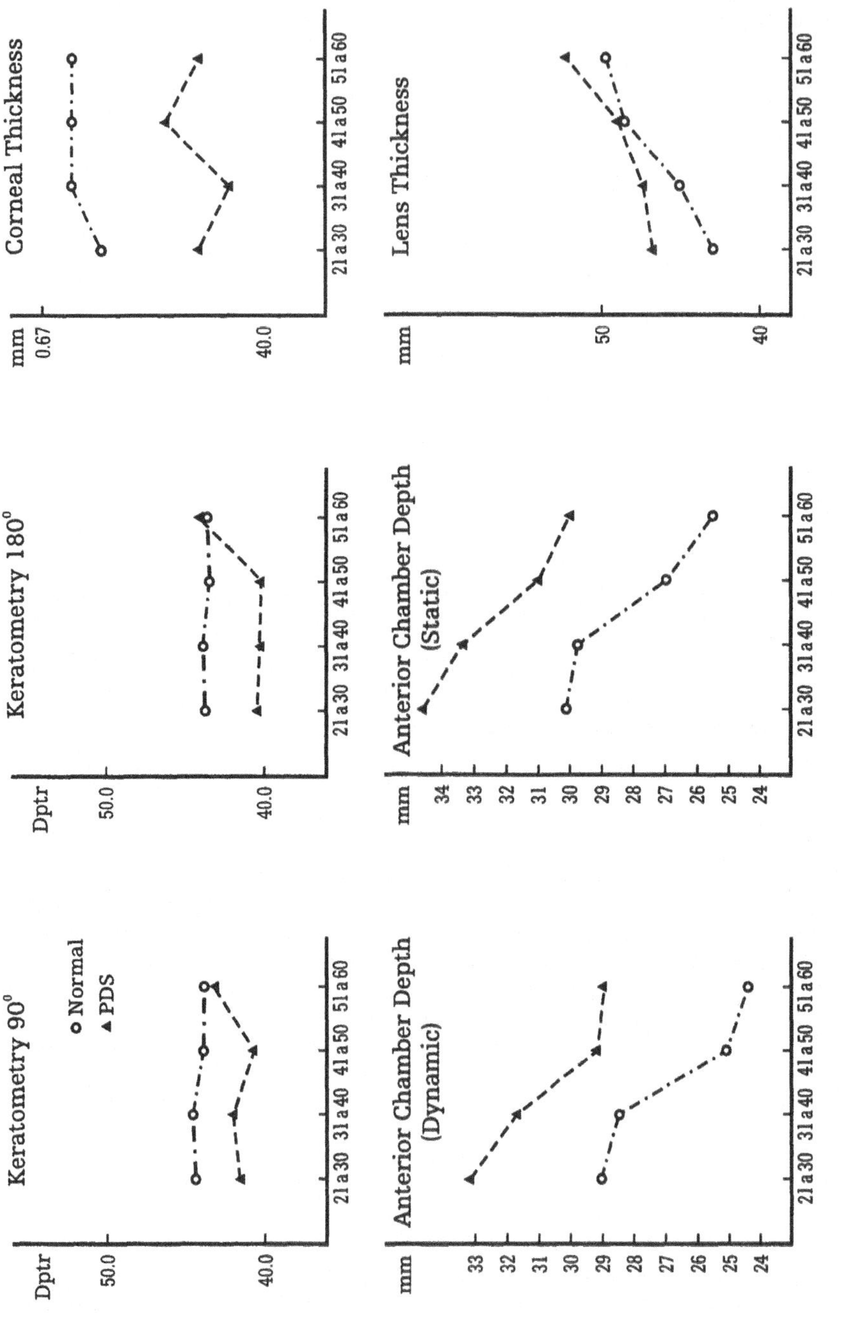

Fig. 5. Keratomety, corneal and lens thickness, and anterior chamber depth (dynamic and static) in different age groups

Table 4. Keratometry (90°)

Age group	Normal sample	Pigment dispersion syndrome	"*t*"	*p*<
No.	20	26		
Mean <30 years	44.32	41.84	4.99	0.001
σ	1.33	1.89		
No.	20	22		
Mean 31–40 years	44.32	40.95	5.77	0.001
σ	1.14	2.37		
No.	20	10		
Mean 41–50 years	43.70	40.63	4.92	0.001
σ	1.46	1.89		
No.	20	15		
Mean >50 years	43.78	43.30	0.77	–
σ	2.00	1.54		

Table 5. Keratometry (180°)

Age group	Normal sample	Pigment dispersion syndrome	"*t*"	*p*<
No.	20	26		
Mean <30 years	43.66	40.71	6.58	0.001
σ	1.28	1.66		
No.	20	22		
Mean 31–40 years	43.76	40.59	5.43	0.001
σ	1.16	2.36		
No.	20	10		
Mean 41–50 years	43.29	40.50	4.92	0.001
σ	1.29	1.76		
No.	20	15		
Mean >50 years	43.41	43.75	–0.54	–
σ	1.73	1.99		

Table 6. Corneal thickness (Pachometer I)

Age group	Normal sample	Pigment dispersion syndrome	"*t*"	*p*<
No.	20	30		
Mean <30 years	0.65	0.62	3.03	0.005
σ	0.04	0.03		
No.	20	31		
Mean 31–40 years	0.66	0.61	5.81	0.001
σ	0.03	0.03		
No.	20	14		
Mean 41–50 years	0.66	0.63	2.15	0.05
σ	0.04	0.04		
No.	20	17		
Mean >50 years	0.66	0.61	4.23	0.001
σ	0.04	0.03		

Table 7. Anterior chamber depth – dynamic pupil (Pachometer II)

Age group	Normal sample	Pigment dispersion syndrome	"t"	p<
No.	20	30		
Mean <30 years	2.89	3.22	-6.08	0.001
σ	0.22	0.26		
No.	20	31		
Mean 31–40 years	2.85	3.18	-3.59	0.001
σ	0.35	0.30		
No.	20	14		
Mean 41–50 years	2.56	2.93	-2.95	0.01
σ	0.33	0.40		
No.	20	17		
Mean >50 years	2.44	2.90	-4.65	0.001
σ	0.30	0.30		

Table 8. Anterior chamber depth – static pupil (Pachometer II)

Age group	Normal sample	Pigment dispersion syndrome	"t"	p<
No.	20	30		
Mean <30 years	3.06	3.46	-6.02	0.001
σ	0.23	0.23		
No.	20	31		
Mean 31–40 years	2.99	3.33	-3.80	0.001
σ	0.33	0.30		
No.	20	14		
Mean 41–50 years	2.70	3.10	-3.28	0.001
σ	0.31	0.40		
No.	20	17		
Mean >50 years	2.56	3.03	-4.92	0.001
σ	0.28	0.30		

Table 9. Lens thickness (Pachometer II)

Age group	Normal sample	Pigment dispersion syndrome	"t"	p<
No.	20	27		
Mean <30 years	4.33	4.62	-4.28	0.001
σ	0.18	0.26		
No.	20	30		
Mean 31–40 years	4.58	4.72	-2.07	0.05
σ	0.24	0.23		
No.	20	13		
Mean 41–50 years	4.85	4.86	-0.14	–
σ	0.22	0.16		
No.	20	17		
Mean >50 years	4.97	5.21	-3.89	0.001
σ	0.20	0.17		

Fig. 6. Amsler-Huber test (hemato-aqueous barrier) in PDS

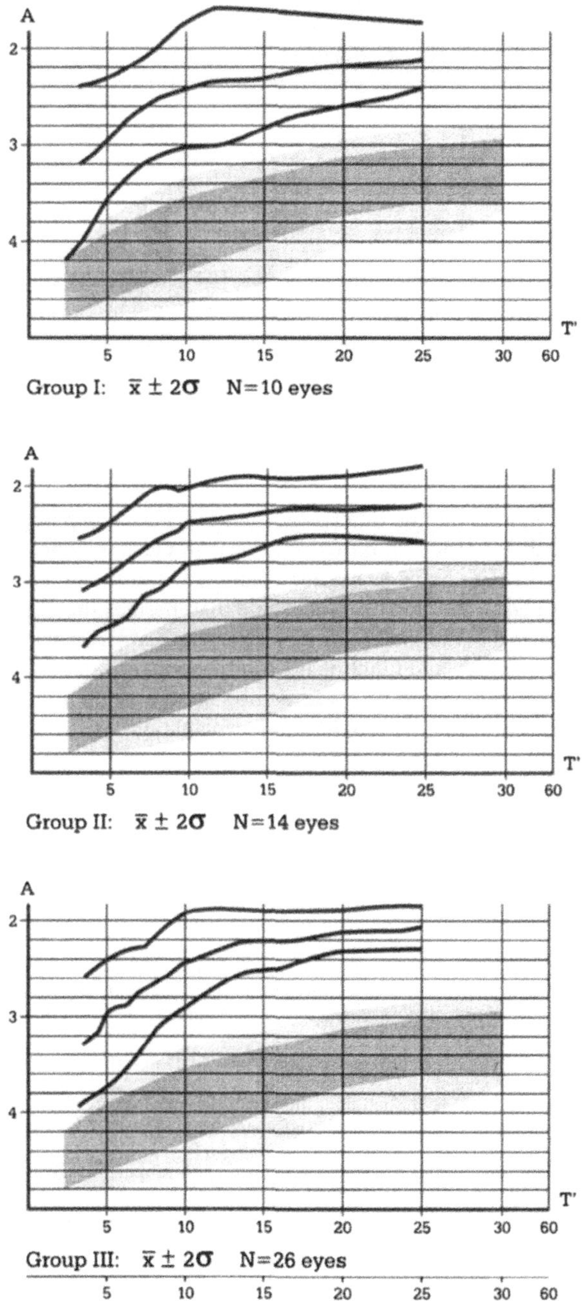

Table 10. Mean ophthalmic artery pressure (OAP) in patients with pigment dispersion syndrome (PDS) compared with mean values obtained by Weigelin and Lobstein (1963)

	No. of patients		OAP	OAP (tabular)	Paired t	$p<$
Group I	20	x	68.39	68.86	–6.50	0.001
	–	σ	12.91	9.61	–	–
Group II	30	x	78.00	79.00	–6.40	0.001
	–	σ	11.26	9.77	–	–

cate that the ophthalmic artery pressure in patients with PDS is low and the perfusion pressure in this group is deficient. This might be one of the reasons to explain the occurrence of optic disc damage and visual field changes in a shorter period of time in patients with this syndrome, especially when the IOP is elevated (Table 10).

Conclusion

In conclusion, the differences found in PDS, compared with a normal sample of the same age group, in terms of corneal and lens thickness, anterior chamber depth and the hemato-aqueous barrier, combined with the differences found in the parameters related to IOP, led us to conclude that, besides the anomalous pigmentation and the changes in the camerular sinus, the whole anterior segment of the eye in PDS is morphologically and functionally distinct from normal eyes. If the low perfusion pressure in the optic nerve is confirmed by more up-to-date techniques of study of the ophthalmic artery, we will have the explanation for the optic disc damage which occurs over a short period of time.

References

Brown JD, Brubaker RF (1989) A study of the relation between intraocular pressure and aqueous humor flow in the pigment dispersion syndrome. Ophthalmology 96(10):1468–1470

Calixto N (1967) Contribuição para o estudo de alguns aspectos da síndrome de dispersão pigmentária do segmento anterior do olho. Tese de Professorado, UFMG

Cardoso RD (1986) O descolamento de retina na sindrome de dispersão pigmentária do segmento anterior do olho. Tese (doutorado). Faculdade de Medicina da Universidade Federal de Minas Gerias, p 119

Farrar SM, Bruce Shields M (1993) Current concepts in pigmentary glaucoma. Surv Ophthalmol 37(4):233–252

Kraupa E (1974) Studien über die Melanosis des Augapfels. Arch F Augenheilk 82:67–93

Krukenberg F (1899) Beiderseitige angeborene Melanose der Hornhaut. Klin Monatsbl F Augenheilk 37:254–258

Lichter PR, Shaffer RN (1969) Diagnostic and prognostic signs in pigmentary glaucoma. Trans Am Acad Ophthalmol Otolaryngol 74:984–988

Malbran J (1957) Le glaucome pigmentaire, ses relations avec le glaucome congénital. Prob Act Ophthalmol 1:132–146

Sampaolesi R (1975) Desprendimiento de retina y glaucoma pigmentario. Arch Oftalmol B Aires 50:375–380

Scheie HG, Fleischhauer HW (1958) Idiopathic atrophy of the epithelial layers of the iris and ciliary body. Arch Ophthalmol 59:216–228

Sugar HS, Barbour FA (1949) Pigmentary glaucoma: a bare clinical entity. Am J Ophthalmol 32:90–92

Weigelin E, Lobstein A (1963) Ophthalmodynamometry, table VIII. Karger, Basel, p 46

CHAPTER 4

Risk Factors in Pigmentary Glaucoma

E. Gramer · H. Thiele · R. Ritch

Abstract. *Purpose:* To evaluate whether family history of glaucoma (FHG) and myopia are risk factors for pigmentary glaucoma (PG) in patients with pigment dispersion syndrome (PDS). To evaluate the relation between age of the patient at the time of the first examination and the stage of the visual field loss. This may allow indirectly to judge the time-dynamic of untreated visual field loss. *Methods:* We evaluated 149 eyes of 149 patients with pigmentary glaucoma (PG) and 43 eyes of 43 patients with pigment dispersion syndrome with ocular hypertension (PDS), who were able to give information about FHG. *Results:* (1) FHG was found in PG and PDS with equal frequency. Overall frequency of FHG was 39.1 % and in one third of the patients with FHG more than one relative suffered from glaucoma. Patients with PG in advanced stages did not have a higher incidence of FHG than patients in early stages of the disease. (2) Patients with PG had a significantly higher myopia than patients with PDS ($p < 0.01$). The higher the myopia in PG, the earlier the disease was diagnosed ($p = 0.008$). (3) PG was diagnosed at a higher age compared to PDS. The mean age of PG-patients at the time of first examination for patients with stage I and II of visual field loss was 42.5±13.2 years, with stage III and IV 46.2±13.8 years and with stage V 51.1±17.3 years. Mean maximum IOP and mean myopia were not significantly different between the three groups. For untreated PG with average maximum IOP-peaks of 34.9±11.5 mmHg the time frame from beginning stages to blindness is only about 8.5 years. (4) Krukenberg spindles in patients on long-term miotic therapy decreased in the upper half of the cornea. *Conclusions:* (1) As PDS is inherited as an autosomal dominant disorder, screening of relatives should be performed beginning in the mid- to late teens. (2) The greater the myopia, the earlier the onset of glaucoma. (3) The age at the time of diagnosis and therefore the height and duration of uncontrolled IOP determines the stage of visual field loss. (4) Early diagnosis and therapy oriented toward decreasing pigment liberation improve the prognosis in this disease.

Introduction

Pigment dispersion syndrome (PDS) is a unique and fascinating entity and far more prevalent than previously suspected (6). The disorder is characterized by disruption of the iris pigment epithelium (IPE) secondary to iridozonular contact with resultant liberation of pigment particles, their dispersion in the aqueous humor, and pigment deposition throughout the anterior segment. The classic diagnostic triad consists of corneal pigmentation (Krukenberg spindle), midperipheral radial slit-like iris transillumination defects and dense trabecular pigmentation. When these findings are present without an increase of intraocular pressure (IOP) and without glaucoma damage of optic disc and visual field, these conditions are defined as PDS. When these findings are associated with IOP elevation, with evidence of optic nerve damage and visual field loss, the condition is referred to as PG.

Eyes with PDS and PG differ from normal in having a larger iris, a midperipheral posterior iris concavity which becomes exaggerated with accommodation, a more posterior iris insertion, increased iridolenticular contact which is reversed by inhibition of blinking, possibly an inherited weakness of the iris pigment epithelium, and an increased incidence of lattice degeneration of the retina [5]. In PG, we have an IOP – dependent glaucomatous damage with quantitative differences in topography of visual field loss and quantitative differences in the correlation of visual field loss and biomorphometric findings of the optic disc compared with normal tension glaucoma (NTG) and primary open angle glaucoma (POAG) [3, 7]. In eyes with NTG, we found a significantly larger cup/disc ratio (CDR) with stages I and II of visual field loss than in eyes with POAG or PG when comparing eyes with no significant differences in visual field loss and disc size [3, 7]. We hypothesized, therefore, that in NTG, there are more often patients with a genetically determined risk factor in the morphology and/or the amount of connective tissue of the lamina cribosa in contrast with PG; in NTG we found, on average, a 20 % larger CDR at the onset of visual field loss compared with PG and POAG and chronic angle closure glaucoma [3, 7].

In patients with PG, we found a family history of glaucoma (FHG) in 39,1 % [4], and while examining 443 patients with ocular hypertension, we found a FHG in 76 patients (17.1 %) [8]. FHG is a risk factor for glaucomas, but whether a FHG in patients with PG is a prognostic indicator is unknown. The purpose of the recent study was, therefore, to evaluate the prevalence of FHG and the influence of FHG on the severity of the disease in PG and PDS and to evaluate the stage-dependence of risk factors in these patients [4]. In the present paper, we attempted to evaluate from these data the relation between the age of the patient and the stage of visual field loss at the time of diagnosis. From the age of the patient at the time of the diagnosis and from the stage of the visual field loss, some conclusions might be drawn about the rate of progression of visual field loss in untreated patients with PG. This may allow some conclusions on the influence of primarily IOP-dependent glaucomatous damage.

Methods

Of 236 patients with PG and PDS , the findings of 207 patients [149 PG, 43 PDS with ocular hypertension (OH), 15 PDS without OH], who were able to give information about FHG were evaluated at the glaucoma services in Würzburg (86 patients) and at the New York Eye and Ear Infirmary (148 patients) by means of a standardized protocol. This contains 61 parameters for all patients and 489 parameters for the 86 patients from Würzburg, for which long-term follow-up was evaluated in addition. Inclusion and exclusion criteria are published in a previous paper in detail [4].

Results

Significance of FHG

FHG was found in 39.1 % of the patients with PG and PDS, and in one-third of the patients more than one relative had the disease. FHG was not more common in PG than in PDS. Patients with PG in advanced stages of the disease did not have a higher incidence of FGH than patients with early damage (Fig. 1).

Cup-to-Disc Ratio

Within the stages I–V of visual field loss, no significant differences were found in the CDR of patients with and without FHG, when comparing the same stages of the disease. There does not appear to be a genetic predisposition in patients with PG to a larger CDR in patients with FGH compared to patients without.

Other Risk Factors

Within the groups PG, PDS with OH, and PDS without OH, patients with and without FHG showed no significant differences with respect to (1) the age of the patient at diagnosis, (2) the age at first examination, (3) the maximum IOP, and (4) the amount of medication for IOP regulation. These and other findings [4] show that FHG does not influence the severity of the disease in PG and PDS.

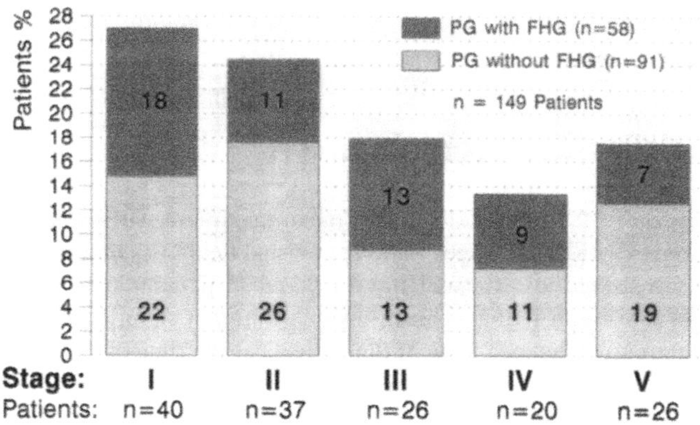

Fig. 1. Frequency of visual field loss stages I–V and incidence of patients with and without a family history of glaucoma (*FHG*) in those stages

Is There Any Difference in the Proportion of Men in patients with PG and PDS With and Without FHG?

Of 207 patients with PG and PDS, 71 % were male and 29 % were female ($p < 0.001$). Of the 81 patients with a FHG, the proportion of men was 64.2 % and not significantly different from 126 patients without a FHG with a proportion of men of 75.4 %. The gender distribution of parents and grandparents having glaucoma was 1:1.

Myopia

The 167 patients with PG had a significantly greater myopia than the 48 patients with PDS ($p < 0.01$). In the PG group, 25 patients had a emmetropia or hyperopia. These patients were, on average, 13.4 years older at the time of diagnosis ($p < 0.001$) than patients with myopia. The higher the myopia, the earlier the disease was diagnosed ($p = 0.008$).

Time of Diagnosis

PG was diagnosed at an older age than PDS (Fig. 2a). In 95 %, PDS was a bilateral. We found reversibility of the Krukenberg spindle in the upper half of the cornea after approximately 2 years of therapy in patients treated with miotics, but no reversibility in patients who did not have miotic therapy. The age at time of diagnosis was under 40 years in 67.4 % of the patients with PDS and 39.8 % of the patients with PG, as shown in Fig. 2a. Within the stages I–V, there were no significant differences in the time interval between the mean age at the time of diagnosis and that at first clinical examination in the university eye hospital in patients with PG, (Fig. 2b). Therefore following conclusions may be drawn.

Conclusions on Visual Field Progression in Untreated PG

Table 1 shows the mean age at the time of diagnosis, mean maximum IOP and mean myopia for 88 eyes/patients with PG in stages I and II of visual field loss compared to 48 eyes/patients with visual field loss stages III and IV, and 25 patients with visual field loss stage V. Mean maximum IOP and mean myopia were not significantly different among the three groups. The mean age of the patients at the time of diagnosis was 42.5±13.2 years for patients with stages I and II of visual field loss, 46.2±13.8 years with stages III and IV and 51.1±17.3 years with stage V. For untreated PG with average maximum IOP peaks of 34.9±11.5 mmHg, the time frame is only about 8.5 years from the beginning stages to blindness. The average onset of the disease is before the age of 40 years. Time of the diagnosis is important for the prognosis of the disease.

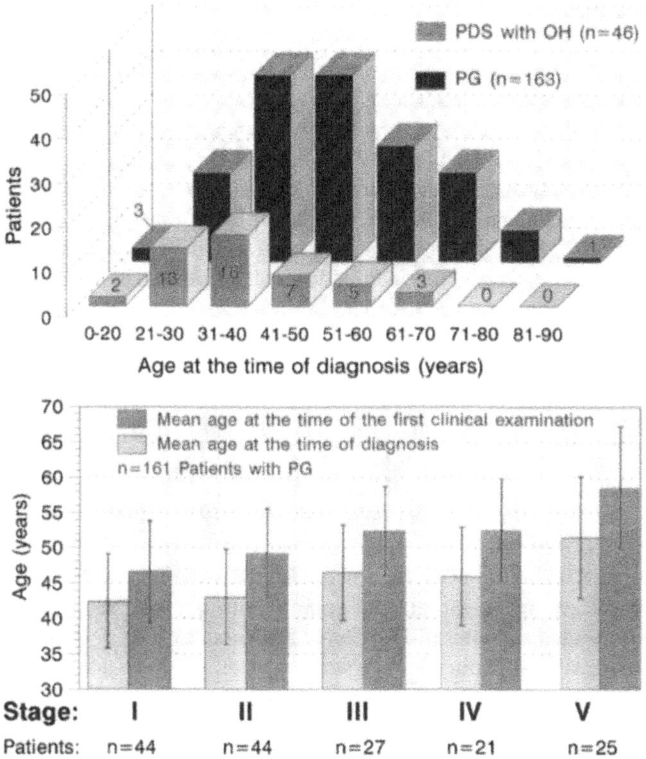

Fig. 2a. Age at the time of diagnosis in 163 patients with pigmentary glaucoma (*PG*) and 46 patients with pigment dispersion syndrome (*PDS*) and ocular hypertension (*OH*) who were able to give information on the family history of glaucoma (top). **b** Mean age at the time of diagnosis and at the first clinical visual field examination of patients with PG (bottom). There is no significant difference in the time interval among stages I–V, allowing the conclusions made in Table 1

Table 1. Stage of visual field loss and mean age at the time of diagnosis in 161 eyes of 161 patients with untreated PG

Patients/eyes Visual field loss	n = 88 Stages I and II	n = 48 Stages III and IV	n = 25 Stage V
Mean IOP (max) (mmHg)	32.5±8.2	35.1±12.9	34.9±11.5
Mean myopia (dpt)	-4.3±3.5	-3.5±3.4	-5.0±5.0
Mean age at time of diagnosis (years; $p<0.05$)	42.5±13.2	46.2±13.8	51.1±17.3

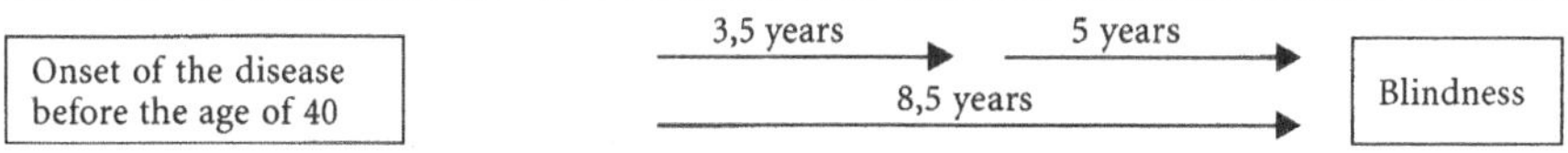

Discussion/Conclusions

Our findings of FHG of 39.1 % demonstrates genetic predisposition for PDS and PG and is consistent with autosomal dominant inheritance. FHG is a risk factor but does not influence the severity of the disease in PG compared to patients without a FHG. In a recent study [1], the gene locus for PDS was identified at the 7q35-q36 region by studying four families, two of which had elevated IOP. In studying three pedigrees with PDS, the possibility of linkage of this phenotype with the juvenile glaucoma (JOAG) locus (GLC1 A) was excluded. These findings suggest that JOAG and PDS are caused by different genetic defects. Study of additional families will determine whether or not PDS is a heterogenous disorder. Eventual characterisation of the genetic defect will allow further elucidation of the pathophysiology of PDS and its relationship with risk factors for glaucomatous damage.

Since PDS has been noted as young as the early teens, we strongly suggest screening siblings and childen of PDS patients starting in the mid-teens and, possibly, in the future, human genetic examination. Screening of relatives of PG patients and the identification of glaucoma-related genes should allow early identification of people at risk from the disease and the ability to direct them towards sight-saving therapy. The frequency of PDS without elevated IOP is equal in men and women. We found in patients with PG, with and without a FHG, that men have twice the frequency of pigmentary glaucoma of women, but in parents and grandparents a gender distribution of 1:1. We would have expected a greater proportion of glaucoma by history in fathers and grandfathers. It is possible that our patients were more aware of disease present in mothers than in fathers or that other glaucomas were present in maternal forebears. From this it can be suggested that the disease is inherited just as much from the mother's side as the father's. The gender distribution of 1:1 for relatives with glaucoma gives us no explanation as to why males have the disease twice as often. The risk factor myopia may be the explanation. Patients with PG had a significantly higher myopia than patients with PDS, and the higher the myopia the earlier the disease was diagnosed in PG. Myopia seems, therefore, to be a risk factor determining the onset of the disease. Myopia is a risk factor and a determinant of phenotypic expression if there is a genetic predisposition for pigment liberation. Ultrasound biomicroscopic findings show that men have a larger axial length and a larger anterior chamber depth than women [4]. This could explain why, in spite of the equal distribution of the genetic risk, PG and PDS were found more often in men and with an earlier onset of the disease. Myopia is a risk factor for both the phenotypic expression of PDS and the development of glaucoma in patients with PDS. It was also discussed that female hormones possibly exert a protective effect against the development of elevated IOP [5].

This study further demonstrates that the later the diagnosis and, therefore, the longer the duration of uncontrolled IOP, the higher is the stage of the visual field loss. Due to the high IOP levels in this disease, there is a high risk of visual field loss progression if the disease is not detected early. The time frame between visual field loss stages I and II to irreversible blindness is only approximately 8.5 years in untreated PG. Early diagnosis and appropriate treatment both to lower IOP and to prevent further pigment loss from the iris determine the prognosis of the disease. Miotic therapy might be doubly therapeutic by improving aqueous outflow and reducing pigment dispersion [2, 4, 5, 9, 10, 11]. The reversibility of the Krukenberg spindle found in this study supports this therapeutic concept. One study has reported that pilocarpine completely inhibits exercise-induced pigment release and IOP elevation, whereas iridotomy does so incompletely [11].

Ultrasound biomicroscopic scanning following administration of pilocarpine shows resolution of the iris concavity leading to a convex iris configuration and elimination of iridozonular contact in all eyes [9]. Pilocarpine seems to produce a convex rather than a planar iris configuration. Laser iridotomy relieves reverse pupillary block [10] by allowing aqueous flow from the anterior to the posterior chamber and produces a planar iris configuration. It seems to prevent in many, but not in all patients, the iris concavity. PDS may become the first common cause of glaucoma for which we are on the verge of a coherent overall explanation of pathogenesis and pathophysiology.

References

1. Andersen JS, Pralea AM, DelBono EA, Haines JL, Gorin MB, Schuman JS, Mattox CG, Wiggs JL (1997) A gene responsible for the pigment dispersion syndrome maps to chromosome 7q35-q36. Arch Ophthalmol 115:384–388
2. Campbell DG, Schertzer RM (1996) Pigmentary glaucoma. In: Ritch R, Shields MB, Krupin T (eds) The glaucomas, clinical science, 2nd edn, vol II. Mosby Year Book, St Louis, pp 975–991
3. Gramer E, Tausch M (1995) The risk profile of the glaucomatous patient. In: Krieglstein GK (ed) Glaucoma: current science, Philadelphia, pp 78–88 (Current opinion in ophthalmology, vol 6, no 2)
4. Gramer E, Thiele H, Ritch R (1998) Family history of glaucoma and risk factors in pigmentary glaucoma. A clinical study. Klin Monatsbl Augenheilkd 212:454–464
5. Ritch R (1996) A unification hypothesis of pigment dispersion syndrome. Trans Am Ophthal XCIV:389–409
6. Ritch R, Steinberger D, Liebmann JM (1993) Prevalence of pigment dispersion syndrome in a population undergoing glaucoma screening. Am J Ophthalmol 115:707–710
7. Gramer E, Gramer G (1999) A new unification hypothesis of the pathogenesis of glaucomas based on clinical studies on disc appearance in relation to the stage of visual field loss in different types of glaucoma. In: Gramer E, Grehn F (eds) Pathogenesis and Risk Factors of Glaucoma, Chapter 20, 170–203 Springer Berlin Heidelberg [in press]
8. Gramer E, Gramer G, Kimmich F, Burkard G (1999) Riskoprofil unbehandelter Patienten am Beginn der Glaukomerkrankung und Änderung von Gesichtsfeld, Augeninnendruck, Blutdruck und Herzfrequenz unter gleichbleibender vierjähriger augeninnendrucksenkender Therapie. Eine prospektive Studie bei 460 Patienten mit okulärer Hypertension und Glaucoma chronicum simplex Stadium I [Submitted for publication] Der Ophthalmologe
9. Potash SD, Tello C, Liebmann J, Ritch R (1994) Ultrasound biomicroscopy in pigment dispersion syndrome. Ophthalmology 101:332–339
10. Karickhoff JR (1992) Pigmentary dispersion syndrome and pigmentary glaucoma: a new mechanism concept, a new treatment, and a new technique. Ophthalmic Surg 23:269–277
11. Haynes WL, Johnson AT, Alward WLM (1990) Inhibition of exercise-induced pigment dispersion in a patient with the pigment dispersion syndrome. Am J Ophthalmol 109:599–601

CHAPTER 5

The Vascular Pharmacology of Ocular Hypotensive Drugs: A New Approach to the Therapy of Visual Loss

M. E. Langham

Loss of autoregulation in the microcirculation and/or the presence of relative ischemia in discrete areas of the optic nerve (most probably in the scleral lamina cribrosa) characterize the onset of glaucoma. Therapy aimed at minimizing visual loss depends on the ability to sustain the autoregulation in the undamaged areas, reduce the intraocular pressure (IOP) and, more importantly, to increase and maintain ocular pulsatile blood flow above 500 μl/min. The characteristics of the autoregulation are reflected in the stability of the short-term differential light sensitivity (DLS), its response to increased IOP and to changes in the ocular perfusion pressure. In this presentation, the heterogeneity of the loss of the autoregulation in glaucoma and the response of the differential light sensitivity to ocular pulsatile blood flow have been used to examine the potential of commonly used ocular hypotensive drugs to protect vascular autoregulation and vision.

With the onset of glaucoma, a fluctuation of the short-term DLS develops in discrete areas of the retina [1]. The presence and spatial distribution of this abnormality may be identified by measurements of the short-term DLS at chosen retinal points (Fig. 1). For example, over a 10-min period, the range (scatter) of the DLS values in healthy eyes is less than 5%, whereas with the onset of glaucoma the fluctuation of the DLS at discrete retinal points is continuous and substantial over the same time period (Fig. 1).

The potential severity of visual impairment at a retinal point may be evaluated from the response of the short-term DLS to experimentally induced increased IOP [1]. In areas with unstable short-term DLS that later develop visual loss, there is frequently a marked and rapid reduction of the DLS when the IOP is experimentally increased by 15–25 mmHg [1]. By comparison, in healthy eyes the DLS remains stable and unchanged when the IOP is increased by more than 30–40 mmHg, i.e., to an IOP of 50–60 mmHg [1].

The independence of the visual threshold in healthy eyes to a reduction of the ocular perfusion pressure by increased IOP also extends to conditions in which the ocular perfusion pressure is decreased by the ophthalmic arterial pressure. This occurs clinically in patients who have suffered a moderate to severe stenosis of the internal carotid artery [2]. In these patients, decreases of 40–50 mmHg in the ocular perfusion pressure are common and may persist for many months without causing visual loss or decreased stability of the short-term DLS (it is to be noted that this autoregulation of the choroidal blood flow develops to its maximum relatively slowly, for it is not seen as an immediate response to experimentally induced decreased perfusion pressure induced by ligation of the common carotid artery).

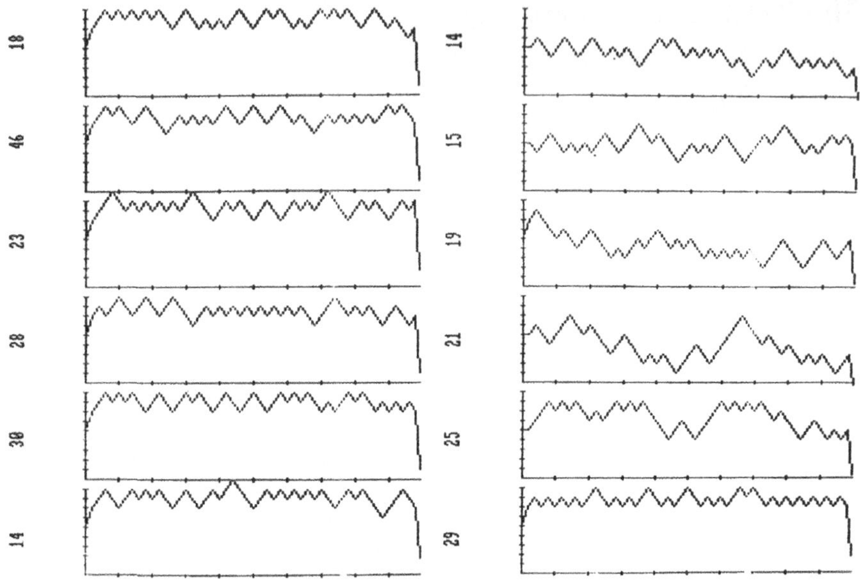

Fig. 1. The short-term differential light sensitivities (DLS) in pairs of eyes of a glaucoma patient with asymmetric visual field loss (*right figure*). Note the stability of the DLS in the left compared with the right eye. The *x* axis is time, where each period is approximately 50 s (the exact time depends on the response time of the patient). The *y* axis is the light intensities at 16 intensity levels, where the ratio of the intensities between each level is 2. The DLS is defined as a light stimulus that can be recognized above background with a probability of 50 %. The numbers at the *side* refer to the position of the test point in the central visual field [1]

The survival of normal vision and the stability of the short-term DLS in healthy eyes when the ocular perfusion pressure is decreased either by increased IOP or decreased ophthalmic arterial pressure indicates the efficacy of the vascular autoregulation to maintain a rate of ocular pulsatile blood flow at a level necessary to sustain vision. The magnitude of this autoregulatory capacity is seen dramatically in subjects with severe stenosis of the internal carotid artery. For example, in a group of ten patients with unilateral stenosis of the internal carotid arteries exceeding 50 %, confirmed by arteriography, the mean ophthalmic arterial pressures in the affected and non-affected eyes were 54.3±2.4 mmHg and 88.6±3.2 mmHg, respectively, and the mean pulsatile blood flows in the corresponding eyes were 695±23 µl/min and 755±16 µl/min. This compares to an ocular pulsatile blood flow of less than 50 % of normal when the ophthalmic arterial pressure is decreased experimentally in conscious rabbits. Following successful surgical endarteriectomy in these patients to relieve the stenosis, the ophthalmic artery pressure on the affected side increased to a mean of 76±5 (10) mmHg.

The stability of the time- and pressure-dependent autoregulation of the DLS becomes impaired with the onset of glaucoma. In the earliest phase of the disease and well before diagnosis has been made by conventional clinical procedures, fluctuation of the DLS develops (Fig. 1). With progression of the disease and increased loss of vision the number of retinal points with unstable time- and pressure-dependent DLS increase. However, even under these conditions, there persists substantial areas of the retina with stable time- and pressure-dependent short-term DLS. The heterogeneity of the glaucoma pathology comprising physiologically intact functioning retinal points with intact autoregulation, coexisting with areas of moderate to severe visual loss and impaired vascular autoregulation, underlines the need to focus therapy on the protection of the vascular autoregulation in the intact areas. The commonly used ocular hypotensive drugs differ significantly in their pharmacological profiles and it is to be anticipated that their action on ocular blood flow and on vascular autoregulation will differ. The ocular hypotensive drugs include β-adrenergic receptor antagonists, such as timolol and betaxolol; the specific β-adrenergic agonist salbutamol; mixed α_1- and α_2-adrenergic agonists, such as epinephrine, Dipivalyl epinephrine, Apraclonidine and Brimonidine; the inhibitors of carbonic anhydrase, Diamox and Trusopt; prostaglandin analogues, such as Latanoprost; and the specific α_2-adrenergic agonists, such as clonidine and Dipivalyl α methylepinephrine.

The β-adrenergic receptor antagonists increase peripheral vascular resistance and decrease pulsatile and total ocular blood flow in the choroid and in the retina [4, 5]. Moreover, this decrease of ocular pulsatile blood flow in long-term studies on glaucoma patients has been found to increase the number of retinal points with instability of the time- and pressure-dependent DLS as well as increasing visual loss [6]. In these long-term studies, the impairment of vascular autoregulation was associated with increased instability of the time- and pressure-dependent DLS [6].

The ability of the β and the mixed α- and β-adrenergic agonists to modulate ocular pulsatile blood flow in man remains to be determined. In conscious rabbits, salbutamol and epinephrine increase and Apraclonidine decreases ocular pulsatile blood flow [3]; Brimonidine has been reported to have a negligible effect on blood flow in the optic nerve and on the pulsatile blood flow in human subjects. The effect of these drugs on vascular autoregulation and on the stability of the DLS remain to be determined.

The action of the carbonic anhydrase inhibitors is of particular clinical interest for they are used systemically (e.g., Diamox) and topically (e.g., Trusopt). Diamox increases the tissue pCO_2 level and, in the dosage used therapeutically, increases cerebral blood flow as a result of the decreased cerebral vascular resistance. In the ocular tissues, the raised pCO_2 also decreases the vascular resistance, but the expected increase of ocular blood flow may not occur due to a "blood-flow steal" to the brain. This vascular "steal" phenomenon is also seen in mountaineers treated with Diamox to ameliorate altitude sickness and improve cerebral blood flow. In these conditions, the ocular pulsatile blood flow decreases despite the vasodilatation and decreased IOP.

The carbonic anhydrase inhibitor Trusopt used topically to treat glaucoma has very little systemic action and therefore has little, if any, effect on cerebral blood flow. Consequently, it is to be anticipated that Trusopt increases ocular pulsatile blood flow. This appears to be true as, in recent studies, Schmidt et al. [7] reported that Trusopt increased the ocular pulse amplitude and lowered IOP in glaucoma patients. An increase in pulse amplitude occurring at the same time as decreased IOP means that the ocular pulsatile blood flow must have increased. The action of Trusopt on the time- and pressure-dependent DLS remains to be evaluated.

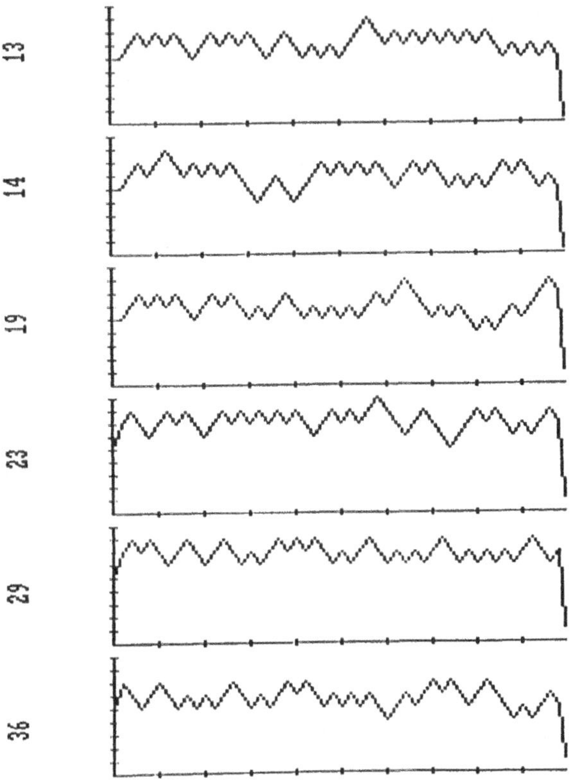

Fig. 2. Improved stabilization of the short-term differential light sensitivity (DLS) in a glaucoma patient with the ocular pulsatile blood flow increased from a mean of 410 µl/min to a mean of 560 µl/min following treatment with topically applied 0.25 % clonidine

The α_2-adrenergic agonists given systemically decrease peripheral resistance and, therefore, may be expected to increase ocular blood flow. These ocular hypotensive drugs include clonidine, α-methyl epinephrine and Dipivalyl α-methylepinephrine. All three compounds increase ocular pulsatile blood flow in animals and man [3]. Furthermore, in long-term treatment of glaucoma patients with topically applied clonidine, it was found that the drug improved the stability of the time- and pressure-dependent DLS, maintained increased ocular pulsatile blood flow and reduced the rate of visual loss in patients treated previously with Timolol (Fig. 2).

In conclusion, the therapy of glaucoma requires that the ocular hypotensive drug protects the vascular autoregulation in the undamaged areas of the retina. The physiologic mechanisms sustaining autoregulation are complex, but it is evident that it requires adequate ocular pulsatile blood flow. Pulsatile blood flow in glaucomatous eyes is abnormally low and, because autoregulation requires optimal pulsatile blood flow, it is important that the ocular hypotensive drug increases ocular pulsatile blood flow. The recording and analysis of the time- and pressure-dependent DLS provide simple and objective means for identifying the progress of the therapy in protecting healthy areas of the retina and in minimizing visual loss.

References

1. Krakau GL, Mullins D, Langham ME (1990) Intraocular pressure-dependent light sensitivity in glaucoma. Invest Ophthalmol Vis Sci 31:2552–2559
2. Langham ME, Preziosi TJ (1984) Non-invasive diagnosis of mild to severe stenosis of the internal carotid artery. Stroke 15:614–620
3. Langham ME (1990) The influence of timolol, clonidine and aminoclonidine on the pulsatile ocular blood flow in the rabbit and human subjects (abstract). Invest Ophthalmol Vis Sci [Suppl] 31:242
4. Yoshida A, Feke GT, Ogasara DG, Murray DL, McMeel JW (1991) Effect of timolol on human retinal, choroidal and optic nerve head circulation. Ophthalmic Res 23:162–170
5. Langham ME (1995) The role of ocular blood flow in the therapy of glaucoma: In: Krieglstein GK (ed) Glaucoma update V, Springer, Berlin Heidelberg New York, pp 271–279
6. Langham ME, McHenry M (1994) The prevention of visual loss by ocular hypotensive drugs. Invest Ophthalmol Vis Sci 36:966
7. Schmidt KG, Dick B, Rückman AV, Pillunat LE (1996) Choroidal perfusion in primary open angle glaucoma patients and healthy controls on Dorzalanide. Invest Ophtalmol Vis Sci 38:440

Genetics

CHAPTER 6

Myocilin Mutations in Families with Late-Onset Primary Open-Angle Glaucoma

R. Rand Allingham · J. L. Wiggs · M. A. de la Paz · D. Vollrath · D. A. Tallett
B. Broomer · K. H. Jones · E. A. Del Bono · J. Kern · K. Patterson · J. L. Haines
M. A. Pericak-Vance

Introduction

Late-onset primary open-angle glaucoma (POAG) is a bilateral disease, which typically has its onset in the fifth or sixth decade of life. The clinical course usually consists of mild to moderately elevated intraocular pressure (IOP), although a significant number of patients may not have a measured IOP greater than the normal range [1]. Optic nerve damage and visual field loss, which may culminate in blindness, occur over many years, usually decades after onset of the disease. The mode of inheritance for late-onset POAG is not known. POAG is considered a complex trait that results from interaction of multiple genes in conjunction with environmental influences.

Juvenile-onset POAG is an uncommon, autosomal dominant form of glaucoma. The age of onset is between the second and fourth decades of life. The clinical course is more severe than late-onset POAG. Recently, mutations in a gene that codes for a newly described protein, called both trabecular meshwork-induced glucocorticoid response (TIGR) protein and myocilin (MYOC), have been identified in families with juvenile-onset POAG [2–4]. The Human Genome Organization Genome Database Nomenclature Committee has recently adopted the term myocilin.

In this paper we report on the presence of mutations in myocilin in families ascertained for late-onset POAG.

Methods

Family Collection and Ascertainment

Families were ascertained through the Departments of Ophthalmology at the Duke University Medical Center (DUMC) in Durham, North Carolina, and Tufts New England Medical Center (NEMC) in Boston, Massachusetts. Some family members were ascertained by referring ophthalmologists. This study was approved through the DUMC and NEMC investigational review boards.

All family members were personally examined or had their medical records reviewed by either JLW (NEMC) or RRA (DUMC). All family members were examined without knowledge of their mutation status. The diagnosis of late-onset POAG in the proband of each family was defined as:

1. Age of onset of more than 35 years
2. IOP measured by applanation tonometry in both eyes of 22 mmHg or more (or 19 mmHg or more while on two glaucoma medications)
3. Glaucomatous optic neuropathy in both eyes
4. Visual field loss consistent with optic nerve damage in at least one eye.

In addition to age of onset, two of three ocular criteria described above (elevated IOP, glaucomatous optic neuropathy, or visual field loss) were used to classify individuals as affected. Individuals with an IOP of 22 mmHg or who had optic nerves which appeared glaucomatous were classified as glaucoma suspects. Individuals who had an IOP in the normal range (<22 mmHg) and normal appearing optic nerves were classified as unaffected. Individuals with a history of incisional surgery, e.g., cataract extraction, prior to documentation of glaucoma status, a history of penetrating or blunt ocular trauma, or any secondary form of glaucoma were not included in the initial screen for mutations in myocilin. Families with any member identified with pseudoexfoliation or pigment dispersion syndrome were excluded from analysis. All families had at least two siblings who were affected with POAG.

DNA was obtained for analysis both from all available family members and from an unrelated group of individuals to be used as controls, with age-related macular degeneration who had no personal or family history of glaucoma.

Single-Strand Conformational Polymorphism and Sequencing Analysis

DNA from all family members and controls was screened for myocilin mutations using single-strand conformational polymorphism (SSCP). All polymorphisms identified by means of SSCP were sequenced. All individuals from families identified to have at least one individual with a myocilin mutation were sequenced regardless of affected status.

Statistical Analysis

The 2-tailed student *t*-test was used for statistical analysis. A value of $p \leq 0.05$ was considered significant.

Results

A total of 83 affected individuals in 29 POAG families (2 African-American and 27 Caucasian) and 104 unrelated Caucasian individuals with age-related macular degeneration ($n = 88$) and their spouses ($n = 16$) with no personal or family history of glaucoma (used as controls) were screened for mutations of the myocilin gene. The mean age of controls was 72.8 years.

Three myocilin mutations were identified in five unrelated families. One family (5039) with mutations in myocilin was of African-American ancestry; the remainders were of Caucasian descent. All mutations were located in the third codon of myocilin.

Two missense mutations were found, one in each of two families. One mutation changes glutamate to lysine at amino acid 352 (Glu352Lys) and the other changes threonine to methionine at amino acid 377 (Thr377Met). A nonsense mutation, Gln368STOP, was identified in three families. A wobble mutation, Tyr347Tyr, was identified in six families and eight controls and did not segregate with the disease phenotype. No other mutations were identified in the control population.

The Thr377Met mutation in family 27 was present in three individuals, one affected and two glaucoma suspects. One affected individual in this family did not have the mutation. The Glu352Lys mutation was found in two members of family 5039, a family of African-American descent. Of the five affected individuals, only one had this mutation. Furthermore, the only unaffected family member also had this mutation. Two glaucoma suspects did not have the mutation. These mutations are discussed elsewhere [5]; the primary focus of this paper will be on families with the Gln368STOP mutation. The Gln368STOP mutation consisted of a CAG to TAG base-pair change at codon 368 in all three families. Pedigrees of these families are depicted in Fig. 1.

A total of 48 individuals were screened. Of these, 26 family members had the Gln368STOP mutation. There were 8 affected individuals, 8 glaucoma suspects, and 10 unaffected individuals with the mutation. The remaining 22 individuals did not have the mutation.

All affected individuals demonstrated elevated IOP, normal and open-angles on gonioscopy, characteristic glaucomatous optic nerve damage, and associated visual field loss. The Gln368STOP mutation was present in all affected individuals. Five of eight affected individuals had moderate to advanced optic nerve damage and visual field loss and five required either laser or incisional surgery in addition to medical management to control their glaucoma.

Twelve family members were glaucoma suspects. Eleven of 12 suspects had elevated IOP in one or both eyes. Eight of 12 suspects had the Gln368STOP mutation. The one glaucoma suspect who was classified on the basis of suspicious optic nerve cupping had a normal IOP and visual fields and did not have the Gln368STOP mutation. There were 28 unaffected family members, of whom 10 had the Gln368STOP mutation and 18 did not.

The mean IOP of those with POAG was 31.1 mmHg. For all glaucoma suspects, the mean IOP was 24.2 mmHg. For those glaucoma suspects with and without the mutation, mean IOP was 25.8 mmHg and 21.1 mmHg, respectively, and were significantly different from each other ($p = 0.05$). The mean IOP of unaffected individuals with and without the mutation was 16.8 mmHg and 16.2 mmHg, respectively, and was not significantly different ($p = 0.25$). The mean age of diagnosis for POAG was 61.8 years (range 41–75 years). The mean age of diagnosis for all glaucoma suspects was 53.8 years (range 39–73 years). Mean age of diagnosis for glaucoma suspects with the mutation was 49.5 years (range 23–72 years) and without the mutation was 62.5 years (range 41–73 years) which was not significantly different ($p = 0.20$). The mean age at the time of examination of unaffected individuals was 47.1 years (range 28–91 years).

Of those with the Gln368STOP mutation who were over age 70 years at the time of their last examination, 100 % (9 of 9) had an elevated IOP, 78 % (7 of 9) were classified as affected.

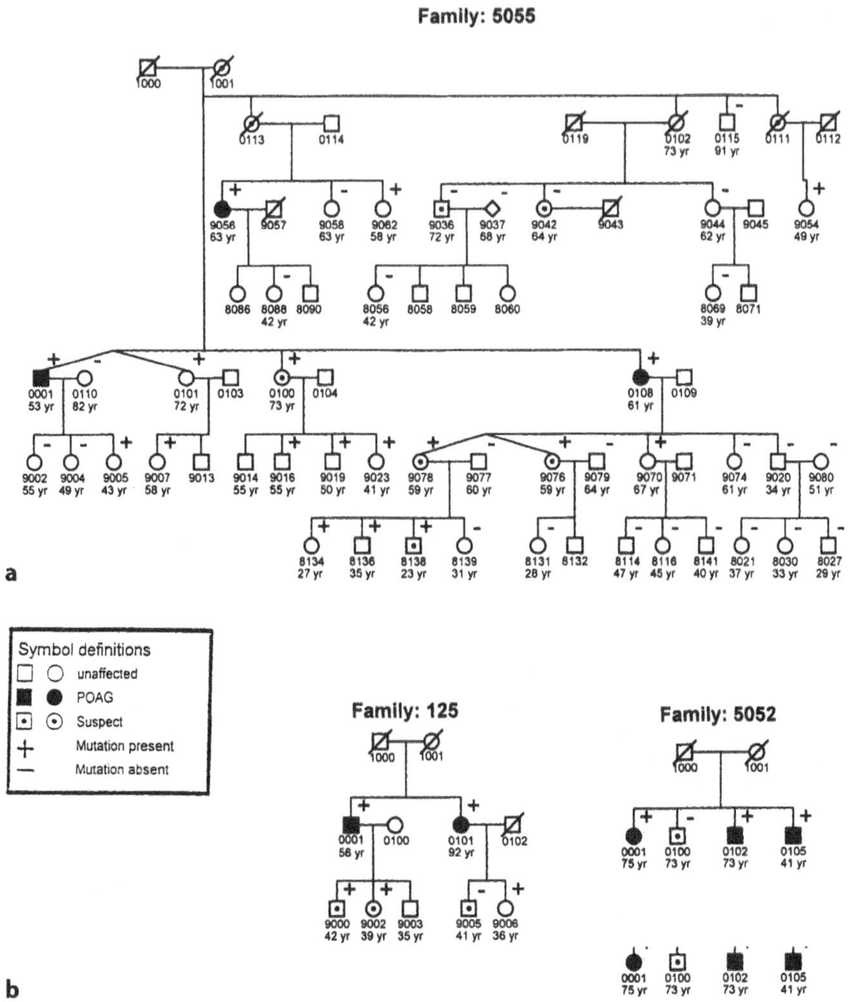

Fig. 1. Pedigrees of late-onset primary open-angle glaucoma (*POAG*) families identified with Gln368STOP myocilin mutation

Discussion

Mutations in the myocilin gene that are associated with the development of POAG, usually of juvenile onset, have been identified [4]. We identified three mutations in myocilin in families screened for late-onset POAG. Two missense mutations (Thr377Met and Glu352Lys) were found in one family each. Interestingly, neither mutation segregated with the POAG phenotype in these families. These mutations have been described by Alward and co-workers [6]. These investigators described the Thr377Met mutation as a glaucoma-associated mutation but felt that the Glu352Lys mutation was unlikely to be associated with glaucoma development. The third mutation was a nonsense mutation (Gln368STOP) and was found in three families. The primary focus of this paper was on the Gln368STOP mutation. All individuals in these families diagnosed with POAG had the Gln368STOP mutation. Furthermore, considering only family members over age 70 years with the Gln368STOP mutation, 100 % had an elevated IOP and 78 % had developed glaucoma.

Classification as a glaucoma suspect alone was a relatively poor predictor of mutation status. Four of 12 glaucoma suspects and 3 of 11 ocular hypertensives did *not* have the Gln368STOP mutation. When one compares glaucoma suspects with and without the Gln368STOP mutation, there are significant differences. Glaucoma suspects with the mutation had significantly higher IOP and were over 10 years younger on average than those without the mutation. Therefore, it appears that factors in addition to the Gln368STOP mutation are playing a role in producing an elevated IOP in these families. It is possible that these unknown factors, which may be genetic or environmental, play an important role in the pathogenesis of POAG.

Interestingly, excluding the Thr377Met and Glu352Lys mutations described above, which do not segregate with the disease phenotype, the mean age of glaucoma diagnosis with missense mutations is under age 35 years (Table 1). In contrast, the age of onset for the Gln368STOP mutation occurs at least three decades after these missense mutations. The reason for this striking difference in the age of onset of POAG between missense mutations and the Gln368STOP mutation is unclear. However, it is reasonable to speculate that this observation is due to differences in expression or function between proteins with amino acid substitutions and those that are prematurely truncated.

We identified the Gln368STOP mutation in over 10 % (3/29) of probands and none of the 104 controls. This association was highly significant ($p = 0.00002$). Stone and co-workers found the Gln368STOP mutation in 2.6 % (6/227) of probands. Since this sample included many families with juvenile-onset glaucoma, this figure may underestimate the number that would have been found in families with late-onset POAG. Therefore, the actual prevalence of the Gln368STOP mutation in families with late-onset POAG may be considerably greater than previously thought.

In summary, we have identified three mutations in the gene coding for myocilin in families with late-onset POAG. Of these, the Gln368STOP mutation is highly associated with the development of the disease phenotype. All individuals with this muta-

Table 1. Current myocilin mutations with mean age of diagnosis

Mutation (type)	Mean age at diagnosis (years)	Source
Gln368STOP	62–64	[4]
Pro370Leu	10–11	[7, 8]
Ile477Ser	33	[7]
Asn480Lys	30–35	[7]
Ile499Phe	31	[7]
Gly246Arg	20	[7]
Tyr437His	22	[4]
Gly364Val	33	[4]
Lys423Glu	30	[7, 9]

tion either developed glaucoma or were glaucoma suspects by the age of 70 years. However, factors in addition to the presence of this mutation appear to play a role in the development of ocular hypertension in these families.

Acknowledgements. The authors would like to gratefully acknowledge the families who have enthusiastically participated in this project. NEI Grant EY10086, the Glaucoma Research Foundation, Research to Prevent Blindness, the American Health Assistance Foundation and the Barkhauser Glaucoma Research Fund supported this research. The authors also acknowledge the use of the resources and staff of the Center for Human Genetics of the Duke University Medical Center.

References

1. Sommer A, Tielsch JM, Katz J, Quigley HA, Gottsch JD, Javitt J et al (1991) Relationship between intraocular pressure and primary open angle glaucoma among white and black Americans. The Baltimore Eye Survey. Arch Ophthalmol 109:1090–1095
2. Nguyen TD, Huang W, Bloom E, Polansky JR (1993) Glucocorticoid (GC) effects on HTM cells: molecular biology approaches. In: Lutjen-Drecoll E (ed) Basic aspects of glaucoma research III. Shattauer, Stuttgart
3. Polansky JR, Fauss DJ, Chen P, Chen H, Lutjen-Drecoll E, Johnson D et al (1997) Cellular pharmacology and molecular biology of the trabecular meshwork inducible glucocorticoid response gene product. Ophthalmologica 211:126–139
4. Stone EM, Fingert JH, Alward WLM, Nguyen TD, Polansky JR, Sunden SLF et al. (1997) Identification of a gene that causes primary open angle glaucoma. Science 275:668–670
5. Wiggs JL, Allingham RR, Vollrath D, Jones KH, de la Paz M, Kern J, et al. (1998) Prevalence of mutations in TIGR/myocilin in patients with adult and juvenile onset primary open-angle glaucoma. Am J Hum Genet 63:1549–1552
6. Alward WL, Fingert JH, Coote MA, Johnson AT, Lerner SF, Junqua D, et al. (1998) Clinical features associated with mutations in the chromosome 1 open-angle glaucoma gene (GLC1A). New Engl J Med 338:1022–1027
7. Adam MF, Belmouden A, Binisti P, Brezin AP, Valtot F, Bechetoille A et al. (1997) Recurrent mutations in a single exon encoding the evolutionary conserved olfactomedin-homology domain of TIGR in familial open-angle glaucoma. Hum Mol Genet 6:2091–2097
8. Suzuki Y, Shirato S, Taniguchi F, Ohara K, Nishimaki K, Ohta S (1997) Mutations in the TIGR gene in familial open-angle glaucoma in Japan. Am J Hum Genet 61:1202–1204
9. Morissette J, Cote G, Anctil JL, Plante M, Amyot M, Heon E et al. (1995) A common gene for juvenile and adult-onset primary open-angle glaucomas confined on chromosome 1q. Am J Hum Genet 56:1431–1442

CHAPTER 7

Characterization of a Large Family with Adult-Onset Primary Open-Angle Glaucoma Caused by a Mutation in the GLC1A Gene

W. L. M. Alward · J.H. Fingert · Y. H. Kwon · A. T. Johnson · S. S. Hayreh
V. C. Sheffield · E. M. Stone

Introduction

In 1997, Stone and colleagues discovered that a gene (GLC1A) on the long arm of chromosome 1 caused a large percentage of autosomal dominant juvenile-onset primary open-angle glaucoma (POAG). GLC1A encodes a 57-kDa protein, known as myocilin, which is expressed in the trabecular meshwork, ciliary body, retina, and 17 of 23 other organs throughout the body (Fingert et al. 1998). In the trabecular meshwork, myocilin production can be induced by corticosteroids, leading some to call it trabecular-meshwork inducible glucocorticoid response (TIGR) protein (Polansky et al. 1997).

To date, a large number of mutations in GLC1A have been identified in populations around the world (Adam et al. 1997; Stone et al. 1997; Alward et al. 1998). While most mutations in GLC1A cause juvenile-onset POAG, a screen of 103 unselected adult-onset POAG patients found three (2.9 %) to have GLC1A mutations (Stone et al. 1997). In a subsequent study, GLC1A mutations were present in 29 (4.1 %) of 716 probands compared with only 1 (0.2 %) of 596 normal subjects and subjects from the general population ($p< 0.0001$) (Alward et al. 1998). Of the 16 mutations reported in GLC1A, there was enough clinical information on six (GLY364VAL, GLN368STOP, THR377MET, 396INS397, TYR437HIS, and ILE477ASN) to characterize their phenotypes (Alward et al. 1998). Five of these mutations caused juvenile-onset POAG with a mean age of onset ranging from 20 years to 37 years. One mutation (GLN368STOP) caused a typical adult-onset POAG with a mean age of onset of 59 years. Of the 716 adult-onset POAG probands, the GLN368STOP mutation was found in 15 (2.1 %). This study describes the phenotype and ancestry of patients with the GLN368STOP mutation in greater detail.

Materials and Methods

This study was approved by the University of Iowa Human Subjects Review Committee, and informed consent was obtained from all of the participating individuals. POAG was defined as an intraocular pressure (IOP) greater than 21 mmHg with optic nerve head cupping and characteristic visual field loss in an eye with open angles by gonioscopy. There could be no secondary cause for glaucoma, such as exfoliation syndrome, pigment dispersion, inflammation, previous surgery, or trauma. Patients were consider to have adult-onset POAG if their disease was diagnosed at age 40 years or older.

To evaluate prevalence, all patients presenting to the clinics of four physicians specializing in glaucoma (WLMA, YHK, ATJ, and SSH) with the diagnosis of adult-onset POAG were recruited. This analysis was performed after 418 consecutive unselected adult-onset POAG patients had been recruited. In addition, DNA samples stored from previous studies of patients with adult-onset POAG were analyzed. Relatives of individuals who harbored mutations in GLC1A were contacted and asked to send medical records and submit blood for DNA testing.

Single strand conformational polymorphism analysis (SSCP) was used to screen the entire coding sequence of the GLC1A gene for mutations. Any SSCP variations were confirmed by sequencing as previously described by Stone et al. (1997).

To determine whether there was a founder effect, the 15 glaucoma probands harboring the GLN368STOP mutation were genotyped using short tandem repeat polymorphisms. Nine markers flanking the GLC1A gene were evaluated, including markers at the 3' and 5' ends of GLC1A.

Statistical comparison of means was performed using an unpaired *t*-test. Two-by-two contingency tables were compared with the Fisher's exact test. Two-tailed analysis was used for both tests. A p value of less than 0.05 was considered to be significant.

Results

Prevalence

Of 418 consecutive unselected adult-onset POAG patients, 14 (3.3 %) had mutations in GLC1A. The GLN368STOP mutation occurred in 10 (71.4 %) of the 14 or 2.4 % of the total population of 418 patients. These 10 probands were evaluated along with 5 probands found in other studies.

Clinical Features

The ten unselected adult-onset POAG patients with the GLN368STOP mutation identified in the consecutive series had a mean age at diagnosis of 56.5±8.5 years. The mean peak IOP was 38.0±8.6 mmHg. Their mean cup-to-disc ratio was 0.8±0.1 and the mean loss of visual field, as measured on the Humphrey Field analyzer, was: mean defect (MD) −2.8±4.7 dB; corrected pattern standard deviation (CPSD) 3.4±1.8 dB. These patients were on a mean of 1.2±0.9 medications. Most patients had undergone laser trabeculoplasty (mean of 1.5 eyes were treated per patient). The patients had undergone a mean of 0.6±0.4 surgeries for glaucoma.

Evaluation of Relatives

DNA specimens were obtained from 77 blood relatives of the 15 GLN368STOP probands. Of these, 36 (46.8 %) had the GLN368STOP mutation. Affection status was available for 33 of the 36 subjects with the mutation. Of these 33, 10 (30.3 %) had glaucoma and 23 (69.7 %) did not.

Age data were available for 28 of the relatives with the GLN368STOP mutation. The mean age of the 8 relatives with glaucoma was 65.4±15.1 years. The mean age of the 20 relatives without glaucoma was 44.7±11.8 years, which was significantly younger ($p = 0.0006$). Of 20 GLN368STOP mutation subjects younger than age 60 years, only 2 (10 %) had a diagnosis of glaucoma, compared with 6 (75 %) of the 8 subjects aged 60 years or older ($p = 0.0018$). Of the 2 GLN368STOP patients aged 60 years or older, who did not have glaucoma, 1 had ocular hypertension and was on medication. Therefore only 1 (12.5 %) of 8 GLN368STOP mutation patients aged 60 years or older had normal IOP.

Shared Haplotype Analysis

None of the 15 probands was aware that they were related to one another. Nine markers around GLC1A were evaluated with short tandem repeat polymorphisms (Fig. 1). All 15 of the glaucoma probands shared alleles of the flanking markers. The degree of allele sharing was high at all markers examined, but was highest (100 %) at the markers closest to the GLC1A gene. There were more alleles shared between individuals than could be explained by chance. This demonstrates that all of the probands and their families inherited the GLN368STOP mutation (and alleles of the flanking markers) from a single progenitor.

The geographic location of known GLN368STOP family members is shown in Fig. 2. These patients have been identified throughout the United States. The clustering around the central United States reflects the referral area of the University of Iowa Hospitals and Clinics.

Discussion

GLC1A mutations were shown to cause approximately 3 % of cases of adult-onset POAG in a previous study (Stone et al. 1997). The present study represents a larger population and confirms that 3.3 % of patients with adult-onset POAG have mutations in GLC1A. The majority (71 %) of patients with adult-onset POAG who harbor

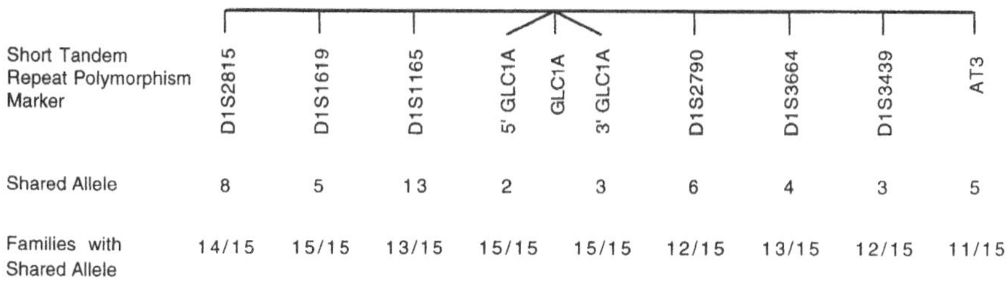

Fig. 1. Diagram of markers on chromosome 1q surrounding the GLC1A gene. The 3' GLC1A and 5' GLC1A markers are very close to both ends of the gene. The most common shared allele is listed along with the number of probands that share that allele. The high correlation of these markers proves that these 15 probands are all related to a common founder

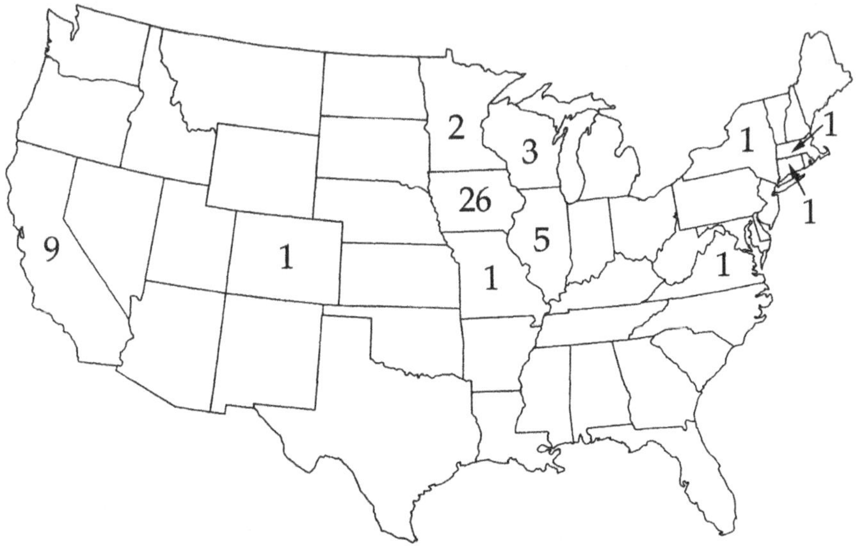

Fig. 2. A map of the United States showing the distribution of the 51 known individuals with the GLN368STOP mutation in the GLC1A glaucoma gene (15 probands and 36 relatives). The clustering around the central states reflects the referral area of the University of Iowa Hospitals

GLC1A mutations have the GLN368STOP mutation; 2.4 % of our adult-onset POAG patients had this mutation. If this prevalence holds throughout the United States, this single mutation could account for 50–70,000 cases of POAG in the United States alone.

The clinical features of patients with the GLN368STOP mutation in GLC1A are similar to ordinary adult-onset POAG, with moderate IOP values, good preservation of visual field, and responsiveness to medical and laser treatment. This is different from the features seen in the GLC1A mutations that cause juvenile-onset POAG, in which the values of IOP are extremely high and poorly responsive to medical and laser treatment (Stone et al. 1997; Alward et al. 1998).

The expression of the glaucoma phenotype in those relatives harboring the mutation is usually only seen late in life. Of the molecularly affected individuals, only 10 % under the age of 60 years had glaucoma, compared with 75 % of those aged 60 years and older (87.5 % had either glaucoma or ocular hypertension). The penetrance of the gene therefore appears to be very high if the patient lives to be age 60 years or older.

Shared haplotype analysis shows that these GLN368STOP patients share genetic material around the GLC1A gene, demonstrating that they are all related to each other and all stem from a common distant founder. Thus, this GLN368STOP mutation family would represent the largest single family ever described with glaucoma.

Acknowledgements. This study was supported in part by the National Institutes of Health EY10564, The Howard Hughes Medical Institute, the Carver Charitable Trust, The Grousbeck Family Foundation, The Glaucoma Research Foundation, and by unrestricted grants from Research to Prevent Blindness, New York.

References

Adam MF, Belmouden A, Binisti P et al. (1997) Recurrent mutations in a single exon encoding the evolutionary conserved olfactomedin-homology domain of TIGR in familial open-angle glaucoma. Hum Mol Genet 6:2091–2097

Alward WLM, Fingert JH, Coote MA et al. (1998) Clinical features associated with mutations in the chromosome 1 open- angle glaucoma gene (GLC1 A). N Engl J Med 338:1022–1027

Fingert JH, Ying L, Alward WLM et al. (1998) Characterization and comparison of the human and mouse GLC1 A glaucoma genes. Genome Res 8:377–384

Polansky JR, Fauss DJ, Chen P et al. (1997) Cellular pharmacology and molecular biology of the trabecular meshwork inducible glucocorticoid response gene product. Ophthalmologica 211:126–139

Stone EM, Fingert JH, Alward WLM et al. (1997) Identification of a gene that causes primary open angle glaucoma. Science 275:668–670

CHAPTER 8

Pitfalls in Mutation Screening for the Gene TIGR/MYOC

P. R. Lichter · S. Shimizu · C. A. Downs · F. W. Rozsa · J. E. Richards

Introduction

Primary open angle glaucoma (POAG) is of great diagnostic concern because it is so common and because often the disease is asymptomatic, even in the presence of irreversible ocular damage. Though assessing known risk factors – including age, race, ocular signs, family and medical history – can aid in calculating a patient's risk for developing glaucoma, there has been no screening/testing available to accurately predict who will develop glaucoma. The advent of DNA diagnostics offers the potential to accurately test for the presence of mutations that lead to the development of glaucoma. As is the case with any diagnostic test, a specificity and sensitivity of less than 100 % means that both false negatives and false positives will occur. In addition, there are potential pitfalls specific to testing for disease-causing genes. In this paper, we discuss testing for the first cloned POAG gene, TIGR/MYOC (trabecular meshwork inducible glucocorticoid response/myocilin) [1, 2], and pitfalls in interpretation of the test results.

Subjects and Methods

Study subjects were defined as affected with POAG if they presented with a typical glaucomatous appearance of the optic disc and/or characteristic visual-field loss, highest reported intraocular pressure (IOP) of 22 mmHg or more, and normal anterior chamber angles on gonioscopy. Subjects were not classified as having POAG if there was evidence of other possible causes of open angle glaucoma, such as pseudoexfoliation. They were also excluded if there was evidence of angle recession, iris abnormalities, or non-age-related corneal endothelial abnormalities. Additional exclusion criteria were history of blunt ocular trauma, intraocular surgery or retinal-buckling surgery prior to diagnosis, corticosteroid use for more than 1 month, or refractive error outside of +8 to −8 diopters.

Informed consent was obtained under a protocol approved by the University of Michigan Institutional Review Board. Screening for TIGR/MYOC was carried out by determination of the DNA sequence of the TIGR/MYOC gene from PCR-amplified fragments by traditional methods that use radioactive labeling and autoradiography, as previously described [3] or by use of an ABI377 semi-automated sequencer to carry out laser scanning of fluorescently labeled sequencing-reaction products, according to the manufacturer's directions. For some individuals, DNA sequencing was carried out using both methods.

Results and Discussion

In general, genetic testing offers the possibility of identifying the presence of disease-causing genes prior to the presence of symptoms and/or clinical signs of disease. This, in turn, allows the clinician to offer early intervention to best treat the disease in question. The patient directly benefits from improved diagnosis, treatment and information regarding prognosis. Genetic testing does, however, have its limitations and, in some cases, test results are uninformative. In addition, in contrast to other medical test results, genetic test results may have an impact on other family members and not just the individual patient. The process of offering genetic testing needs to include efforts to ensure that patients deciding whether to be tested at this time understand the scope and limitations of test results prior to taking the test. In addition, physicians who will be offering such testing and communicating test results to patients need to be aware of the complex ethical and legal issues associated with interpretation of genetic testing results and communication of those interpreted results to the patient [4].

There are arguments to be made for and against TIGR/MYOC genetic testing. There are some large families with early onset of severe POAG, in which early detection and intervention can greatly improve prognosis and in which TIGR/MYOC test results will most likely be unambiguous. This is combined with the fact that TIGR/MYOC is a small enough gene with a simple enough gene structure (1512 bp divided into three exons) that screening it is technically not very difficult. However, mutation screening of TIGR/MYOC is expected to give negative results even in most cases of patients who have or will develop POAG, since TIGR/MYOC is responsible for only a small fraction of POAG. An additional confounding factor will be the occurrence of novel mutations in small families; confirmation of the presence of the mutation in the other affected relatives will be required as one of the more important forms of validation of the mutation finding. To date, there is not yet any identified function for TIGR/MYOC and so there are no biochemical tests as an alternative method to confirm changes in function in apparently altered forms of the protein.

Some of the ambiguities in genetic testing result from failure to detect mutations. However, even in cases where an altered DNA sequence has been found, we do not always know what it means. Two of the most important pitfalls in genetic testing are sequence changes that look harmless, but actually have a functional impact, and sequence changes that appear to cause a change in the protein but that actually have no functional effect.

Testing of one of our juvenile-glaucoma families brought out several of the problem situations in current TIGR/MYOC testing. Testing seemed likely to give a reasonable return on investment, since about 64 % (7/11) of our juvenile-glaucoma families have TIGR/MYOC mutations. In a Panamanian family, onset of glaucoma in children and young adults was linked to the GLCIA locus on chromosome 1q, which has since been shown to be the TIGR/MYOC gene. We expected the screening and interpretation of results to be relatively easy. We were surprised that we did not find a mutation that could explain the POAG and the GLC1A linkage. However, we had to consider one of the pitfalls of genetic testing – that none of the current testing technologies, not even DNA sequencing, has a 100 % detection rate.

When we screened this family again, we did find a mutation that was barely detectable when traditional radioactively labeled sequencing reactions were carried out, but that turned out to be very clear and easily detected by the fluorescence-labeled sequence reactions (in which more than just the labeling method differs). The mutation found, Glu323Lys, passed the additional tests performed: it co-segregates with POAG in the Panamanian family; it is a missense mutation at residue 323 that results in a change in charge at that position in the protein; and it is not present in a panel of 43 normal individuals ranging in age from 35 years to 83 years (mean 55 years).

Undiagnosed family members might anticipate that they would receive clear-cut results if they were screened for the Glu323Lys mutation. They might expect that those with the mutation would develop glaucoma and those without the mutation would remain free of the disease. However, we find two more pitfalls of TIGR/MYOC testing: (1) individuals found to have the mutation would not have their original 50 % risk of glaucoma altered to 100 %. Because of observed non-penetrance in GLC1A glaucoma, there is a small chance that they would never develop glaucoma, even though they would potentially pass the disease along to their children, and (2) an individual found to not have the known family mutation would not have their glaucoma risk drop to 0 %. Instead, their risk would become that of the general population (with adjustment for other identifiable risk factors).

In adult-onset POAG, there are three major factors that confound interpretation of test results. First, at this still relatively early stage of TIGR/MYOC testing, most of the sequence changes are novel and we cannot look to information from other families to help clarify our understanding of a novel mutation. The next limiting factor is the small size of most adult-onset POAG families, which prevents us from using co-segregation information from the patient's own family to assist in interpretation of the TIGR/MYOC test results. Finally, the fraction of glaucoma cases with TIGR/MYOC mutations is very low (4 %–5 %), so there will be a low yield of results which will not tell us any more than we knew before doing the test.

In one of our adult-onset POAG families, a Lys398Arg sequence variant was identified. Since we also found Lys398Arg in one of the normal individuals who we screened, might we conclude that Lys398Arg is not a mutation? No. Here we hit another one of the pitfalls that must concern us. The normal individuals used in these studies, even if well characterized, might go on to develop glaucoma later in life. Thus, the presence of Lys398Arg does not rule out a significant mutation. However, when we review the literature, we see that Alward and colleagues [5] have reported the presence of Lys398Arg in multiple normal and unexamined individuals in addition to POAG cases. Thus, although we cannot tell it from the family we screened, Lys398Arg is unlikely to be a disease-causing mutation.

In many POAG families, there are not enough family members available to allow us to test for co-segregation of TIGR/MYOC and POAG; and, for many of the novel sequence changes detected, we find that no one else has the same change, neither POAG cases nor normal individuals. What can we do in such cases? If we could test for a change in the protein function it might tell us something more about the mutation, but that is not possible. However, it is possible to make some predictions about the protein that can help shed some light on the test results. For instance, we can predict a variety of points within the protein where modifications, such as phosphorylation or addition of carbohydrate groups, are expected. In the case of a Thr377Met mutation in one of our JG families, there are not enough affected relatives to allow us to test for co-segregation of mutation and disease. However, we do see that this mutation causes a predicted (and only predicted) change in the protein structure near a casein kinase 11 modification point, with minor changes to the actual protein structure in close proximity to more than a half dozen different mutations that cluster near position 377. Without co-segregation in the family, there is concern about whether this is really a disease-causing mutation that we could use in testing of unaffected family members. We rely on another piece of information to provide insights into the possibility that this might truly be a causative mutation. Since the Thr377Met mutation turns up in a region of the molecule in which other mutations are clustered, and "hits" one of the four amino acids of the CK2 phosphorylation recognition sequence, we suspect that this might be causing POAG. However, we have hit another problem: we can make models of the protein structure and ways in which it is modified, but the absence of a true TIGR/MYOC functional assay prevents us from translating our predictions into information that is clinically useful at this time.

What would improve this situation? If we had a long list of mutations that have already been shown to cause POAG, we could tell that some of our screening "hits" were validly mutations because of their presence on such a list, even if we could not get enough information from our family data alone. If we knew the function of TIGR/MYOC, we could make the mutant form of the protein and perform a biochemical test for altered function. Our efforts to correctly assess risk would also be improved if we knew what causes non-penetrance in GLCIA glaucoma. If we had the rest of the POAG genes available for screening, we could provide more useful information to the ~95 % of the POAG population who do not have TIGR/MYOC mutations.

Eventually, genetic testing in glaucoma will be very useful to patient and clinician both. As we try to carry out TIGR/MYOC testing during this early stage, when we still do not know enough to make all results unambiguous and helpful, we need to keep in mind the limitations in the interpretation of test results. It is especially important to be sure that the patient understands the limitations of the test before deciding whether to have the test done. As long as we are cautious in our interpretations and take care that the patient does not misinterpret the test results, TIGR/MYOC testing can be useful, especially for the juvenile-glaucoma population.

Acknowledgements. This study was supported in part by grants EY09580 (JER), EYI 1671 (JER) from the National Eye Institute of the National Institutes of Health, Bethesda, Maryland, USA; by an unrestricted grant from Research to Prevent Blindness, Inc., New York, New York, USA; by the Glaucoma Research Foundation, San Francisco, California, USA; and by the Helen van Arnam Glaucoma Research Fund of the University of Michigan Department of Ophthalmology, Ann Arbor, Michigan, USA.

References

1. Nguyen TD, Chen P, Huang WD, et al. (1998) Gene structure and properties of TIGR, an olfactomedin-related glycoprotein cloned from glucocorticoid-induced trabecular meshwork cells. J Biol Chem 273:6341–6350
2. Kubota R, Noda S, Wang Y, et al. (1997) A novel myosin-like protein (myocilin) expressed in the connecting cilium of the photoreceptor: molecular cloning, tissue expression, and chromosomal mapping. Genomics 41:360–369
3. Richards JE, Scott KM, Sieving PA (1995) Disruption of conserved rhodopsin disulfide bond by Cysl87Tyr mutation causes early and severe autosomal dominant retinitis pigmentosa. Ophthalmol 102:669–677
4. The American Society of Human Genetics Social Issues Subcommittee on Familial Disclosure (1998) ASHG statement: professional disclosure of familial genetic information. Am J Hum Genet 62:474–483
5. Alward WL, Fingert JH, Coote MA, et al. (1998) Clinical features associated with mutations in the chromosome 1 open-angle glaucoma gene (GLCIA). New Engl J Med 338:1022–1027

References

CHAPTER 9

TIGR/MYOC Gene Mutations Found in Japanese POAG Patients

S. Shirato · Y. Suzuki · F. Taniguchi · A. Tawara

Abstract. Mutations in the trabecular-meshwork inducible/induced glucocorticoid response (TIGR) gene, also known as myocilin (MYOC) gene, were screened in 155 Japanese primary open-angle glaucoma (POAG) patients and 12 steroid responders. Fifty-nine POAG patients of 53 pedigrees with a family history of POAG, 102 POAG patients without no family history and 12 steroid responders were examined for the mutation in a portion (nucleotides corresponding to amino acid residue 317–476) of the TIGR/MYOC gene. No mutations were found other than the two which have been reported previously (Gly367Arg and Leu370Pro) in the POAG patients with a family history. The trabeculectomy specimen from a patient with the Leu370Pro mutation in the TIGR/MYOC gene was examined immunohistologically. The TIGR/MYOC protein was identified in the trabecular meshwork in the patient, and the immunoreactivity seemed more intense than that from the patient without the mutation.

Introduction

The trabecular-meshwork inducible/induced glucocorticoid response (TIGR) gene is the first identified gene whose mutation causes the development of juvenile-onset and adult-onset primary open-angle glaucoma (POAG) [1]. This gene is also called MYOC because its product, myocilin, was to be found as the protein specifically expressed in the retina by Kubota et al. [2]. In 1997, Stone et al. identified that the gene whose locus had been designated as GLC1A was in fact TIGR and reported that three mutations in the gene were responsible for the development of not only juvenile open-angle glaucoma, but also adult-onset type POAG [1]. Since this first report, several other mutations in the TIGR/MYOC gene have been reported. We have reported two new mutations in the TIGR/MYOC gene that caused the development of POAG in Japanese familial POAG pedigrees [3].

The identification of the TIGR/MYOC gene has the potential to lead to the development of a screening test for identifying mutations in this gene and a strategy for early detection of POAG development. To validate this screening strategy, it is important to determine the prevalence of the TIGR/MYOC gene mutations in POAG patients. In this report, we screened mutations in a portion of the TIGR/MYOC gene in Japanese POAG patients with or without a family history of glaucoma. We also screened the mutations in some steroid responders as well. In addition, we describe the histological findings and the expression pattern of TIGR/MYOC protein in the specimen obtained by trabeculectomy in a patient with Pro370Leu mutation in the TIGR/MYOC gene.

Subjects and Methods

Included in this study were 59 POAG patients in 53 pedigrees with a family history of POAG (including 52 patients of 50 pedigrees which we reported elsewhere [3]), 102 POAG patients without any familial background of glaucoma, and 12 patients who had at least one episode of intraocular pressure (IOP) elevation of more than 5 mmHg with the application of steroid eye drops (steroid responder). Ten normal volunteers were included as controls. All subjects were Japanese. POAG patients were diagnosed by ocular and systemic examinations. All POAG patients had an elevated IOP (> 21 mmHg), open-angle (Schaffer grade III or IV), visual field defect characteristic of glaucoma and glaucomatous optic disk damage. The family history was obtained by direct interviews with the patients. Patients were defined as having a family history when they had at least one relative with POAG within the third degree of relationship.

Peripheral blood samples were obtained with informed consent, and genomic DNA was extracted from total blood. A DNA fragment encoding a peptide of the TIGR/MYOC protein (amino acid residue 317–476) was amplified by the polymerase chain reaction (PCR) method and directly sequenced with an automatic DNA sequencer (model 3733S, Perkin Elmer Applied Biosystems, Foster City, Calif.). The primers used were ATACTGCCTAGGCCACTGGA (5'-sense direction) and CATGCTGCTGTACTTATAGCGG (3'-antisense direction). Mutation was recognized by the approximately equal peak intensity of two fluorescent dyes at the mutation site.

An 18-year-old patient who carried a heterozygous mutation of cytosine to thymine at the position of the 1109th nucleotide sequence of the TIGR/MYOC gene, which induced an amino acid change of proline to leucine at the 370th amino acid residue (Pro370Leu), underwent trabeculectomy on her right eye because of uncontrollably high IOP. The trabecular specimen was immediately immersed in ▪ O.C.T. compound using liquid nitrogen. Cryosections was fixed and stained immunohistochemically by means of the avidin–biotin complex method. The anti-TIGR antibody was generously presented by Dr. Plansky and Dr. Ngyen, Department of Ophthalmology, Cellular Pharmacology and Molecular Biology Laboratories, University of California at San Francisco Medical Center. As a control, a trabeculectomy specimen obtained from a 74-year-old woman with capsular glaucoma was treated using the same procedure.

Results

No mutations were found other than the two mutations [3] (Gly367Arg and Leu370Pro) in familial POAG patients. Examination of steroid responders also revealed no mutation in the screened portion of the TIGR/MYOC gene. The prevalence of TIGR/MYOC gene mutations was calculated as 3.8 % (2 of 53 pedigrees) in POAG patients with family history and 0 % (0 of 102) in POAG patients with no family history.

Figure 1 shows the immunohistochemical demonstration of TIGR/MYOC protein in the trabeculectomy specimen. TIGR/MYOC protein was identified in the trabecular meshwork. There was no notable difference in staining throughout the meshwork. The trabecular meshwork from the capsular glaucoma patient also showed a positive

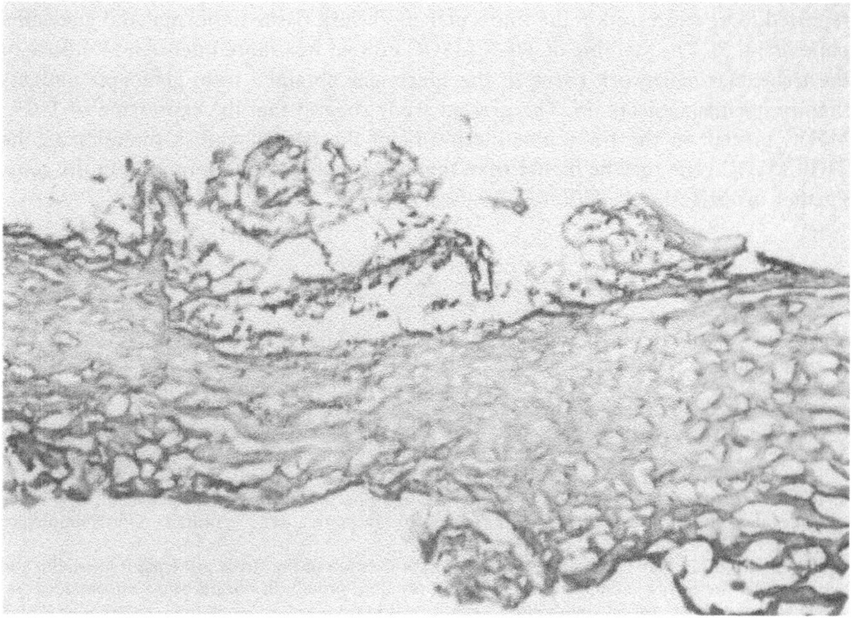

Fig. 1. The immunohistochemical demonstration of TIGR/MYOC protein in the trabeculectomy specimen obtained from a patient with Pro370Leu mutation in the TIGR/MYOC gene. Sagittal section shows marked staining of TIGR/MYOC protein in the trabecular meshwork. There is no notable difference in staining throughout the meshwork

TIGR/MYOC protein immunoreactivity, but the staining seemed less intense than that from the patient with the mutation.

Discussions

In this study, no mutations were found in the examined portion of the TIGR/MYOC gene in non-familial POAG patients. Although we screened the mutations in only a limited portion of the gene, this finding was compatible with other previous reports. This may indicate the strong penetrance of the mutations in the TIGR/MYOC gene for the POAG development.

We could not detect any mutations in steroid responders, as well. TIGR/MYOC protein has been reported to be induced by stress such as that produced by glucocorticoid and superoxide [4]; therefore, it was expected that there was some relationship between the steroid response and the mutations in the TIGR/MYOC gene. This study, however, could not show any relationship between steroid responsiveness and the mutations in the TIGR/MYOC gene.

The trabeculectomy tissue investigations proved that the TIGR/MYOC protein was expressed in the trabecular-meshwork tissue and the immunoreactivity seemed more intense than that from the capsular glaucoma patient. TIGR/MYOC protein was reported to be expressed in the trabecular-meshwork tissue in normal and glaucoma patients [4, 5]. The staining of TIGR/MYOC protein was more intense and diffuse in the trabecular-meshwork tissue in the specimens obtained from glaucoma patients than in normal subjects [5]. The present study suggest that the expression of TIGR/MYOC protein in the trabecular meshwork of the patient with a mutation in the TIGR/MYOC gene may be higher than that of patients with no mutation in the gene. Further investigation is definitely necessary.

References

1. Stone EM, Fingert JH, Alward WLM et al. (1997) Identification of a gene that causes primary open angle glaucoma. Science 275:668–670
2. Kubota R, Noda S, Wang Y et al. (1997) A novel myosin-like protein (myocilin) expressed in the connecting cilium of the photoreceptor: molecular cloning, tissue expression and chromosomal mapping. Genomics 41:360–369
3. Suzuki Y, Shirato S, Taniguchi F et al. (1997) Mutations in the TIGR gene in familial primary open-angle glaucoma in Japan. Am J Hum Genet 61:1202–1204
4. Polansky JR, Fauss DJ, Chen P et al. (1997) Cellular pharmacology and molecular biology of the trabecular meshwork inducible glucocorticoid response gene product. Ophthalmologica 211:126–139
5. Lütjen-Drecoll E, May CA, Polansky JR (1998) Localization of the stress proteins? B-crystallin and trabecular meshwork inducible glucocorticoid response protein in normal and glaucomatous trabecular meshwork. Invest Ophthalmol Vis Sci 39:517–525

CHAPTER 10

Gene Therapy of Cultured Rat Retinal Ganglion Cells

R. Polk · R. Varma

Retinal ganglion cells (RGCs) are selectively damaged in patients with glaucoma or other optic neuropathies. The mechanisms causing the selective ganglion-cell death are not completely understood; however, it is thought that a decrease in axonal transport due to axonal injury plays a key role. Obstruction of axonal transport at the lamina cribrosa may block retrograde neurotrophic signaling, leading to apoptotic cell death. Apoptosis is the normal active process of cells controlling their numbers by a genetically programmed process of cell death and is associated with distinct morphological changes, including cell shrinkage, cytoplasm membrane blebbing, nuclear fragmentation, and DNA degradation.

The introduction of the anti-cell-death proto-oncogene *Bcl-2* and/or the gene for *Bcl-2*-binding protein *BAG-1* into RGCs may prevent cell death following glaucoma and other optic neuropathies. *Bcl-2* is an intracellular membrane-associated protein shown to inhibit cell death induced by a variety of apoptotic stimuli [2]. *BAG-1* is a novel *Bcl-2*-binding protein that interacts physically and functionally with Bcl-2 and can enhance the anti-apoptotic activity of *Bcl-2* in co-transfection assays [3]. Although the mechanism by which *Bcl-2* and *BAG-1* protect cells from programmed cell death is still being determined, several transgenic mouse studies have shown that *Bcl-2* overexpression prevents developmental and injury-induced apoptosis and that co-expression of *Bel-2* and *BAG-1* is more protective than *Bcl.-2* alone.

Adenoviral vectors provide a potential means for transfer of the *Bcl-2* and *BAG-1* genes to RGCs. Adenovirus containing the *lacZ* reporter gene can be used to monitor transduction efficiency and determine optimal transfection conditions for adenovirus gene delivery. The expression of the *lacZ* reporter gene, coding for β-galactosidase, permits the visualization of infected cells. A major advantage to using adenoviral vectors for gene delivery is their ability to infect terminally-differentiated cells, such as ganglion cells. In addition, adenoviruses and can be prepared at high titers.

Cultured rat RGCs provide a good in vitro system for the study of adenoviral-mediated gene transfer. While previous studies have examined adenovirus-mediated gene transfer to retinal cells in vivo and in vitro through whole retinal cultures, culturing the ganglion cells alone allows the delivery of genes directly to and only to our target cells, allowing us to determine the efficiency of adenoviral transfer to these cells.

Methods utilized in these studies include RGC purification and culture, immunostaining, adenoviral transfection, X-gal assay and TdT-mediated dUTP nick-end labeling (TUNEL) assay. The immunopanning technique was used to isolate RCGs from new born Sprague Dawley rats. Briefly, retinal tissue was dissociated and triturated to yield a suspension of single cells. RGCs were then immunopanned using Thy-1 a RGC surface marker. Purified RGCs were cultured and maintained in serum-free medium containing trophic factors. The purity of cultured RGCs was confirmed by immunostaining with anty-Thy1.1, anti-neurofilament, anti-MAP2 for dendrites and anti-tau for axons.

To test the effectiveness of Bcl-2 and BAG-1 in increasing survival, the cultured RGCs were incubated with adenovirus containing the *Bcl-2* and/or *BAG-1* and the *lacZ* genes driven by a cytomegalovirus (CMV) promoter (AdCMV/*Bcl-2* and AdCmV/*BAG-1* and AdCmV/*lacZ*) at varying concentrations. The expression of the *lacZ* reporter gene, coding for β-galactosidase, permits the visualization of infected cells and thereby serves as a control. All cells were maintained in serum-free medium with growth factors for up to 3 weeks with daily cell counts taken to monitor survival. Multiple counts of surviving cells in each sample were taken daily, beginning 1 h after plating and using a microscope fitted with an eyepiece grid. In order to verify transfection, AdCMB/*Bcl-2* and AdCmV/*BAG-1* infected cells were immunostained with primary antibodies to *Bcl-2* and a *BAG-1*, followed by fluorescently labeled secondary antibodies. In order to monitor apoptosis in the cultured RGCs, TUNEL assays were performed on both infected and non-infected cells up to 14 days post-infection.

Cotransfecton with AdCMV/*Bcl-2* and AdCMV/*BAG-1* increases survival of the purified rat RGCs. The daily cell counts indicated that survival in the *Bcl-2/BAG-1* samples was significantly greater than *BAG-1* only or *lacZ* control samples from day 6 onwards, as was survival in *Bcl-2*-only samples. Immunostaining showed that less than 20 % of total cells were expressing either *Bcl-2* and/or *BAG-1* with an overlapping pattern of distribution. TUNEL assays demonstrated that fewer *Bcl-2/BAG-1*-infected cells were likely to undergo early apoptotic cell death. Although we see an increasing number of *Bcl-2/BAG-1*-infected cells dying apoptotically over time, these cells clearly remain viable longer than in non-infected cells. Up to 3 days post-infection with *Bcl-2/BAG-1*, we see virtually no infected cells positive for TUNEL. After 7 days, some of the *Bcl-2/BAG-1* infected cells are positive for TUNEL and after 14 days, still more. However, even after 14 days, half of the infected cells still remain negative for the TUNEL assay.

This study demonstrates that adenovirus can effectively mediate the transfer and expression of a gene to cultured rat RGCs. We have also found the anti-cell-death gene *Bcl-2* alone significantly increases both the number of surviving cells and the time of survival. *Bcl-2* and *BAG-1* co-infection produces even greater survival rates, lending further evidence that there is a synergistic effect between the two genes. These results are consistent with previous findings showing that not only does *BAG-1* interact with *Bcl-2*, but that co-expression of *Bcl-2* and *BAG-1* is more protective than either protein alone in response to apoptotic stimuli. The pathways through which these anti-cell-death genes work remain to be elucidated.

Viral gene therapy has been suggested as one method to reduce apoptosis of RGCs in glaucoma and other optic neuropathies. By introducing anti-cell-death genes, such as *Bcl-2* and *BAG-1*, into RGCs via adenoviral vectors, it may be possible to inhibit apoptosis resulting from damage causing obstruction of neurotrophic signaling.

References

1. Quigley HA, Nickells RW, Kerrigan LA, Pease ME, Thibault DJ, Jack DJ (1995) Retinal ganglion cell death in experimental glaucoma and after axotomy occurs by apoptosis. Invest Ophthalmol 36:774–786
2. Reed JC (1994) Bcl-2 and the regulation of programmed cell death. J Cell Biol 124:1–6
3. Takayama S, Sato T, Krajewski S, et al. (1995) Cloning and functional analysis of BAG-1; a novel bcl-2-binding protein with anti-cell death activity. Cell 80:279–284
4. Chen DF, Schneider GE, Martinou JC, Tonegawa S (1997) Bcl-2 promotes regeneration of severed axons in mammalian CNS. Nature 385:434–439
5. Bonfanti L, Strettoi E, Chierzi S, et al. (1996) Protection of retinal ganglion cells from natural and axotomy-induced cell death in neonatal transgenic mice overexpressing bcl-2. J Neurosci 16:4186–4194

Blood Flow

CHAPTER 11

Optic Nerve Head Blood Flow Measured by Laser-Doppler Flowmetry

S. S. Hayreh · B. L. Petrig · C. E. Riva

Abstract. The optic nerve head (ONH) is supplied by two main sources of blood flow: the superficial layers by the central retinal artery (CRA) and the deeper layers by the posterior ciliary arteries (PCAs). Using a fundus camera-based laser-Doppler flowmetry (LDF) technique to measure blood flow in the ONH tissue, we conducted a study in rhesus monkey eyes to obtain a better understanding of which part of the ONH circulation is measured by LDF. LDF measurements were taken at baseline, then after experimental occlusion of CRA (12 eyes), all the PCAs (9 eyes) and combined occlusion of CRA and all the PCAs (9 eyes). ONH, choroidal and retinal circulations following the various arterial occlusions were investigated by fluorescein fundus angiography. Average LDF flow during CRA occlusion alone was highly significantly decreased ($p< 0.001$) by 39±21 % (mean±95 % confidence interval) compared with normal baseline. Combined occlusion of CRA and PCAs reduced LDF flow even more markedly by 57±27 % ($p< 0.0005$), but the difference between this flow reduction and that with CRAO alone was not significant ($p> 0.20$). After PCA occlusion alone, however, measurements showed a non-significant increase in LDF flow of 17±37 %. Thus, the findings of this study suggest that the LDF technique is predominantly sensitive to flow changes in the surface layer of the ONH and less sensitive to those in the deeper layers of the ONH.

Introduction

Recently, there has been mounting evidence that vascular insufficiency in the optic nerve head (ONH) may play an important role in glaucomatous optic neuropathy [1–11]. All this has naturally resulted in the current major thrust of research to explore the various aspects of ONH circulation and vascular insufficiency of the ONH. This, in turn, has led to a proliferation of methods to evaluate the state of circulation in the ONH. The ONH tissue is supplied by two main sources of blood flow: (1) the superficial layers of the ONH, i.e., the nerve fiber layer on the surface of the optic disc, by the central retinal artery (CRA) circulation, and (2) the deeper layers, i.e., prelaminar, lamina cribrosa and retrolaminar regions, by the posterior ciliary artery (PCA) circulation (Fig. 1) [12, 13]. Available evidence indicates that the primary site of lesion in glaucomatous optic neuropathy and other ischemic disorders of the ONH is in the part of the ONH nourished by the PCA circulation and not by the retinal circulation [2, 3, 5, 7, 10, 12]. Thus, any method used to evaluate the role of the ONH circulatory disorders in glaucomatous optic neuropathy must give reliable information

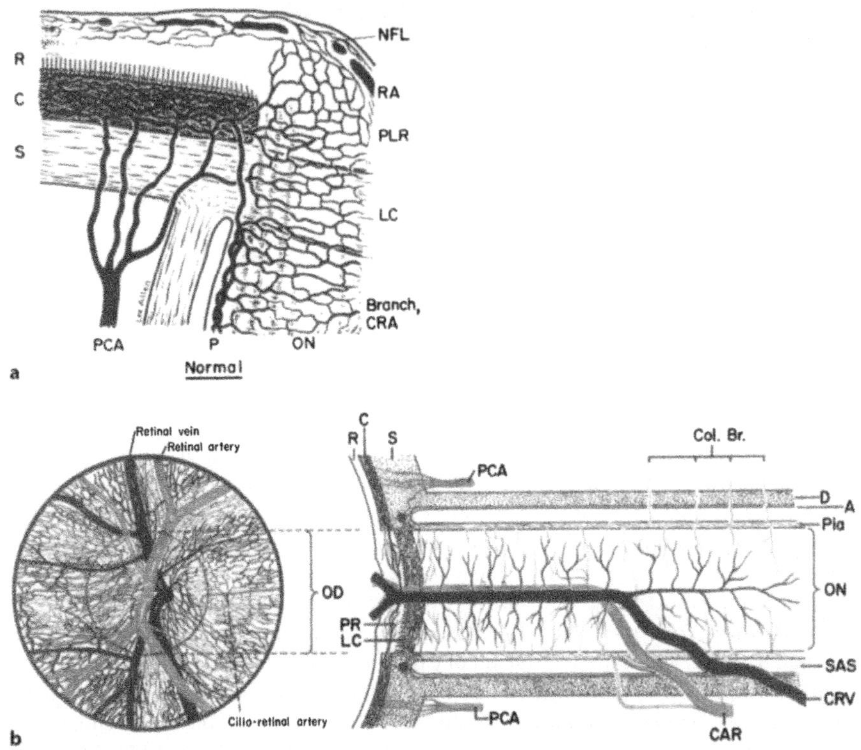

Fig. 1A, B. Schematic representation of blood supply of optic nerve head (A), and entire optic nerve (B). **B** The *right* diagram is a schematic representation of blood supply of the optic nerve and of anastomoses established by the central retinal artery; the *left* is an ophthalmoscopic view of the vessels on the optic disc and surrounding fundus. **A** Reproduced from [28]. **B** Modified from [29]. *A* arachnoid; *C* choroid; *CAR* and *CRA* central retinal artery; *Col. Br.* collateral branches; *CRV* central retinal vein; *D* dura; *LC* lamina cribrosa; *NFL* surface nerve fiber layer of the disc; *OD* optic disc; *ON* optic nerve; *P* pia; *PCA* posterior ciliary artery; *PR* and *PLR* prelaminar region; *R* retina; *RA* retinal arteriole; *S* sclera; *SAS* subarachnoid space

about flow in the deeper part of the ONH tissue. This fact is highly critical in the evaluation of the ONH ischemic disorders.

One of the many methods currently used to evaluate the ONH blood flow is the laser-Doppler flowmetry (LDF) technique. This is a non-invasive method and was first described in 1992 by Riva et al. [14]. There is no definite study showing whether LDF measures the retinal, posterior ciliary or both components of the ONH blood flow. The present study was designed to investigate systematically, in eyes of rhesus monkeys, which part of the ONH circulation is actually measured using the LDF technique. When the CRA, PCA or both of these sources of the ONH circulation are selectively eliminated, the expected effect on LDF flow measurements would be a reduction proportional to the amount that each source contributed to the total measured blood flow within the LDF sampling volume, unless flow from other sources compensated for the missing flow during occlusion of the CRA and/or PCAs. This study is reported in detail elsewhere [15] and the following is an abbreviated account of that.

Materials and Methods

This study was conducted in 17 eyes of normal, healthy, adult rhesus monkeys. The animals were first sedated with intramuscular ketamine hydrochloride (8–10 mg/kg body weight), then anesthetized with pentobarbital, 20 mg/kg, intravenously. Both pupils were dilated using cyclopentolate hydrochloride (1 %) eye drops. All procedures for animal care and experimentation conformed to the University of Iowa Guidelines on Animal Research.

Studies Performed

By lateral orbitotomy, the occlusion of CRA and/or PCA were performed in different combinations. All eyes had fluorescein fundus angiography and LDF flow measurements performed, first before the occlusion to obtain baseline data, then, after the various types of occlusion, to evaluate the state of the ONH circulation.

Experimental Occlusion of CRA and/or PCAs

By lateral orbitotomy, the following types of CRA and/or PCA occlusions were performed.

Central Retinal Artery Occlusion Alone

Central retinal artery occlusion (CRAO) alone was produced by placing a microclamp on the CRA at its site of entry into the optic nerve sheath in four eyes. After a variable length of time, the clamp was removed from the CRA (in an attempt to restore the retinal circulation to normal). The CRAO was carried out in an attempt to eliminate the retinal source of blood flow to the ONH, so that LDF would be measuring, presumably, the blood flow of the deeper ciliary circulation with no masking effect of the overlying retinal circulation.

Posterior Ciliary Artery Occlusion Alone

Posterior ciliary artery occlusion (PCAO) alone was achieved by cutting all the PCAs near their site of entry into the eyeball in four eyes. The PCAO procedure was carried out to eliminate the posterior ciliary source of blood flow to the deeper parts of the ONH, so that LDF would measure presumably the blood flow in the surface retinal circulation with no effect from the underlying ciliary circulation.

CRAO and PCAO in Different Combinations

CRAO and PCAO in different combinations were carried out in the following order in nine eyes on the same day in acute sequential experiments. Eight eyes belonged to four animals who were sacrificed at the end of the experiment.

CRAO Alone. At first, CRA only was clamped in eight of nine eyes; this provided further information from these eight eyes for the study of CRAO alone described above, making a total of 12 eyes with CRAO alone.

Table 1. Retinal and choroidal filling on fluorescein fundus angiography. Negative numbers indicate retina filling before the choroid

Parameter	Circulation time (s) Interval between the start of filling in choroid and retina*	Complete retinal filling	Complete choroidal filling
Normal circulation:			
Minimum	0	1	3
Maximum	1	2	5
Mean	0.12	1.35	3.4
SD	0.3	0.5	0.6
Median	0	1	3
With CRAO alone:			
Minimum	1	13	2
Maximum	19	290	6
Mean	7.5	105	3.5
SD	6	98	1
Median	7.5	70.5	3.5
With PCAO alone:			
Minimum	-1	1	Never
Maximum	-50	2	Never
Mean	-13	1.4	Never
SD	-15	0.5	Never
Median	-11	1	Never

* Choroid usually starts to fill before the retina.
CRAO, central retinal artery occlusion; PCAO, posterior ciliary artery occlusion.

Unclamping of CRA. Then, the clamp on the CRA was removed to restore the retinal circulation. In three of the eight eyes, the clamping had produced thrombosis of the CRA so that it either did not reopen at all, or its circulation was markedly delayed.

Posterior Ciliary Artery Occlusion. Next, in all eight eyes, all the PCAs were cut. Because in three of these eight eyes the CRA did not reopen after removal of the CRA clamp, information about LDF measurements with PCAO alone was available in only five of these eyes. Thus, LDF information in PCAO alone was available in these five eyes and the four eyes mentioned above, making a total of nine eyes in this group.

CRAO and PCAO Combined. Finally, CRA was once again clamped in the eight eyes with PCAO. In a ninth eye, LDF measurements were available only while the PCAs were cut and the CRA was clamped. This provided information on LDF measurements in nine eyes with combined CRAO and PCAO.

Thus, LDF measurements in the above experiments collectively gave the following total number of eyes in the three different occlusion paradigms (Table 1): CRAO alone in 12 eyes, PCAO alone in 9 eyes, and CRAO and PCAO combined in 9 eyes.

LDF Flow Measurements

Before any of the above occlusions was induced, baseline LDF measurements were recorded to obtain the reference flow information. Subsequently, LDF measurements were repeated after each of the above experimental interventions, for which surgery lasted between 30 min and 45 min. LDF measurements began approximately 5–10 min after the surgery and lasted 10–15 min.

LDF Technique

The standard, fundus camera-based LDF technique was used, as described in detail elsewhere [14, 16]. LDF measurements were taken at five locations on the optic disc, away from any visible large vessel. One site was near the center, the other four were at the rim of the optic disc. At each site, the probing laser beam was positioned and then the detection fiber was first centered over it to take an LDF reading in on-beam mode. Then the detection fiber was displaced by one diameter to take a second reading in off-beam mode. The rationale behind separating the detection fiber from the probing laser spot is that more scattered laser light originating from deeper tissue layers is expected to reach the photodetector [17]. For each LDF reading, the fundus camera operator continuously checked that the laser beam remained at the same location for the measurement duration of about 10 s. When the laser beam was steady on target, the Doppler signal was analyzed and the LDF flow parameter recorded. If the eye moved during this time, the measurement was repeated. On the first occasion, the exact location of the measurement was documented on a fundus photograph or a hand-drawn sketch, to be able to later return to the same point of measurement.

LDF provides three relative flow parameters commonly referred to as *flow, volume* and *velocity* of red blood cells. The instantaneous LDF flow parameter is proportional to the product of the other two parameters, volume and velocity, which are proportional to the number and the average speed of moving red blood cells, respectively.

LDF Analysis

To determine and compare the changes induced by the various occlusions, the *normalized* LDF flow at each measurement point was calculated as: the ONH flow value measured during the occlusion divided by the corresponding baseline LDF flow value measured at the same point, e.g., a normalized LDF flow value of 1.0, 0.5, or 1.2 indicates no change, 50 % decrease, or 20 % increase in LDF flow at that point, respectively. For each eye, the normalized LDF flow values at all the measured points were then averaged. Then, the mean normalized LDF flow value was calculated for each group of eyes with the same occlusion type. All means are given with the corresponding 95 % confidence interval unless indicated otherwise.

To compare the measurements in the center of the disc with those at the rim, the normalized LDF flow values for all the rim points and those for the center points were also averaged separately for each group of eyes with the same occlusion type. To compare the measurements obtained with the fiber placed on the laser spot (on-beam mode) with those obtained with the fiber off the spot (off-beam mode), two sets of normalized LDF flow values were calculated and averaged separately for the two detection modes.

Data Analysis

LDF data were analyzed in a masked fashion by two of us (BLP and CER) not knowing the nature of the procedure done on different eyes. The extent of retinal, optic disc and PCA perfusion following the various types of occlusion was evaluated from the fluorescein fundus angiography by one of us (SSH), also masked with respect to the procedure done and to the findings of the other two (BLP and CER). The data were later collated. The 95 % confidence interval of the mean, linear regression analysis and Spearman's rank correlation test were used to assess the statistical significance of the results. p values of less than 0.05 were considered significant.

Results

Fluorescein Fundus Angiography Data During CRAO and/or PCAO

We evaluated the effect of CRAO or PCAO on the filling pattern of the retinal and choroidal vascular beds by fluorescein fundus angiography. During CRAO, the retinal vasculature eventually filled in all cases, but with a relatively long and highly variable time delay. After PCAO, as expected, the choroid usually started to fill after a variable interval from the start of filling of the CRA and almost never filled completely. There was a marked interocular variation seen in the speed and amount of filling of residual retinal and choroidal circulations after the various types of occlusions, due to marked interocular differences in the amount of anastomoses. Table 1 summarizes the findings following the various types of occlusions on the three parameters: choroid to retina filling delay, retinal filling time and choroidal filling time. Baseline values for these parameters were 0 s (0–1), 1 s (1–2) and 3 s (3–5), respectively [median (minimum–maximum)].

LDF Data During CRAO and/or PCAO

The results of LDF during CRAO and/or PCAO are summarized in Table 2.

In Normal Control Eyes

Table 2 summarizes the LDF results in the nine contralateral eyes available as controls during various types of CRAO and/or PCAO. None of the LDF parameters changed significantly during re-test, as seen from the confidence intervals given in Table 2. When averaged separately, the LDF parameters measured at the rim and center points did not change significantly.

Table 2. Laser-Doppler flow (LDF) results for various groups

Parameter	Normalized LDF parameters								
	Flow			Volume			Velocity		
	All points	Rim points	Center point	All points	Rim points	Center point	All points	Rim points	Center point
LDF results for control eyes:									
Mean	1.04	1.09	0.79	1.06	1.09	0.93	1.07	1.05	1.16
Standard Deviation	0.24	0.25	0.30	0.29	0.32	0.71	0.12	0.11	0.26
Confidence Interval	0.19	0.19	0.23	0.23	0.25	0.54	0.09	0.08	0.20
LDF results for CRAO alone:									
Fiber On Beam:									
Mean	0.61	0.61	0.59	0.86	0.87	0.81	0.96	0.97	0.89
Standard Deviation	0.33	0.32	0.45	0.76	0.81	0.69	0.57	0.58	0.61
Confidence Interval	0.21	0.20	0.29	0.49	0.51	0.44	0.37	0.37	0.39
Fiber Off Beam:									
Mean	0.72	0.73	0.74	0.97	1.01	0.83	0.84	0.81	1.03
Standard Deviation	0.37	0.37	0.79	0.61	0.68	0.82	0.48	0.41	0.83
Confidence Interval	0.34	0.34	0.83	0.56	0.63	0.86	0.44	0.38	0.87
LDF results for PCAO alone:									
Fiber On Beam:									
Mean	1.17	1.18	1.07	1.03	1.03	0.99	1.24	1.24	1.29
Standard Deviation	0.48	0.55	0.42	0.46	0.53	0.80	0.41	0.41	0.69
Confidence Interval	0.37	0.42	0.32	0.35	0.41	0.61	0.32	0.31	0.53
Fiber Off Beam:									
Mean	0.95	0.86	1.25	0.86	0.82	1.07	1.16	1.15	1.18
Standard Deviation	0.56	0.66	0.81	0.58	0.72	0.75	0.23	0.24	0.18
Confidence Interval	0.69	0.82	1.00	0.72	0.89	0.93	0.28	0.30	0.22
LDF results for combined CRAO and PCAO:									
Fiber On Beam:									
Mean	0.43	0.43	0.41	0.99	0.98	1.02	0.75	0.75	0.74
Standard Deviation	0.36	0.33	0.49	0.99	0.90	1.48	0.61	0.58	0.86
Confidence Interval	0.27	0.25	0.38	0.76	0.69	1.14	0.47	0.45	0.66
Fiber Off Beam:									
Mean	0.43	0.44	0.40	1.06	1.11	0.79	0.71	0.71	0.69
Standard Deviation	0.42	0.41	0.49	1.03	1.13	0.65	0.56	0.53	0.75
Confidence Interval	0.39	0.38	0.45	0.95	1.05	0.60	0.52	0.49	0.69

CRAO central retinal artery occlusion; *PCAO* posterior ciliary artery occlusion.

During CRAO Alone

Measurement during CRAO alone was done in a total of 12 eyes. With on-beam detection mode, only the LDF flow parameter was significantly decreased during CRAO ($p < 0.001$), with the rim and center points showing similar behavior. The ONH volume and velocity results, however, were not significantly decreased. Results for the off-beam detection mode followed a similar pattern as the on-beam results, but showed a smaller decrease in LDF flow of 0.72±0.34 (not significant because of the smaller number of eyes).

After removal of the CRA clamp, taking into account only those eyes where patency of the CRA was confirmed by angiography, normalized LDF flow, volume and velocity were 1.13±0.48, 1.05±0.47 and 1.02±0.20, respectively, for on-beam detection mode. These data indicate that these parameters had returned to the normal baseline values.

During PCAO Alone

In the nine eyes in this category, rim and center points showed no significantly different behavior under this experimental condition compared with the baseline.

During Combined CRAO and PCAO

For the entire group of nine eyes, the average LDF flow was significantly decreased both for on-beam ($p< 0.001$) and off-beam ($p< 0.01$) detection modes – with the rim and center points showing similar behavior – whereas the ONH volume and velocity values were not significantly decreased.

Follow-Up Clinical Evaluation of Eyes With PCAO

Of the nine eyes with permanent PCAO alone, only four eyes in four animals were followed for many weeks after the occlusion, while the remaining five eyes were part of the acute experiment only. All four of them developed marked anterior ischemic optic neuropathy, with pale swollen optic disc and complete loss of vision when evaluated the day after the occlusion. One of these four eyes also developed signs of anterior segment ischemia.

Discussion

Our group average LDF results show that LDF flow during CRAO alone is highly significantly decreased ($p< 0.001$) compared with the normal baseline, by an average of 39±21 % (mean±95 % confidence interval). Combined CRAO and PCAO reduced LDF flow even more markedly, by 57±27 % ($p< 0.0005$). After PCAO alone, however, our measurements showed a non-significant increase in LDF flow of 17±37 %. Thus, on average, CRAO alone did significantly reduce LDF flow, but PCAO alone did not. With the CRA and all the PCAs occluded, LDF flow was reduced more than with CRAO alone, but the difference between the flow reductions was not significant ($p>0.20$). The remaining LDF flow after combined CRAO and PCAO, however, was highly significantly greater than zero ($p< 0.005$).

Previous work demonstrated that LDF flow was detectable in vitro behind unperfused layers of excised cat ONH tissue with thicknesses of up to 600 μm, that the sensitivity of LDF measurements decreased with increasing thickness and that, in vivo, twice as much light was backscattered by the cat optic nerve [18]. Table 11 from a report by Delori and Pflibsen [19] shows that a large portion of light at 675 nm penetrates the ONH tissue, reaches the lamina cribrosa and is reflected there – about 50 % at the rim and 90 % in the cup. This suggests that photons detected by LDF have been scattered in all layers of the ONH tissue, before and after being reflected by the lamina. This was confirmed by our own observation that the entire surface area of the ONH lit up with diffuse red laser light, although only a small fraction of its surface was actually illuminated by the incident laser beam (spot size diameter of 150 μm). The same report demonstrates the presence of an absorption "signature" characteristic of hemoglobin [19]. This indicates that, at the wavelength used by the LDF method, many photons are scattered not only by the ONH tissue, but at least once by a moving red cell, giving rise to a Doppler shift.

Based on these optical considerations, we had expected to find significant LDF flow changes in all types of arterial occlusions. Unexpectedly, however, we found no LDF flow decrease in PCAO alone, which could be either due to a substitution of the flow missing from the PCAs after PCAO by flow from other sources, or to a masking of the Doppler signal originating from the deep layers by the signal originating from the surface layers.

Interpretation of LDF Flow Findings in the ONH Following CRAO and/or PCAO

The surface nerve fiber layer is mostly supplied by the CRA and the deeper prelaminar, lamina cribrosa and retrolaminar regions mainly by the PCAs (Fig. 1) [12, 13]. To understand where the LDF flow measurement originates, we need explanations for the following three findings of our LDF flow measurements:

(1) If the LDF sampling volume comprises only the surface nerve fiber layer, then why was 61 % LDF flow still recorded when the CRA alone was clamped?
(2) Why did LDF flow not go to zero when both the CRA and all the PCAs were occluded simultaneously?
(3) Why did occlusion of all the PCAs alone not significantly decrease the LDF flow?

Why Was 61% LDF Flow Still Recorded When the CRA Alone Was Clamped?

Our results indicate that the PCAs and/or other sources substituted 61 % of the original flow to the surface layer in our group of eyes. This is due to constant presence of a highly variable amount of residual circulation in the surface nerve fiber layer of the ONH, in spite of complete occlusion of the CRA at its site of entry into the dural sheath of the optic nerve; this residual circulation was always shown by fluorescein fundus angiographic studies in the present as well as in previous studies [20]. There are two mechanisms for this residual circulation in the superficial layers of the ONH even after complete occlusion of the CRA.

Via Cilio-Retinal Capillary Anastomoses Within the ONH

The capillary bed in the entire ONH is continuous (Fig. 1A). When the CRA is occluded, invariably there is a sluggish and highly variable amount of flow of blood from the normally filling deeper capillaries (supplied by the PCA circulation) to the adjacent empty superficial capillaries in the ONH [12, 20, 21].

Via Pial and Intraneural Anastomoses of the CRA

The CRA gives out prominent pial branches in 95 % of eyes near the point of entry into the optic nerve and a variable number of intraneural (within the optic nerve) branches in 75 % [22] (Fig. 1B). The great majority of the pial branches of the CRA establish very conspicuous anastomoses with pial branches from other orbital arteries [22] ("collateral branches" in Fig. 1B). When the site of CRAO is outside the optic nerve dural sheath, as in the present study, all the pial anastomoses are still functioning, and that results in slow filling of the CRA and the retinal vascular bed from its intraneural course at the optic disc to a variable extent (Table 1) [12, 20]. The speed and extent of the filling of the CRA depend on the magnitude of the anastomoses [20].

From this, it follows that the amount of residual retinal circulation in the superficial nerve fiber layer of the ONH following CRAO, shown by fluorescein angiography, varies widely, depending on the marked interindividual variability in the amount and efficiency of these anastomoses (Table 1) [20]. This can account for both the variability and the remaining average of 61 % of LDF flow measured in the present study during CRAO.

Why Did LDF Flow Not Go to Zero When Both the CRA and All the PCAs Were Occluded Simultaneously?

Following combined occlusion of the CRA and all the PCAs, a group average of 43 % of LDF flow was still present, although in two of nine eyes we found only 8 % of baseline LDF flow remaining. The following sources provided the variable amount of residual LDF flow in this situation.

Pial and Intraneural Anastomoses of the CRA

As discussed above, these anastomoses helped in filling of the intraneural part of the CRA and consequently of capillaries in the surface nerve fiber layer of the ONH to a variable degree.

Peripapillary Choroidal Anastomoses

The peripapillary choroid can fill via two types of anastomotic connections: (1) recurrent pial branches of the peripapillary choroid anastomose with the other optic nerve pial branches derived from other orbital arteries; in eyes with PCAO, the peripapillary choroid can fill via these anastomoses (Fig. 1B) [23]; and (2) during PCAO there is a retrograde filling of the vortex veins [23, 24], and that in turn causes a slow and highly variable filling of the peripapillary choroid. Since the peripapillary choroid is the main source of blood supply to the prelaminar region of the ONH, this filling of the prelaminar region, though very slow and minimal, may also contribute in some cases with CRAO to a certain amount of the residual circulation in the surface nerve fiber layer capillaries via the cilioretinal anastomoses, as discussed above; however, the amount of cilioretinal flow with PCAO is bound to be much less than that occurring normally, and that would account for the change in average LDF flow decrease from 39±21 % during CRAO alone to 57±27 % during combined CRAO and PCAO.

Therefore, it is not at all surprising that, in spite of combined occlusion of the CRA and PCAs, a variable amount of flow is still present in the surface nerve fiber layer of the ONH, which can account for the remaining average of 43 % of LDF flow in these eyes. With combined occlusion of the CRA and all the PCAs, LDF flow was reduced more than with CRAO alone, i.e., 57±27 % vs 39±21 %, but the difference in flow reduction was not significant ($p > 0.20$).

Why Did Occlusion of All the PCAs Alone Not Significantly Decrease the LDF Flow?

After PCAO alone, we found a non-significant increase (17±37 %) in LDF flow compared with the baseline. This indicates that, unlike the restoration of residual circulation in the surface nerve fiber layer following CRAO, there is no mechanism available to produce residual circulation in the deeper layers of the ONH following PCAO. This is further shown by the fact that, in the present study, all four of the eyes with PCAO, followed for many weeks, were found to have fulminant anterior ischemic optic neuropathy the next day when they were first examined after the PCAO. All experimental [24, 25] and clinical [26] studies with PCAO have shown the development of anterior ischemic optic neuropathy, which is a clear sign of ischemia of the deeper layers of the ONH [27]. This clearly indicates that all the eyes in the present study with PCAO must have had marked ischemia of the deeper layers of the ONH, in spite of no significant decrease in the LDF flow measurement from baseline and normally filling capillaries in the superficial layer of the ONH from the CRA.

Conclusions

The ONH blood circulation is highly complex, and its measurement remains very challenging. The results of this study, using a standard, fundus camera-based LDF technique to measure blood flow in the ONH tissue during various occlusions of its blood supply sources, suggest that this LDF technique is predominantly sensitive to flow changes in the surface nerve fiber layer and less sensitive to those in the prelaminar and laminar regions. That may limit its usefulness in evaluation of ONH blood flow in glaucomatous optic neuropathy and other ONH ischemic disorders. The same may be applicable to the scanning LDF technique.

Acknowledgements. The authors thank Ms. D. McAllister and Mr. S. Cranstoun for their help with the experimental part of the study. Dr. Hayreh is a Research to Prevent Blindness senior scientific investigator. This work was supported by Grant EY1576 from the U.S. National Institutes of Health and, in part, by unrestricted grants from Research to Prevent Blindness, Inc., New York (to SSH), Man Singh Foundation and the Dreiseszun Family Foundation. It was also supported in part by the Swiss National Fund for Scientific Research (#32-043157) and the Pennsylvania Lions Sight Conservation & Eye Research Foundation (to CER).

References

1. Hayreh SS (1963) Blood supply and vascular disorders of the optic nerve. Ann Inst Barraquer 4:7–109
2. Hayreh SS (1970) Pathogenesis of visual field defects: role of the ciliary circulation. Br J Ophthalmol 54:289–311
3. Hayreh SS, Revie HIS, Edwards J (1970) Vasogenic origin of visual field defects and optic nerve changes in glaucoma. Br J Ophthalmol 54:461–472
4. Spaeth G (1977) The pathogenesis of nerve damage in glaucoma: contributions of fluorescein angiography. Grune & Stratton, New York
5. Hayreh SS (1978) Pathogenesis of optic nerve damage and visual field defects. In: Heilmann K, Richardson KT (eds) Glaucoma. Conceptions of a disease. Thieme, Stuttgart, pp 103–138

6. Lambrou GN, Greve EL (1989) Ocular blood flow in glaucoma: means, methods and measurements. Kugler & Ghedini, Amstelveen
7. Geijssen HC (1991) Studies on normal pressure glaucoma. Kugler & Ghedini, Amstelveen
8. Drance SM (1992) International symposium on glaucoma, ocular blood flow and drug treatment. Williams & Wilkins, Baltimore
9. Hayreh SS (1993) Die Bedeutung vaskulärer Faktoren in der Pathogenese des Glaukomschadens. In: Pillunat LE, Stodtmeister R (eds) Das Glaukom. Springer, Berlin Heidelberg New York, pp 34–58
10. Hayreh SS (1994) Progress in the understanding of the vascular etiology of glaucoma. Curr Opin Ophthalmol 5(2):26–35
11. Kaiser HJ, Flammer H, Hendrickson P (1996) Ocular blood flow: new insights into the pathogenesis of ocular diseases. Karger, Basel
12. Hayreh SS (1969) Blood supply of the optic nerve head and its role in optic atrophy, glaucoma and oedema of the optic disc. Br J Ophthalmol 53:721–748
13. Hayreh SS (1995) The 1994 Von Sallmann lecture: the optic nerve head circulation in health and disease. Exp Eye Res 61:259–272
14. Riva CE, Harino S, Petrig BL, Shonat RD (1992) Laser Doppler flowmetry in the optic nerve. Exp Eye Res 55:499–506
15. Petrig BL, Riva CE, Hayreh SS (1999) Laser doppler flowmetry and optic nerve head blood flow. Am J Ophthalmol 127:413–425
16. Petrig BL, Riva CE (1996) Optic nerve head laser Doppler flowmetry: principles and computer analysis. In: Kaiser HJ, Flammer J, Hendrickson P (eds) Ocular blood flow. New insights into the pathogenesis of ocular diseases. Karger, Basel, pp 120–127
17. Bonner RF, Nossal R (1990) Principles of laser Doppler flowmetry. In: Shepherd AP, Oberg PA (eds) Laser-Doppler blood flowmetry. Kluwer Academic Publishers, Boston, pp 17–46
18. Koelle JS, Riva CE, Petrig BL, Cranstoun SD (1993) Depth of tissue sampling in the optic nerve head using laser Doppler flowmetry. Laser Med Sci 8:49–54
19. Delori FC, Pflibsen KP (1989) Reflectance properties of the optic disc. In: Noninvasive assessment of the visual system. (Technical digest series, vol 7) Optical Society of America, Washington DC, pp 154–157
20. Hayreh SS, Weingeist TA (1980) Experimental occlusion of the central artery of the retina. 1. Ophthalmoscopic and fluorescein fundus angiographic studies. Br J Ophthalmol 64:896–912
21. Hayreh SS (1974) Central retinal vascular occlusion: morphology and pathogenesis. In: Brancato F, Pratesi F (eds) International symposium on ocular angiology, Centro Minerva Medica, pp 15–40
22. Singh S, Dass R (1960) The central artery of the retina 11. Distribution and anastomoses. Br J Ophthalmol 44:280–299
23. Hayreh SS, Baines JAB (1972) Occlusion of the posterior ciliary artery. 1. Effects on choroidal circulation. Br J Ophthalmol 56:719–735
24. Hayreh SS, Chopdar A (1982) Occlusion of the posterior ciliary artery. V Protective influence of simultaneous vortex vein occlusion. Arch Ophthalmol 100:1481–1491
25. Hayreh SS, Baines JAB (1972) Occlusion of the posterior ciliary artery. III Effects on the optic nerve head. Br J Ophthalmol 56:754–764
26. Hayreh SS, Podhajsky PA, Zimmerman B (1998) Ocular manifestations of giant cell arteritis. Am J Ophthalmol 125:509–520
27. Hayreh SS (1996) Acute ischemic disorders of the optic nerve: pathogenesis, clinical manifestations and management. Ophthalmol Clin North Am 9:407–442
28. Hayreh SS (1978) Structure and blood supply of the optic nerve. In: Heilmann K, Richardson KT (eds) Glaucoma: concepts of a disease. Thieme, Stuttgart, pp 78–96
29. Hayreh SS (1974) Anatomy and physiology of the optic nerve head. Trans Am Acad Ophthalmol Otolaryngol 78:OP240–OP254

CHAPTER 12

Change in the Optic Nerve Head Caused by Endothelin-1-Induced Chronic Ischaemia

I. Azuma · H. Oku

Introduction

Endothelin (ET-1) is the most potent and long-acting of the vasoconstrictor peptides and was originally produced by endothelial cells to control vascular tone and regulate blood flow by modulating Ca-channel activity [1] We have previously shown that the plasma ET-1 level was increased in patients with normal-tension glaucoma (NTG). Recently, Orgul, Cioffi and their colleagues demonstrated reduction of optic-nerve blood flow induced by continuous delivery of ET-1 to the perineural region of the anterior optic nerve of rabbits with an osmotically driven minipump [2]. In the present study, to investigate the effects of chronic ischaemia on the optic nerve, we produced continuous ischaemia of the optic-nerve head by injecting ET-1 directly into the posterior vitreous of rabbits twice per week for 4 weeks and examined the functional and morphological changes of the optic-nerve head.

Materials and Methods

We injected ET-1 (10^{-6} M, 10 µl) into the posterior vitreous of one eye in pigmented rabbits from the pars plana using a Hamilton syringe and a 30-gauge needle under local anaesthesia with 4 % lidocaine twice per week for 4 weeks ($n = 7$). The vehicle for the ET-1 was injected into the contralateral eye as a control ($n = 7$). The subsequent observation period was set at 8 weeks. Capillary blood flow in the optic-nerve head was noninvasively measured using the recently developed laser-speckle circulation analyser. The normalised-blur (NB) value obtained using this method indicates blurring of the speckle pattern formed by scattered light, which was originally regarded as a quantitative index of blood velocity. The NB value was measured serially in the same field (0.42·0.42 mm) of the optic-nerve head [3]. Measurements were carried out once per week before intravitreal injection. To evaluate the changes of visual function, we used visual-evoked potentials (VEPs). The first negative peak, with a latency of 20 ms, was defined as N1 and its latency was measured as an indicator of visual function [4]. The intraocular pressure (IOP) was measured using a pneumatonometer (Alcon, Tokyo, Japan) under local anaesthesia twice per week. The morphology of the optic-nerve head was analysed using fundus pictures taken from different angles before and 8 weeks after treatment. The pictures were digitised, stored in a microcomputer, and arranged to provide a stereograph of the optic-nerve head. Data are expressed as the mean and the standard error of the mean. Two-way interactions were analysed using repeated-measures analysis of variance (ANOVA), and statistical comparisons between two groups were performed using Student's *t*-test. Differences were accepted as significant at $p < 0.05$ (Fig. 1).

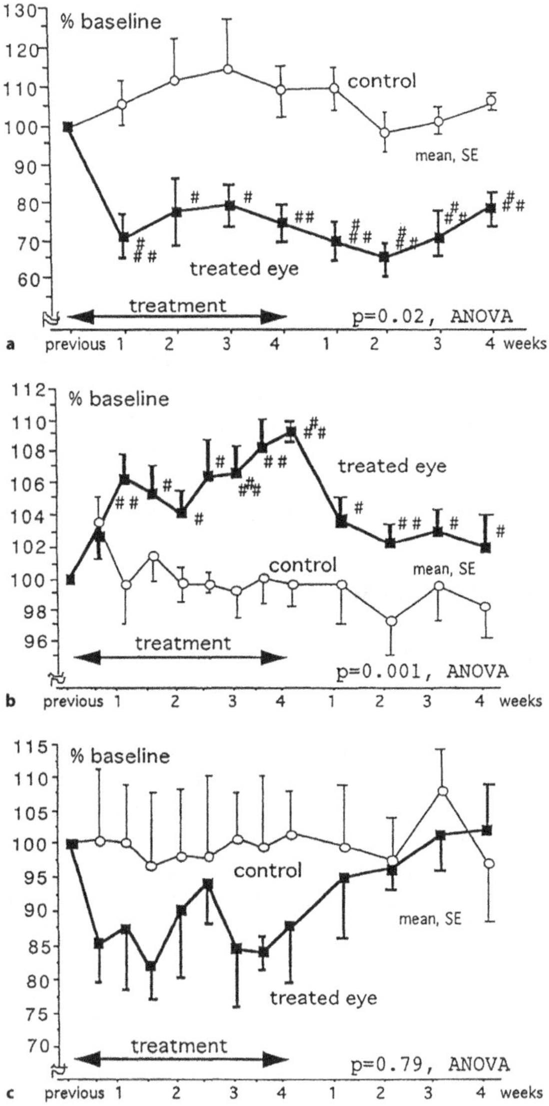

Fig. 1. a Normalised-blur (NB) value in the optic nerve. **b** Visual-evoked potential (VEP) latency. **c** Intraocular pressure

Results

In the ET-1-treated eyes, the NB value was continuously below 80 % of the baseline during treatment, while the vehicle did not decrease the NB value (control). The two-way interaction was significant by repeated-measures ANOVA ($p = 0.02$), and there were significant differences between the ET-1-treated and control eyes at every time of assessment ($p < 0.05$, Student's t-test).

Repeated ET-1 treatment prolonged the N1 latency, which gradually became closer but did not return to the pretreatment level 4 weeks after the completion of treatment, while the control N1 latency remained stable throughout the study. The two-way interaction was significant by repeated-measures ANOVA ($p = 0.001$), and there were significant differences between ET-1-treated and control eyes at every time of assessment except the first ($p < 0.05$, Student's t-test). The IOP tended to be lower in the ET-1-treated eyes, but the two-way interaction was insignificant ($p < 0.05$, ANOVA). In ET-1-treated eyes, the area of the disc cup increased and the cup became more excavated. Cup enlargement occurred mainly towards the edge of the medullary rays. Such changes were not observed in the control eyes. The central area/dorsal area ratios before and after treatment were, respectively, 23.8 (3.78) and 30.5 (3.33) for ET-1-treated eyes, while they were 24.9 (3.78) and 25.3 (3.59) for control eyes. The percentage change relative to the baseline was 135.9 % (12.7) for ET-1-treated eyes, while it was 102.4 % (2.29) for control eyes, and there was a significant difference between them ($p = 0.024$, Student's t-test). Repeated exposure to ET-1 caused loss of axons as well as demyelination affecting the prelaminar portion of the optic nerve.

Discussion

It is well known that blood supply to the retina and the optic-nerve head is controlled via an autoregulatory mechanism that can lower vascular resistance to maintain blood flow when an increase of IOP or a decrease of blood pressure reduces the perfusion pressure to the eye. Autoregulation may be controlled by locally released vasoactive substances, among which nitric oxide and ET-1 are considered to be the most important endothelium-derived relaxing and contracting factors, respectively. Injection of ET-1 into the rabbit vitreous constricted retinal vessels in a dose-dependent manner and impaired VEP responses, while electroretinogram responses were relatively well preserved, suggesting that ET-1 not only acted on retinal vessels but also on the optic-nerve-head blood supply mainly derived from the posterior ciliary artery. Indeed, intravitreal ET-1 caused pallor of the optic-nerve head [4]. Therefore, it seems possible that vascular tone limits autoregulatory dilatation in the optic-nerve-head circulation as a result of elevated ET-1 production [5]. Accordingly, we consider that our method of ET-1 administration produced an animal model of chronic optic-nerve ischaemia.

The most striking finding in this study was that optic-nerve-head ischaemia contributed to enlargement and excavation in the disc cup. Ocular circulation largely depends on the IOP and blood perfusion pressure. Although the difference was not statistically significant, IOP was lower in the ET-1-treated eyes than the control eyes.

Since neither ganglion cell loss nor remarkable defects of myelinated nerve-fibre bundles were observed, chronic ischaemia induced by repeated ET-1 exposure mainly affected the optic-nerve head. This finding was quite similar to that observed with glaucomatous optic neuropathy, in which optic-nerve fibres show the earliest damage at the lamina cribrosa. With longer ischaemic stress, the nerve-fibre bundles and the ganglion cells may have been lost. Further study will be needed to clarify the mechanism of the cup enlargement seen in this study, including abnormalities of the extracellular matrix at the lamina cribrosa caused by ET-1.

Conclusion

Ischaemia might contribute to disc cupping, which is quite similar to that seen in people with chronic glaucoma. This model may be useful for understanding the pathophysiology of NTG and for developing treatment.

References

1. Yanagisawa M, Kurihasi H, Kimura S, Tomobe Y, Kobayashi M, Mitsui Y, Yazaki Y, Goto K, Masaki T (1988) A novel potent vasoconstrictor peptide produced by vascular endothelial cells. Nature 332:411–415
2. Orgul S, Cioffi GA, Wilson DJ, Bacon DR, Van-Buskin EM (1996) An endothelin-1 induced model of optic nerve ischaemia in the rabbit. Invest Ophthalmol Vis Sci 37:1860–1869
3. Sugiyama T, Utsumi T, Azuma I, Fujii H (1996) Measurement of optic nerve head circulation: comparison of laser speckle and hydrogen clearance methods. Jpn J Ophthalmol 40:339–343
4. Oku H, Sugiyama T, Moriya S, Hamada J, Azuma I (1993) Effects of intravitreal injection of endothelin on the visual system. Nippon Ganka Gakkai Zasshi 97:467–473
5. Sugiyama T, Moriya S, Oku H, Azuma I (1995) Association of endothelin-1 with normal tension glaucoma: clinical and fundamental studies. Surv Ophthalmol 39[Suppl 1]:S49–S56

CHAPTER 13

Effects of Ifenprodil on Aqueous Dynamics and Ocular Circulation

M. Araie · K. Muta

Abstract. Ifenprodil is a drug used in patients with cerebrovascular insufficiency with vasodilating activity attributable to α-blocking and papaverine-like activities, inhibitory effects on platelet aggregation and noncompetitive *N*-methyl-D-aspartic acid-receptor antagonistic activity. Effects of this drug on aqueous dynamics and iris, posterior choroid and optic-nerve head-tissue circulation in rabbits were studied. A single unilateral instillation of 0.5 % ifenprodil (50 μl) significantly reduced the intraocular pressure (IOP) for 4 h, with a maximum reduction of 3.5 mmHg without any contralateral effect. It significantly increased the uveoscleral flow from 0.06±0.45 μl/min to 0.96±0.31 μl/min (mean±SE, $n = 20$), but showed no effects on the fluorescein permeability to the blood–aqueous barrier, the aqueous flow rate or the outflow facility to the general circulation. Effects on ocular circulation were studied using the noninvasive laser-speckle method in rabbits receiving 20-day unilateral instillation of 0.5 % ifenprodil twice daily. Two hours after the first instillation in the ifenprodil-treated eye, the normalized blur (NB), an index of tissue blood velocity, showed no change in any of the tissues studied; however, the NB after 3 days or 20 days of instillation twice daily showed a small but significant increase of 5–8 % in all tissues studied. The IOP in the ifenprodil-treated eye showed about 2.5 mmHg reduction at all time points of measurement, while no change was seen in either the IOP or NB in any tissues in the vehicle-treated eye. In addition to the ocular hypotensive effect, topical ifenprodil may have beneficial effects on ocular circulation which are probably not related to the IOP reduction or systemic absorption.

Introduction

Ifenprodil is a relatively old drug which has been used clinically as a cerebral vasodilating drug in patients with cerebrovascular insufficiency. Due to its α-blocking and papaverine-like activities [1], it has vasodilating activity relatively selective for vertebral arteries, and it inhibits platelet aggregation [2]. Further, ifenprodil was known to show *N*-methyl-D-aspartic acid (NMDA)-receptor antagonistic and neuroprotective activities almost equipotential to that of MK801 in vitro, which is attributable to ifenprodil's antagonism of the polyamine modulatory site of the receptor complex [3].

Ifenprodil may have the potential to reduce the intraocular pressure (IOP) through its α-blocking activity, and its vasodilating activity may be beneficial to ocular circulation. Further, if it can reach the retina after long-term use, its NMDA antagonistic activity may be advantageous. The present study was carried out to examine the effects of topical ifenprodil on the aqueous-humor dynamics and ocular circulation in rabbits.

Materials and Methods

To study the effects on the aqueous-humor dynamics, male Japanese albino rabbits weighing 2.0–2.6 kg were conditioned to a schedule of 12 h of light and 12 h of dark for at least 3 weeks before the experiment, and all experiments were carried out in the dark phase using conscious rabbits. An ifenprodil solution of 0.5 % was prepared using distilled water containing a small amount of glycerin, and its pH and osmolarity were about 6.5 and 300 mOsmol, respectively.

Effects on the aqueous-humor dynamics were studied as previously reported [4]. IOP was measured using a calibrated pneumatonograph. The blood–aqueous barrier (BAB) permeability was determined by measuring the fluorescein concentration in the anterior chamber 30 min after intravenous injection of fluorescein (0.02 mg/kg). The aqueous flow rate was measured according to the fluorophotometric method of Jones-Maurice (method II) [5], and the outflow facility to the general circulation and uveoscleral flow was measured according to the fluorophotometric method of Hayashi et al. using systemic Diamox instead of topical levobunolol [6].

The effect of topical ifenprodil (0.5 %) on ocular circulation was studied using male Dutch rabbits weighing 1.7–2.3 kg conditioned to a schedule of 12 h of light and 12 h of dark for at least 3 weeks before the experiment by means of the noninvasive laser-speckle method. With this method, the normalized blur (NB) value is obtained as a quantitative index of the status of tissue circulation [7, 8]. NB is primarily a quantitative index of tissue blood velocity [7, 8], but it also shows correlation with the number of red blood cells in the sampling volume [9]. In the iris or posterior choroid, the NB value showed good correlation with the microsphere technique under any of the following conditions: when blood flow was artificially changed via a step-wise increase in IOP [7], on instillation of unoprostone, which causes inflammation in the rabbit anterior uvea [10], on instillation of carteolol [11] or on injection of nicardipine, a calcium antagonist [12]. In the optic-nerve head (ONH), the NB value showed good correlation with the blood flow rate determined with the hydrogen-gas clearance method under any of the following conditions: when blood flow was artificially changed by injection of a small amount of endothelin-1 [13], on inhalation of carbon-dioxide [13], on injection of nilvadipine, a calcium-antagonist (Araie et al., unpublished result) or on intravitreal injection of a NO donor (Kojima et al., unpublished result).

Measurement of the NB in the iris, posterior choroid and the ONH were carried out as previously described (Fig. 1) [7, 10]. All measurements were carried out by a masked investigator in rabbits under general anesthesia induced by intravenous injection of pentobarbital (15 mg/kg). Absence of eye movement during the measurement was checked by the method previously described [14, 15].

At 10:00 p.m., the IOP was measured in both eyes and, immediately thereafter, the NB measurement in the iris was carried out and the pupil dilated with 0.4 % tropicamide in both eyes. The NB measurements in the posterior choroid and ONH were carried out in both eyes 20 min after tropicamide instillation. At 8:00 p.m. the next

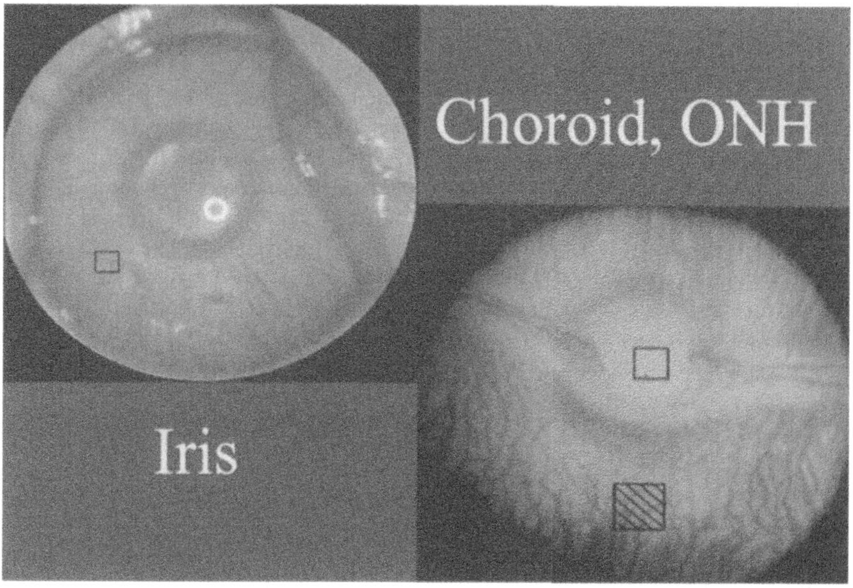

Fig. 1. Measurement site in the iris, posterior choroid and optic-nerve head (ONH). The measurement field was about 0.6·0.6 mm^2 (corresponding to 100·100 pixels on the sensor plane) in the iris and posterior choroid and 0.4·0.4 mm^2 (70·70 pixels) in the ONH

day, 50 μl of 0.5 % ifenprodil and the vehicle were instilled in one eye and the fellow eye, respectively, and the IOP and NB measurements in the iris, posterior choroid and ONH were carried out between 10:00 p.m. and 10:20 p.m., as described above, according to the same time schedule. In another three separate groups of rabbits, a further instillation of 0.5 % ifenprodil and the vehicle was carried out twice daily at 8:00 a.m. and 8:00 p.m., beginning the next day for 1 day (1-day group), for 3 days (3-day group) or for 20 days (20-day group). The IOP measurement and the NB measurements in the iris, choroid and ONH were carried out as above at the same time on the day after the last instillation; that is, 2 days after the baseline IOP and NB measurements for the 1-day group, 4 days after the baseline measurements for the 3-day group, and 21 days after the baseline measurements for the 20-day group.

Results and Discussion

Effect on the Aqueous-Humor Dynamics

A single instillation of 50 μl of 0.5 % ifenprodil solution and the vehicle in one eye and the fellow eye, respectively, showed IOP reduction only in the ipsilateral treated eye, with a maximum effect of about 3.5 mmHg, and its hypotensive effect lasted about 4 h. The fluorescein concentration in the anterior chamber 0.5 h after intravenous fluorescein injection and 2 h after a single instillation of 50 μl of 0.5 % ifenprodil or vehicle was 4.27±0.54·10^{-8} g/ml (mean±standard error [SE], n = 14) in the drug-treated eye and 4.91±0.54·10^{-8} g/ml in the vehicle-treated eye. Averaged aqueous flow rate between 0 h and 4 h after a single instillation of 0.5 % ifenprodil or vehicle was 2.48±0.23 μl/min (mean±SE, n = 15) in the drug-treated eye and 2.89±0.22 μl/min in the vehicle-treated eye. The fluorophotometrically determined outflow facility to general circulation was 0.19±0.03 μl/min/mmHg (mean±SE, n = 20) in the drug-treated eye and 0.23±0.05 μl/min/mmHg in the vehicle-treated eye, respectively, and the fluorophotometrically determined uveoscleral flow was 0.96±0.31 μl/min (mean±SE, n = 20) in the drug-treated eye and 0.06±0.45 μl/min in the vehicle-treated eye, respectively. No significant bilateral difference was seen in the aqueous flow rate, the outflow facility to general circulation, or in the fluorescein concentration in the anterior chamber after intravenous fluorescein injection, while significant bilateral difference was seen in the uveoscleral flow ($p < 0.05$). Topical ifenprodil reduced the IOP in the rabbit eye by increasing uveoscleral outflow, which is thought to be, at least partly, attributable to ifenprodil's α-blocking activity [4], but its ocular hypotensive effect was not so remarkable.

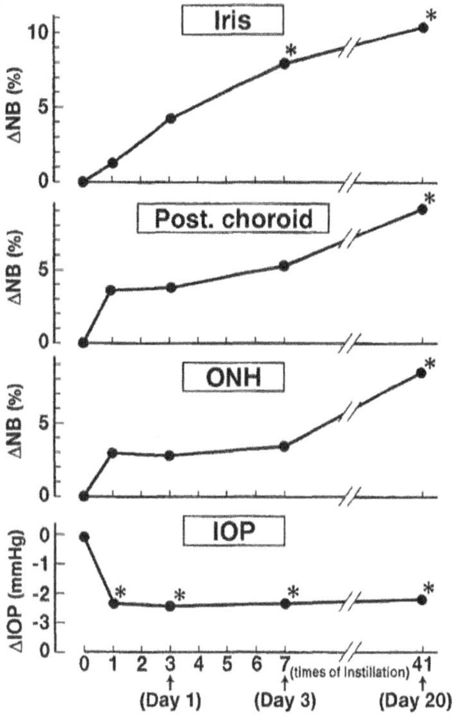

Fig. 2. Bilateral difference (Ifenprodil-treated side minus vehicle-treated side) in the normalized blur and intraocular pressure. *, Statistically significant bilateral difference ($p < 0.05$)

Effect on Ocular Circulation

The results of the IOP measurement and the NB in the iris, posterior choroid and ONH obtained in a total of four groups of rabbits are combined and summarized in Fig. 2. Since results obtained in four separate groups were combined, the NB obtained at each time point of measurement was normalized to the corresponding baseline value. The bilateral difference in the IOP was about 2.5 mmHg without showing any reduction in the contralateral eye and was, therefore, significant at all time points of measurements except for the baseline measurement. The bilateral difference in the NB gradually increased in the all tissues examined, and difference was significant on day 3 and on day 20 in the iris and only on day 20 in the posterior choroid and ONH.

These results are thought to indicate that topical ifenprodil has a significant effect on the iris, posterior choroid and ONH circulation after repeated instillation. The absence of any effect in the vehicle-treated eye speaks against the possibility of effects attributable to systemically absorbed ifenprodil. Secondary effects attributable to the reduced IOP seem rather unlikely since no apparent correlation between the bilateral difference in the IOP and that in the NB was seen. A gradual increase in the bilateral difference in the NB was seen in all tissues examined as the total times of instillation increased. This finding may suggest that the NB-increasing effect of topical ifenprodil presently observed is attributable to local penetration of the drug. The increase in the NB, primarily a quantitative index of tissue blood velocity, is known to correlate well with increase in the blood flow rate determined by the microsphere method or hydrogen-gas clearance method after administration of vasodilating agents such as Ca^{2+}-antagonists [12] or carbon dioxide [13]. Thus, it is possible that topical ifenprodil, a vasodilating drug, increased not only the tissue blood velocity, but also the blood flow rate in the ipsilateral iris, posterior choroid and ONH. The present findings suggest that ifenprodil may have the potential to be used for treatment of ocular diseases associated with local circulatory disturbances and possibly for treatment of some types of glaucoma [16].

References

1. Mizusawa H, Fujihara H (1974) Effect of ifenprodil on isolated arteries. Folia Pharmacol Jpn 70:785–799
2. Irino O, Saito K, Hayashi T, Ohkubo K (1985) Inhibitory mechanism of ifenprodil on rabbit platelet aggregation. Folia Pharmacol Jpn 85:379–385
3. Tamura Y, Sato Y, Yokota T, Akaike A, Sasa M, Takaori S (1993) Ifenprodil prevents glutamate cytotoxicity via polyamine modulatory sites of N-methyl-d-aspartate receptors in cultured cortical neurons. J Exp Pharmacol Ther 265:1017–1025
4. Kanno M, Araie M, Tomita K, Sawanobori K (1998) Effect of topical nipradilol, a beta-blocking agent with alpha-blocking and nitroglycerin-like activities, on aqueous humor dynamics and fundus circulation. Invest Ophthalmol Vis Sci 39:736–743
5. Jones RF, Maurice DM (1966) New methods of measuring the rate of aqueous flow in man with fluorescein. Exp Eye Res 5:208–220
6. Hayashi M, Yablonski ME, Novack GD (1989) Trabecular outflow facility determined by fluorophotometry in human subjects. Exp Eye Res 48:621–625
7. Tamaki Y, Araie M, Kawamoto E, Eguchi S, Fujii H (1995) Non-contact, two-dimensional measurement of tissue circulation in choroid and optic nerve head using laser speckle phenomenon. Exp Eye Res 60:373–374
8. Fercher AF, Briers JD (1981) Flow visualization by means of single exposure speckle photography. Opt Commun 37:326–330

9. Nagahara M, Tamaki Y, Araie M, Fujii H (1997) Measurements of blood flow velocity in human retinal veins using laser speckle flowgraphy system. J Jpn Ophthalmol Soc (Nippon Ganka Gakkai Zasshi) 102:173–179
10. Tomidokoro A, Araie M, Tamaki Y, Tomita K (1998) In vivo measurement of iridial circulation using laser speckle phenomenon. Invest Ophthalmol Vis Sci 39:364–371
11. Tomidokoro A, Tamaki Y, Araie M, Tomita K, Muta K (1998) Effect of topical carteolol on iridial circulation in pigmented rabbit eyes. Jpn J Ophthalmol 42:180–185
12. Tamaki Y, Araie M, Tomita K, Tomidokoro T (1996) Time change of nicardipine effect on choroidal circulation in rabbit eyes. Curr Eye Res 15:543–548
13. Sugiyama T, Utsumi T, Azuma I, Fujii H (1996) Measurement of optic nerve head circulation: comparison of laser speckle and hydrogen clearance methods. Jpn J Ophthalmol 40:339–343
14. Tamaki Y, Araie M, Kawamoto E, Eguchi S, Fujii H (1994) Noncontact, two-dimensional measurement of retinal microcirculation using laser speckle phenomenon. Invest Ophthalmol Vis Sci 35:3825–3834
15. Tamaki Y, Araie M, Tomita K, Nagahara M, Tomidokoro A, Fujii H (1997) Real-time measurement of human optic nerve head and choroid circulation, using laser speckle phenomenon. Jpn J Ophthalmol 41:49–54
16. Fechtner R, Weinreb RN (1994) Mechanism of optic nerve damage in primary open angle glaucoma. Surv Ophthalmol 39:23–42

CHAPTER 14

Perfusion-Map Variations Demonstrate the Activity of the Retinal Autoregulation System in the Human Retina

J. R. Sampaolesi · R. Sampaolesi

Abstract. Optic-nerve head and retinal perfusion were measured in 26 normal volunteers, in 28 hypertensive patients (in the preperimetric period of the evolution of glaucoma) and in 24 patients with advanced glaucoma (perimetric period). Patients were examined with the Heidelberg Retina Flowmeter, and flow, volume and velocity indices were assessed in each report. Perfusion maps were reconstructed based on 12 different acquisitions of each optic-nerve head and adjacent retina in order to cover a larger area. *Results:* Normal patients showed relatively normal perfusion indices, while hypertensive eyes (glaucomatous patients in the preperimetric period) showed significantly increased perfusion values in relation to the control group ($p< 0.001$). Patients with advanced glaucoma (in the perimetric period) showed significantly decreased values ($p< 0.001$) in relation to both groups. *Conclusions:* (1) During exposure to high intraocular pressure, retinal blood flow increases due to stimulation of autoregulation. (2) When this exposure is longer, autoregulation might not be able to preserve blood flow, thus leading to its decrease. (3) Autoregulation seems to have a "point of no return" if intraocular pressure is too high or if exposure is too long.

Introduction

The purpose of this paper is to study optic-nerve flow and its correlation with intraocular pressure (IOP) in three groups of patients: normals, hypertensives (those in the preperimetric period) and those with advanced glaucomas with severe visual field loss (those in the perimetric period). Many papers in the literature worldwide have studied the normal and pathological values of flow both in the optic nerve and in the retina and have described the activity of autoregulation under different conditions [1–5].

Materials

Group 1 consisted of 26 normal patients (12 males, 14 females; mean age 41±12.4 years, range 29–53 years) under no general or local medical therapy. Group 2 consisted of a total of 28 hypertensive patients (17 males, 11 females; mean age 52±8.23 years, range 46–60 years) not treated with local therapy. Group 3 consisted of 24 advanced glaucoma cases with severe visual field loss (14 males, 10 females; mean age 60±11.53 years, range 59–71 years), of which 13 regulated their IOP and 11 failed to regulate it with medical therapy. Only one eye was studied from each patient.

Method

The flow was measured by means of the Heidelberg Retina Flowmeter (HRF), a confocal, scanning, laser-Doppler flowmetry system with a wavelength range corresponding to the red spectrum. A trigger is automatically pressed according to the readings of three electrodes placed on the patient (two subclavicular and a third on the apex). The exact flow is thus measured in a systolic and diastolic heart cycle. Six measurements are performed: one temporal and one nasal, at the horizontal area of the neuroretinal rim, and four at the retina adjacent to the optic disc; the mean of these values is calculated.

Three IOP measurements were performed with Goldmann applanation tonometry attached to the slit lamp, and the mean value was also calculated. The visual fields were examined with computerized perimetry (Octopus 1-2-3 perimeter), and each patient was the subject of at least three visual-field examinations.

Results

The flow values obtained have a good correlation with the IOP values in each eye. The correlation is thus high in normals and preperimetric hypertensives and low in advanced glaucomas (Fig. 1, Table 1).

The flow values found in each group show a marked differentiation between the groups. Analyzed with the Kruskal Wallis test and compared using the Dunn test, the

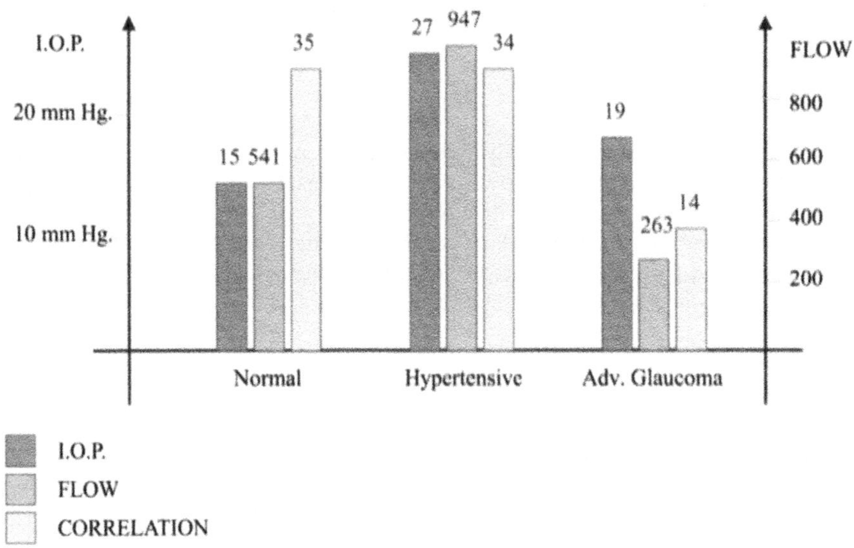

Fig. 1. This graph shows a good correlation between flow and intraocular pressure in normal patients and preperimetric hypertensives; the correlation is low in advanced glaucoma. See values in Table 1

three samples belong to different populations (Fig. 2, Table 2). The normal flow range is consistent with the values obtained by Michelson [1].

As revealed by linear-regression analysis (least-square method), the correlation between flow and IOP was linear in the normal and hypertensive groups and non-linear in the group with advanced glaucomas; there was a significant correlation in the normal and hypertensive groups and no significant correlation in the group with

Table 1. Correlation between flow and intraocular pressure in normal patients, preperimetric hypertensives and those with advanced glaucoma

	Normal	Hypertensive	Advanced glaucoma
Flow (relative units)	541±98.5	947±161.6	263±95.1
Intraocular pressure (mmHg)	15.3±1.79	27.1±2.97	19.7±3.33
Correlation	35.3±4.81	34.8±2.75	14.0±6.02

Table 2. Results were analyzed using Kruskal Wallis test and compared by means of the Dunn test. The three samples belong to different populations

	Normal and hypertensive	Hypertensive and advanced glaucoma	Advanced glaucoma and normal
Flow (relative units)	$p< 0.001$	$p< 0.001$	$p< 0.001$

Table 3. Linear regression analysis according to least-square method ($r+r^2$)

	Normal	Hypertensive	Advanced glaucoma
Linear regression	$p< 0.001$	$p< 0.001$	N.S.
Runs test	Linear correlation	Linear correlation	Non-linear correlation
r	0.63	0.92	0.21
r^2	0.40	0.86	0.04

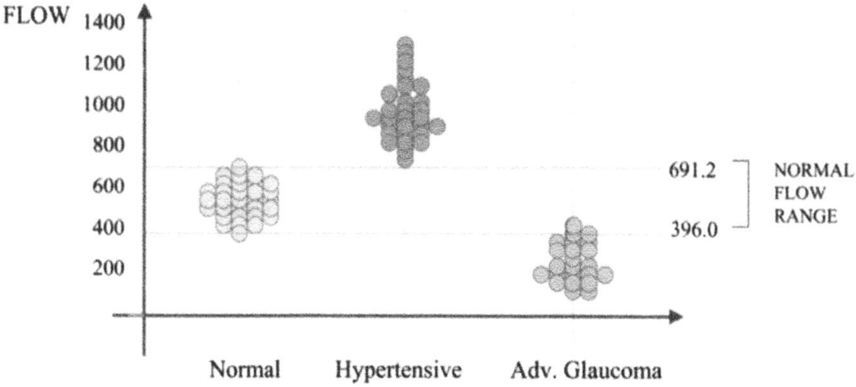

Fig. 2. Flow values found for each group. These values are correlated with the normal flow range described by Michelson [1]

advanced glaucomas. Interestingly, the values of the r and r2 variables were high for the first two groups compared with the third group. In brief, it can be concluded that for normal IOP values, the flow was normal in the normal group; in the hypertensive

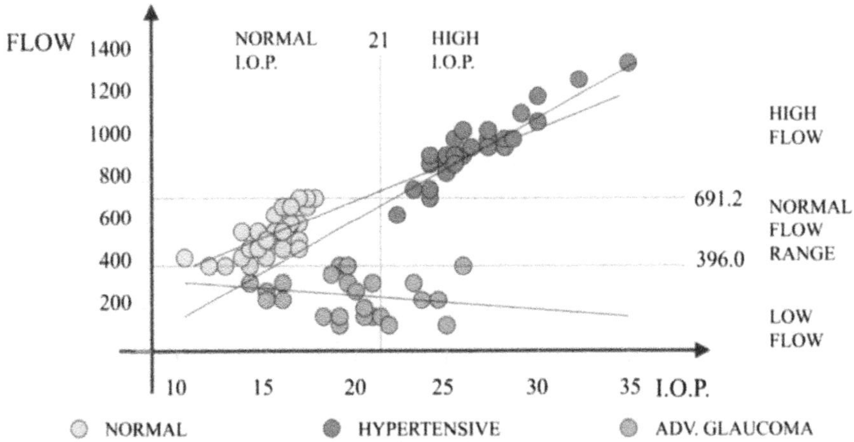

Fig. 3. Linear regression graph showing a good linear correlation between intraocular pressure and flow in normal and hypertensive patients, while the group with advanced glaucoma shows a nonlinear correlation (low flow for different pressure levels)

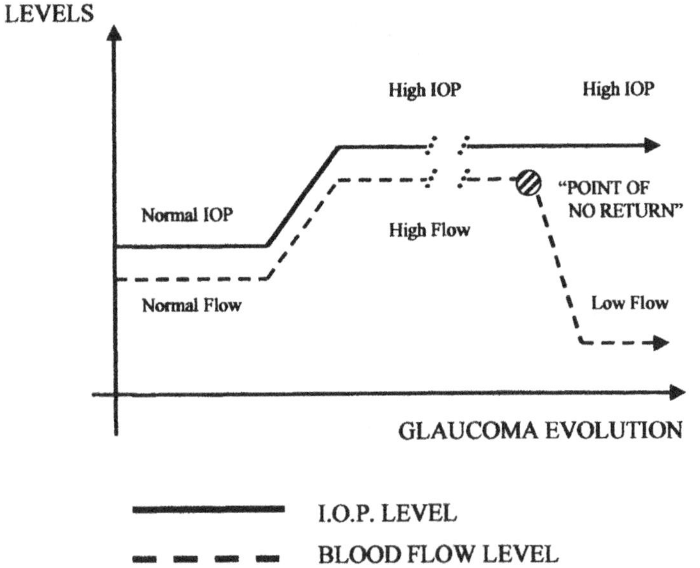

Fig. 4. Activity of autoregulation. The "point of no return" is shown, where the system may not be able to preserve blood flow, with the consequent decrease in retinal perfusion. This phenomenon may occur when the intraocular pressure is too high or the exposure to a high intraocular pressure is too long

group, IOP values correlated with high flow values, while in those with advanced glaucomas, the flow was always low, independent of IOP readings (Fig. 3, Table 3).

The prognostic value of flow can be inferred from the sensitivity, specificity, predictive value and accuracy found for each group. As shown in Fig. 5 and Table 4, when differentiating between the groups, the values for these indicators are always higher than 70 %.

As an illustration of this behavior, Fig. 4 shows how, in the evolution of glaucoma, normal IOP values correspond to normal flow values. As the IOP rises, so does the flow. Nevertheless, this situation seems to reach a point of no return, when it cannot be sustained and, therefore, the IOP remains high and the flow decreases.

Figure 6 shows an example of each group. The normal perfusion map shows homogeneity between large vessels and capillaries. The perfusion map for the example from the hypertensive group shows a marked increase of flow at the capillary

Table 4. Sensitivity, specificity, predictive value and accuracy of the method to differentiate groups

	Differentiation between normal and hypertensive	Differentiation between hypertensive and advanced glaucoma	Differentiation between advanced glaucoma and normal
Sensitivity	74.87	85.75	78.88
Specificity	80.36	86.77	80.36
Predictive value	79.65	86.75	78.88
Accuracy	84.05	92.89	86.29

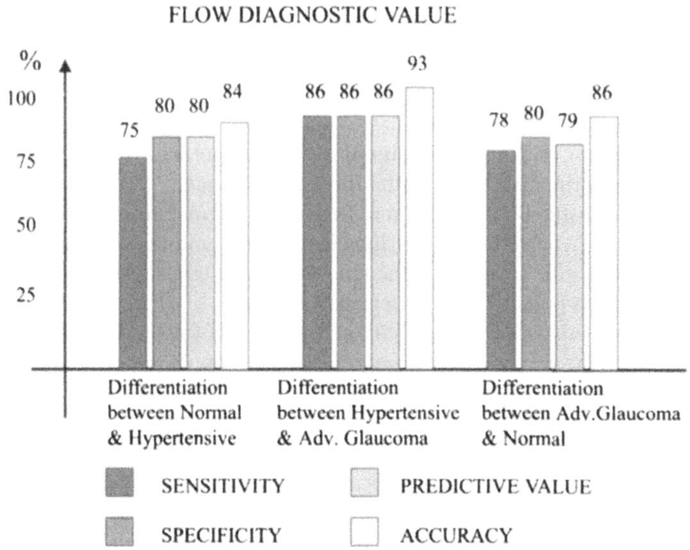

Fig. 5. Sensitivity, specificity, predictive value and accuracy of the method to differentiate groups

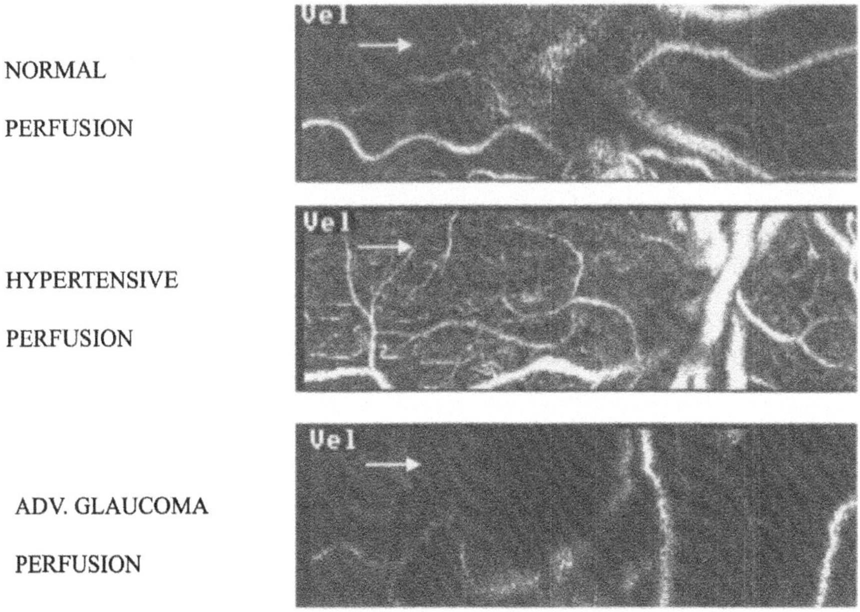

Fig. 6. Three examples. The patient with normal intraocular pressure presents a normal perfusion map. The patient with hypertension shows a perfusion map with increased capillary density and high flow values. The patient with advanced glaucoma shows a perfusion map with an absence of capillary images, low-flow values and basal flow on the central retinal artery and vein. The prepapillary capillary plexus seems to have no circulation at all

level. Finally, the perfusion map of an advanced glaucoma shows the persistence of large vessels in contrast to the absence of capillaries.

Conclusions

1. The flow values found for each group are significantly different, i.e., flow measurement enables one to distinguish between the three populations.
2. There is a linear relationship between IOP and flow in the normal group and in the group of preperimetric hypertensives (the slope is not zero), and the correlation is not linear in the group with advanced glaucomas (the slope tends to zero).
3. This relationship is even higher in the hypertensive group.
4. Flowmetry reveals high sensitivity, specificity and predictive values. This method has a high diagnostic accuracy in differentiating among the three evolutionary periods of glaucoma.
5. During exposure to high IOP, retinal blood-flow values increase due to stimulation of autoregulation.
6. When exposure is longer (or if IOP is significantly increased) autoregulation may not be able to preserve blood flow, thus leading to its decrease.
7. Autoregulation seems to have a "point of no return", if IOP is too high or if exposure is too long (Figs. 5, 6).

Discussion

Based on the results obtained in this study, it is interesting to stress the following possibilities:

1. Though there is extensive argument as to whether flow variations are the cause or effect of optic-nerve-head damage in glaucomatous patients, the flow seems to have a key role in the development of this phenomenon.
2. Circulation of the optic-nerve head is maintained under different conditions (high IOP). This happens up to a point beyond which autoregulation fails to preserve this situation.
3. The most interesting points to be resolved are to determine the factors on which the point of no return depends and where exactly it is located within the evolution of glaucomatous optic-nerve-head neuropathy.

References

1. Michelson G, Schmauss B, Langhans MJ, Harazny J, Groh MJM (1996) Principle, validity and reliability of scanning laser Doppler flowmetry. J Glaucoma 5:99–105
2. Pournaras CJ (1996) Autoregulation of ocular blood flow. In: Kaiser HJ, Flammer J, Hendrickson P (eds) Ocular blood flow. Glaucoma meeting, 1995. Basel, Karger, pp 40–50
3. Haefliger IO, Anderson DR (1996) Pericytes and capillary blood flow modulation. In: Kaiser HJ, Flammer J, Hendrickson P (eds) Ocular blood flow. Glaucoma meeting, 1995. Basel, Karger, pp 74–78
4. Petrig BL, Riva CE (1996) Optic nerve head laser doppler flowmetry: principles and computer analysis. In: Kaiser HJ, Flammer J, Hendrickson P (eds) Ocular blood flow. Glaucoma meeting, 1995. Basel, Karger, pp 120–127
5. Pillunat LE, Anderson DR, Knighton RW, Joos KM, Feuer WJ (1996) Effect of increased intraocular pressure on optic nerve head blood flow. In: Kaiser HJ, Flammer J, Hendrickson P (eds) Ocular blood flow. Glaucoma meeting, 1995. Basel, Karger, pp 138–144

Discussion

CHAPTER 15

The Primate Optic Nerve Following Chronic Ischemia

G. A. Cioffi · P. Sullivan · E. M. Van Buskirk · L. Wang

Abstract. *Purpose:* To examine the effect of chronic ischemia to the primate optic nerve. *Methods:* Chronic optic-nerve ischemia was induced in one eye of five rhesus monkeys using sustained infusion of the potent vasoconstrictor, endothelin-1. Endothelin-1 (0.2 μg/day) was delivered to the perineural region in the retrobulbar space via an osmotically driven minipump. Following 2–6 months of induced optic-nerve ischemia, the eyes were perfusion fixed and sectioned. Optic-nerve histology and axon counts were performed using the contralateral untreated eyes as controls. *Results:* Total axon-count estimates of the optic nerves from the control eye ranged from $1.31 \cdot 10^6$ to $1.47 \cdot 10^6$ (mean±SD; $1.37 \cdot 10^6 \pm 6.8 \cdot 10^4$). In four of the ischemic eyes, the axon counts decreased significantly ($p \leq 0.05$), with a range of $0.77 \cdot 10^6$–$1.31 \cdot 10^6$ (mean reduction of 17 %). The distribution of axonal loss was uniform throughout the nerves. The fifth endothelin/ischemic optic nerve demonstrated severe histological changes, with gross swelling of the extracellular, intra-axonal spaces and increase of the transectional nerve area (approximately 36 % increase, compared with control). *Conclusions:* Ischemia of the anterior optic nerve results in diffuse axonal loss with apparent extracellular-matrix changes.

Introduction

In addition to high intraocular pressure, abnormalities of the circulation to the anterior optic nerve have been implicated in the pathogenesis of glaucomatous optic neuropathy [1]. The principle evidence to support a vascular involvement in the development of glaucoma has come from human epidemiological studies. Diseases associated with hemodynamic compromise, such as systemic hypertension, diabetes mellitus, peripheral vascular disease, and various vasospastic disorders, are considered risk factors for the development of glaucoma. While these associations increase the likelihood that vascular insufficiency is an important factor in glaucomatous optic neuropathy, they do not demonstrate causality.

The development of an in vivo model of chronic optic-nerve ischemia may enhance our understanding of the role of vascular insufficiency in the development of glaucomatous optic neuropathy [2, 3]. A surgically implanted, osmotically driven minipump enabled continuous microapplication of endothelin-1 (ET-1), a potent polypeptide vasoconstrictor of endothelial origin, to the retrobulbar optic nerve of both rabbits and rhesus monkeys. In rabbits, this resulted in a large (38 %) decrease in optic-nerve blood flow with corresponding focal narrowing of vessels supplying the optic nerve, optic disc excavation, and histological evidence of ischemic changes. Studies in rhesus monkeys demonstrated a similar decrease in optic-nerve blood flow.

Quigley has demonstrated a non-uniform loss of axons in human glaucomatous optic nerves, with greater loss in a vertically oriented hourglass distribution [4]. However, clinical studies examining the optic-nerve appearance have demonstrated diffuse loss of the nerve-fiber layers and cup enlargement in as many as half of patients with glaucoma [5]. This may indicate that initial axonal loss may be diffuse in some patients and localized in other patients with glaucoma. The present study was designed to examine the effects of chronic optic-nerve ischemia in the primate eye and to compare these changes with glaucomatous optic neuropathy. Chronic optic-nerve ischemia was induced in one eye of rhesus monkeys, and the relative magnitude and distribution of optic-nerve-axon damage was determined.

Methods

Minipump Implantation

Five adult Rhesus monkeys (*Macaca mulatta*) were used for this experiment. All experiments conformed to the Association for Research in Vision and Ophthalmology resolution on the use of animals in research. ET-1 (0.2 μg/day) was delivered to the perineural region of the respective retrobulbar optic nerve for 2–6 months via osmotically driven minipumps. The minipumps continually delivered the test agent at a controlled and constant flow rate (0.25 μl/h) over a 4-week period. The distal end of the delivery tube was placed adjacent to the optic nerve and its vascular supply.

Axon Counts

At the end of each experiment, the monkey was euthanized and the eyes were perfusion fixed, then enucleated with approximately 1–2 cm of optic nerve intact. The optic nerves were marked for orientation, transected 1–2 mm behind the globe, and immersed in fixative. The optic nerves were processed, sectioned, and stained. Multiple photographs of each optic-nerve cross-section were taken, and a montage of the complete optic nerve was constructed (Fig. 1). Each montage was divided into 16 roughly equal areas (sectors). Using an IBAS image processing system, manual counts of approximately 5 % of the optic-nerve axons were made. Using the area of each field and an estimate of the cross-sectional area for each nerve, estimates of the total axon count and axon density were made. The mean axon number was calculated for each of the sixteen sectors using the average sector area (the optic-nerve cross-sectional area divided by 16).

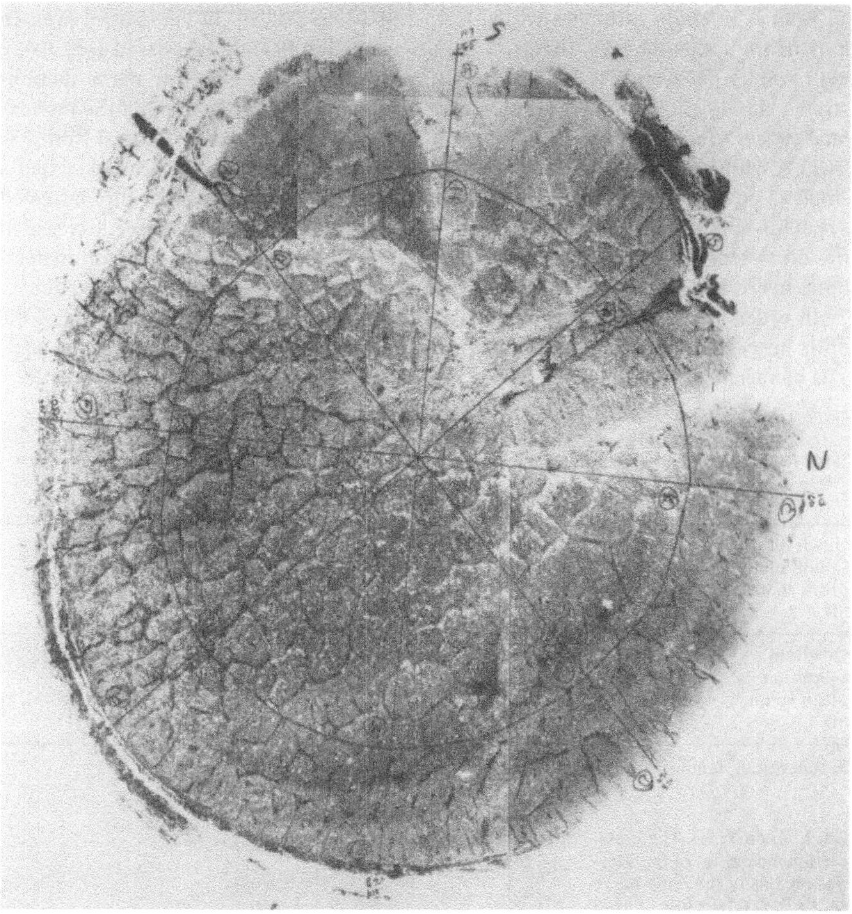

Fig. 1. Photomicrograph montage of an optic-nerve cross-section in a primate eye following endothelin-1-induced ischemia. The nerve has been subdivided into 16 approximately equal regions for regional axon counts

Statistical Analysis

A paired *t*-test was performed to determine whether the total axon number in the ET-1-treated and the control eyes from five monkeys was statistically different. In addition, statistical comparisons of the axon counts within the various regions of the optic nerve were performed.

Results

Of the five monkeys, two were monitored for 2 months, one for 4 months, and two for nearly 6 months. Throughout the course of each experiment, the intraocular pressure measurements were not significantly different from baseline measurements.

Total axon count estimates varied from $1.31 \cdot 10^6$ to $1.47 \cdot 10^6$ in the control eyes. In four of the ischemic eyes, the axon counts were significantly decreased ($p \leq 0.05$), with counts between $0.77 \cdot 10^6$ and $1.31 \cdot 10^6$. The remaining ischemic nerve demonstrated significant retrobulbar optic-nerve swelling, with engorgement of the interaxonal spaces (Table 1). The degree of axon loss in the four monkeys ranged from 7 % to 42 %, with an average axonal loss of approximately 17 %. The fifth monkey had a small (2 %) increase in axon count in the treated eye compared with the untreated eye. This optic nerve demonstrated significant enlargement, with a large increase in the cross-sectional area of the retrobulbar optic nerve relative to the contralateral optic nerve and the optic nerves of the other animals (9.73 mm^2 vs 6.74±0.80 mm^2).

In order to determine whether there was preferential regional axonal loss of the optic nerve, optic-nerve-axon counts from eight regions were evaluated with an analysis of variances (Fig. 2). There was no evidence for regionalization of axonal loss.

Table 1. Quadrant axonal loss in ischemic [endothelin-1 (ET-1)-treated] eyes versus control eyes

	Regional axon distribution analysis			
Quadrant	S	S	N	N
Condition	Control	ET-1	Control	ET-1
Mean count	336497.722	273307.1099	333106.8243	293110.4659
SD	43238.86683	34904.92285	51447.76208	69967.88336
Quadrant	I	I	T	T
Condition	Control	ET-1	Control	ET-1
Mean count	357075.1331	335929.3346	348168.7628	284964.7154
SD	54752.7373	72907.68913	37448.55606	80063.15713

S, superior; T, temporal; I, inferior; N, nasal.

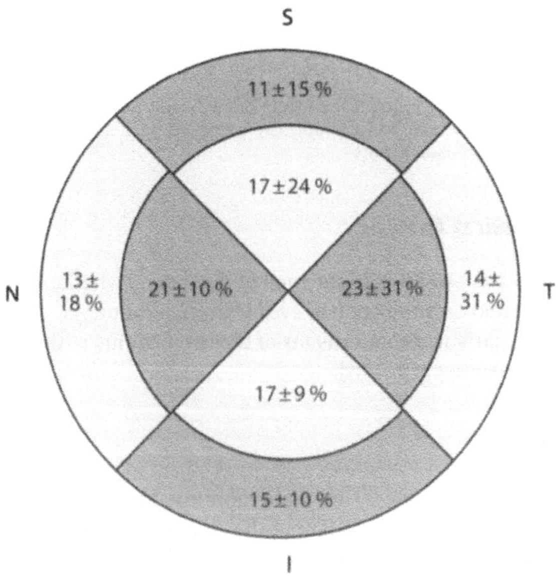

Fig. 2. Axonal loss. The cross-sectional diagram of the various regions of the optic nerve shows the average loss of axons (mean loss±SD) in the ischemic eye compared with the control eyes (*S*, superior; *T*, temporal; *I*, inferior; *N*, nasal)

Summary

Ischemia of the anterior optic nerve results in predictable, diffuse axonal death. In the future, this model of chronic optic-nerve ischemia will allow comparison with other forms of optic-nerve insult.

References

1. Van Buskirk EM, Cioffi GA (1992) Glucomatous optic neuropathy. Am J Ophthalmol 113:447–452
2. Orgül S, Cioffi GA, Wilson DJ, Bacon DR, Van Buskirk EM (1996) An endothelin-1 induced model of optic nerve ischemia in the rabbit. Invest Ophthalmol Vis Sci 37:1860–1869
3. Orgül S, Cioffi GA, Bacon DR, Van Buskirk EM (1996) An endothelin-1-induced model of chronic optic nerve ischemia in rhesus monkeys. J Glaucoma 5:135–138
4. Quigley HA, Addicks EM (1981) Regional differences in the structure of the lamina cribrosa and their relation to glaucomatous optic nerve damage. Arch Ophthalmol 99:137–143
5. Tuulonen A, Airaksinen PJ (1991) Initial glaucomatous optic disk and retinal nerve fiber layer abnormalities and their progression. Am J Ophthalmol 111:485–490

Visual Function

CHAPTER 16

Multifocal Electroretinogram and Visual-Field Defects in Patients with Glaucoma

H. Abe · S. Hasegawa · T. Usui · A. Ooshima · M. Takagi · R. Takada

Abstract. To clarify the correlation between the waveforms of multifocal electroretinograms (M-ERGs) and visual field defects in patients with glaucoma, the visual-evoked-response imaging system (VERIS; Tomey, Nagoya, Japan) was used for M-ERG recording. The signals were analyzed by a VERIS Science 3.0.1 (Electrodiagnostic Imaging, San Mateo, Calif.). Static visual field was measured using a Humphrey Visual-Field Analyzer (Program 30–2). The amplitude and peak latency of M-ERG were measured and compared with mean sensitivity values (in dB) of the corresponding quadrant area of static perimetry. Sixteen eyes of eight patients with glaucoma and 17 eyes of ten normal subjects were examined. Statistically significant negative correlation was found in the peak latency of P2 and N2 components of the first-order kernel M-ERG and in the peak latency of N1, P2, N2 and P3 components of the second-order kernel M-ERG. No significant correlations between averaged M-ERG amplitudes of first- and second-order kernels and averaged sensitivity values of static perimetry were found except for first-order P1–N1 amplitude. The prolongation of the peak latencies of the first-, and second-order kernel responses of M-ERG was observed as the progression of visual-field defects in patients with glaucoma. These results suggest that M-ERG is a response with multiple origins and is composed of retinal and optic-nerve components.

Introduction

Primary open-angle glaucoma or normal-tension glaucoma is a syndrome of progressive optic neuropathy, with characteristic optic-nerve damage and defects in retinal sensitivity leading to loss of visual function. Retinal ganglion cells are lost in glaucoma as optic-nerve damage progresses.

Pattern electroretinogram (P-ERG) has been thought to be a sensitive tool for detection of ganglion cell dysfunction in patients with glaucoma [1]. However, the origin of P-ERG is still controversial and many studies have suggested that P-ERG has responses of multiple origins [2]. Recently, Sutter et al. [3] developed a method for multifocal electroretinograms (M-ERG), and it has been reported [4] that the M-ERG is useful for detection of retinal dysfunction in various ophthalmological diseases. However, little is known about M-ERG components derived from patients with optic-nerve diseases.

In this study, we investigated the relationship between the waveform changes of the M-ERG and glaucomatous optic-nerve dysfunction, as well as the influence of glaucomatous optic-nerve damage on the M-ERG and visual field.

Subjects and Methods

Sixteen eyes of eight glaucomatous patients (mean age ±SD 47.8±7.4 years) and 17 eyes of ten normal subjects (mean age ±SD 45.2±10.9 years) were examined. The patients had clear media and no eye diseases except for glaucoma, and their corrected visual acuity was more than 20/20. The intraocular pressure of these subjects was well controlled: less than 20 mmHg with or without medication. The visual field of these subjects was classified from stage 1 to 5 according to Aulhorn's classification.

The visual-evoked-response imaging system (VERIS; Tomey, Nagoya, Japan) was used for M-ERG recording. The stimulus matrix consisted of 103 hexagonal elements displayed on a cathode-ray tube color monitor driven at a 75-Hz frame rate. At a viewing distance of 27 cm, the radius of stimulus array subtended approximately 25-30°. Each hexagon was independently alternated between black and white, according to a pseudorandom sequence called "binary". A bipolar contact-lens electrode (Kyoto Contact Lens, Kyoto, Japan) was used for signal derivation, and a ground electrode was attached to the earlobe. Mean stimulus luminance was adjusted to approximately 110 cd/m^2. A recording session consisted of eight 30-s segments separated by resting time. The subjects were optically corrected after insertion of the contact-lens electrode. The pupil was fully dilated with 0.5 % tropicamide. The signal amplification was 50,000 and the filter was a bandpass of 6–100 Hz (Nihonkoden, Tokyo, Japan). The signals were analyzed using VERIS Science 3.0.1 (Electro Diagnostic Imaging Inc., San Mateo, Calif.). The static visual field was also measured using a Humphrey Visual-Field Analyzer (Program 30–2).

The first-order kernel was defined as the difference between the mean response to all white frames and the mean response to all black frames for each stimulus area in the sequence. The second-order kernel was defined as the interaction between two consecutive focal flashes (stimulus base interval was 13.3 ms). To improve the signal-to-noise ratio, 103 focal responses of first-, and second-order M-ERGs were averaged.

We named the first positive peak P1, the second positive peak P2, the first trough N1 and the second trough N2 in the first-, and second-order kernels, respectively. Latencies (P1, N1, P2 and N2) and peak-to-trough amplitudes (P1–N1, N1–P2 and P2–N2) were measured. Then, the data of the M-ERG were compared with the mean deviation (MD) and mean sensitivity values (in dB) of the corresponding quadrant area of static perimetry.

Results

In the first-order kernels of M-ERG, a significant negative correlation was found between the peak latencies of P1 and N2 components of averaged M-ERG and the mean sensitivity (dB) of static perimetry (Fig. 1). The correlation coefficients and statistically significant levels of peak latency of P1 and N2 components and static perimetry were $R = -0.531$ ($p < 0.005$) and $R = -0.704$ ($p < 0.01$), respectively. Significant negative correlation ($R = -0.376$, $p < 0.01$) was found between the N1–P1 amplitude of averaged M-ERG and the mean sensitivity of static perimetry. No significant correlation was found between P1–N2 amplitude and the mean sensitivity of static perimetry (Fig. 2).

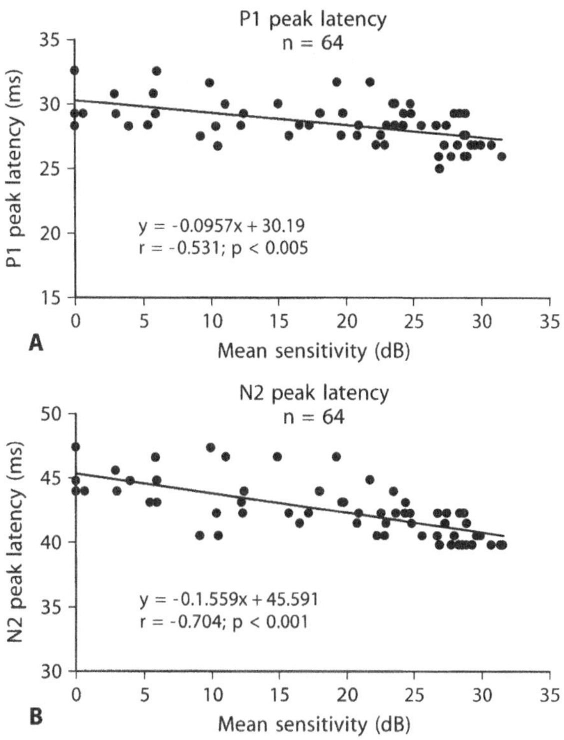

Fig. 1a, b. Correlation between peak latency of the first-order kernels of multifocal electroretinogram and average sensitivity value of static perimetry. **a** Correlation of P1 peak latency ($R = -0.531$, $p < 0.005$). **b** Correlation of N2 peak latency ($R = -0.704$, $p < 0.001$)

In the second-order kernels of M-ERG, a significant negative correlation was found between the peak latencies of N1, P2, N2 and P3 components of averaged M-ERG and the MD of static perimetry. However, no significant correlations were found between the amplitudes of N1–P2, P2–N2 and N2–P3 and the MD of static perimetry.

Discussion

The question of whether ERGs derived from the patients with optic-nerve diseases show abnormality or not has been controversial for a long time. Abnormalities in oscillatory potentials of photopic ERG [5] and scotopic P2 [7] were reported in patients with glaucoma. However, Wanger et al. [8] reported that flash ERGs and oscillatory potentials indicated no reduction of amplitude in patients with unilateral glaucoma. Moreover, Gills [9] found supernormal ERG after sectioning of the optic nerve.

Recently, Sutter et al. [3] developed a method for M-ERG, and it has been reported that this is useful for detection of retinal dysfunction in various ophthalmological diseases. However, little is known about M-ERG components derived from patients with optic-nerve disorders. Recently, Bearse et al. [10] reported a method for extracting

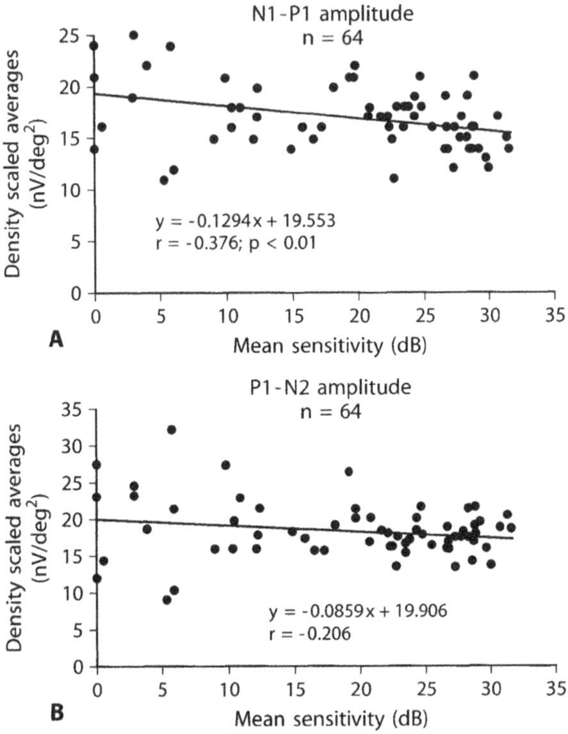

Fig. 2a, b. Correlation between trough-to-peak amplitude of the first-order kernels of multifocal electroretinogram and averaged sensitivity value of static perimetry. **a** Correlation of trough-to-peak amplitude of N1-P1 ($R = -0.376$, $p < 0.01$). **b** Correlation of trough-to-peak amplitude of P1-N2 ($R = -0.206$, not significant)

the optic-nerve head component from M-ERG that is presumed to originate from ganglion cells and tried to show abnormalities in optic-nerve diseases using M-ERG. Bearse et al. [10] also reported abnormal second-order kernels of M-ERG in eyes with glaucoma. They extracted the optic-nerve-head component (ONHC) from M-ERG using a latency-adjusted algorithm. They presumed that the ONHC was generated by retinal ganglion cells and found that the second-order ONHC was reduced or extinguished in patients with glaucoma.

In this study, we investigated the relationship between the waveform changes of the M-ERG and glaucomatous optic-nerve dysfunction and demonstrated the influence of the glaucomatous optic-nerve damage on the first and second-order responses of M-ERG. Our results show that the peak latencies of M-ERG, both in the first- and second-order kernels, were well correlated with the MD and mean sensitivity values (in dB) of static perimetry. Peak latencies of M-ERG components (N1, P1 and N2) increased linearly when the glaucomatous visual field deteriorated. A negative significant correlation was also found between the amplitude of the first-order M-ERG component (N1-P1) and the MD of static perimetry. The tendency of negative correlation was also evident in the N1–P1 amplitude of second-order M-ERG. These results indicate that glaucomatous optic-nerve dysfunction changes the second-order M-ERG almost to the same extent as it changes the first-order M-ERG.

The second-order kernel represents the temporal interactions of the retina between two flashes and is related to photo-adaptation of the retina. Therefore, the second-order M-ERG should exhibit abnormal responses due to retinal dysfunction. If the M-ERG contains post-receptal responses of the various layers from the retinal ganglion cell to the optic nerve, which are damaged by optic nerve atrophy, the second-order M-ERG should change in the same way as the first-order M-ERG.

This study also showed the contradictory finding that the M-ERG amplitude increased as optic-nerve damage progressed. The results of this study suggest the existence of components that vary with glaucomatous optic-nerve dysfunction. Retinal ganglion cells are lost in glaucoma as optic-nerve damage progresses. We suppose that the optic-nerve component of M-ERG is a component which decreases with optic atrophy and that the reduction of the optic-nerve component of M-ERG results in the prolongation of peak latency and the increase of amplitude of first- and second-order M-ERG. Further studies should be required to clarify the origin of the optic-nerve component of M-ERG.

References

1. Wanger P, Persson HE (1985) Pattern-reversal electroretinograms in ocular hypertension. Doc Ophthalmol 61:27–31
2. Holder GE (1987) Significance of abnormal pattern electroretinography in anterior visual pathway dysfunction. Br J Ophthalmol 71:166–171
3. Sutter EE, Tran D (1992) The field topography of ERG components in man. I. The photopic luminance response. Vision Res 32:433–446
4. Kondo M, Kiyake Y, Horiguchi M, et al. (1995) Clinical evaluation of multifocal electroretinogram. Invest Ophthalmol Vis Sci 36:2146–2150
5. Gur MZ, Bielik M, Neumann E (1987) Changes in oscillatory potentials of the electroretinogram in glaucoma. Curr Eye Res 6:451–466
6. Vaegan ■, Graham SL, Goldberg I, et al. (1991) Selective reduction of oscillatory potentials and pattern electroretinograms after retinal ganglion cell damage by disease in humans or by kainic acid in cats. Doc Ophthalmol 77:237–253
7. Korth M, Nguyen NX, Horn F, Martus P (1994) Scotopic threshold response and scotopic PH in glaucoma. Invest Ophthalmol Vis Sci 35:619–625
8. Wanger P, Persson HE (1983) Pattern electroretinograms in unilateral glaucoma. Invest Ophthalmol Vis Sci 24:749–753
9. Gills JP Jr (1966) The electroretinograms after section of the optic nerve in man. Am J Ophthalmol 62:287–291
10. Bearse MA, Sutter EE, Sim D, et al. (1996) Glaucomatous dysfunction revealed in higher order components of the electroretinogram. In: Vision science and its applications. (OSA technical digest series, vol 1) Optical Society of America, Washington, pp 104–107

CHAPTER 17

Association of Blue-on-Yellow Visual Field with Optic Disc and Retinal Nerve Fiber Layer

P. Teesalu · P. J. Airaksinen · A. Tuulonen

Introduction

Glaucoma is a progressive optic neuropathy with characteristic changes of optic nerve head (ONH), retinal nerve fiber layer (RNFL) and visual field. The anatomic loss of neural tissue goes along with deterioration of function, and any of these three may be the first to reach the threshold of clinical recognition. However, the detectable RNFL and optic disc abnormalities usually precede criteria referred to as typical glaucomatous field loss in conventional perimetry (Sommer et al. 1991; Tuulonen et al. 1993). However, over the past 10 years, there has been a large accumulation of evidence that short-wavelength automated perimetry (SWAP) or blue-on-yellow (B/Y) perimetry is superior to standard achromatic (white-on-white, W/W) automated perimetry for assessing early functional glaucomatous damage (Johnson 1996). On these bases we evaluated the relationship between quantitative ONH, semi-quantitative RNFL and B/Y visual-field test results in normal individuals and patients with glaucoma and ocular hypertension.

Materials and Methods

One randomly chosen eye from 40 normal subjects and 37 patients with ocular hypertension and different stages of glaucoma was evaluated. The B/Y and W/W visual fields were obtained using a Humphrey perimeter. The lens autofluorescence measurements were used to separate the optical and neural sources of short-wavelength-sensitivity loss (Teesalu et al. 1997). The age- and lens-adjusted total and hemifield mean deviations (MDs) were calculated as the difference between the obtained and expected mean-sensitivity values predicted by the regression model fitted in normal subjects. The optic discs were measured using the Heidelberg Retina Tomograph (HRT) with software version 1.11. Monochromatic RNFL photographs of 32 normal subjects and 29 patients with ocular hypertension and different stages of glaucoma were assessed in a masked fashion.

Results

The B/Y visual-field total and hemifield MDs showed a statistically significant correlation with respective ONH parameters such as cup shape measure (CSM), rim volume, rim area, mean RNFL thickness and RNFL cross-sectional area. The highest coefficient of correlation (Pearson's $R = -0.65$; $p < 0.0001$) was found between B/Y visual field total MD and CSM (Fig. 1). Most of the HRT parameters were better correlated with the B/Y hemifield data than with the W/W hemifield data. Furthermore, when the data acquired from the advanced glaucoma subjects was omitted, the differences between the correlation coefficients of B/Y and W/W visual fields with the HRT parameters increased, suggesting that B/Y perimetry might add information to that acquired using W/W perimetry, particularly in early stages of glaucoma.

We performed logistic regression analyses with B/Y hemifield MD values and HRT parameters as covariates to test the sensitivity and specificity of the model and to correctly identify normal W/W hemifields of the healthy individuals and glaucomatous W/W hemifields of the glaucoma patients. A W/W hemifield of normal subjects with hemifield MD better than -2 dB was considered normal, and a W/W hemifield with MD worse than -2 dB of glaucomatous subjects was considered abnormal. The B/Y term was selected by the first step of the regression analysis, showing a sensitivity of 93.7 %, specificity of 84.9 % and an overall correct identification of 90.6 %. Of 63 hemifields of normal subjects, 4 were considered as abnormal, and of 33 abnormal W/W hemifields, 5 were considered normal on the basis of B/Y results. The CSM term was entered on the second step of the regression analysis. The sensitivity was 95.2 % with B/Y and CSM terms together in the model, the specificity was 87.9 %, and the

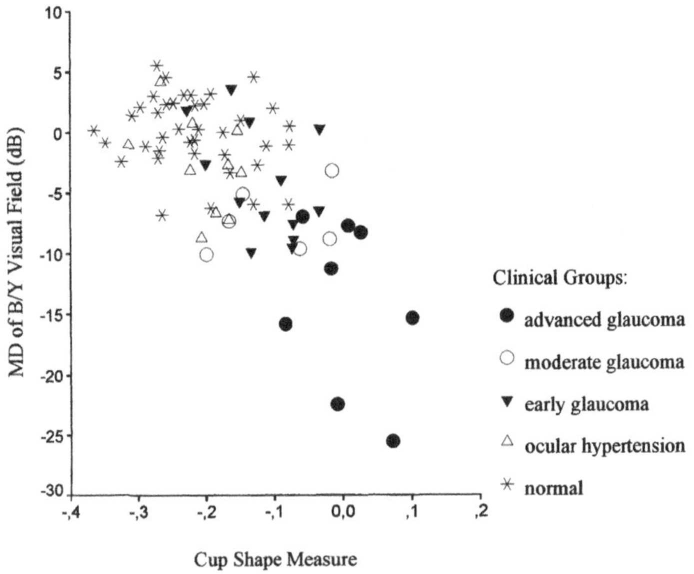

Fig. 1. Scatter plot of the association of the lens- and age-adjusted blue-on-yellow (*B/Y*) visual field mean deviation (*MD*) values with the cup shape measure in the five clinical groups

overall correct identification was 92.7 %. Other HRT terms did not add significantly to the model.

"Normal" W/W Hemifield of Glaucomatous Eyes

In early glaucoma, the visual field defects often develop in one hemifield only. The question arises, is the "healthy" hemifield really unaffected by the disease or does conventional perimetry not detect the functional loss associated with early optic nerve abnormalities? It was therefore interesting to determine how the B/Y visual field test results and ONH measurements label the hemifields of patients with glaucoma and ocular hypertension found to be "normal" on W/W perimetry. For this purpose, a forward stepwise analysis was made where "normal" W/W hemifields of glaucomatous subjects were considered normal and "abnormal" W/W hemifields of glaucomatous subjects abnormal. The B/Y term was entered on step one and 8 of 21 (38 %) cases with normal W/W hemifield were labeled as abnormal. None of the HRT parameters added significantly to the model. With only the HRT parameters in the model, the CSM was entered on step one. This variable classified 11 of 21 (52 %) patients with normal W/W hemifields as abnormal. Although 5 of 33 patients with abnormal W/W hemifields were considered normal by the B/Y as well as the CSM term, and the chosen criterion for W/W hemifield normality or abnormality is conservative, these results suggest that in many cases the seemingly "healthy" W/W hemifield may in fact already be affected by glaucoma.

B/Y Visual Field and RNFL Assessment

The evaluation of the RNFL using black-and-white photographs is found to be a sensitive and useful method with good reproducibility. Therefore, we investigated a relationship between results of B/Y visual field and RNFL assessment in the next stage of our study. We found that the B/Y visual field mean deviation value showed a statistically significant correlation with respective diffuse and overall RNFL loss scores (Pearson's $R = -0.73$ and -0.71, respectively; $p < 0.0001$).

In patients with glaucoma, the RNFL overall loss score indicated abnormality in 16 of 19 (84 %) hemispheres with respect to the "normal" W/W hemifield (Fig. 2). Further, the score of RNFL loss in these 19 hemispheres was well correlated with the MD value of the corresponding B/Y hemifields (Pearson's $R = -0.56$). This suggests that the RNFL and B/Y visual field defects may in many cases reach the boarder of clinical detection before the W/W visual field abnormalities. In addition, our results seem to indicate that in the progression of glaucoma, the changes of B/Y visual field and the RNFL follow each other more closely than do changes of the W/W visual field.

Experimental studies have shown that localized RNFL defects can be clinically detected if more than 50 % of the thickness of the retinal nerve fiber layer is lost (Quigley and Addicks 1982). Therefore, the patients with ocular hypertension may have an impaired function of the ganglion cells in spite of clinically normal-looking RNFL. In our study, the difference between the hemifield MD values of B/Y perimetry

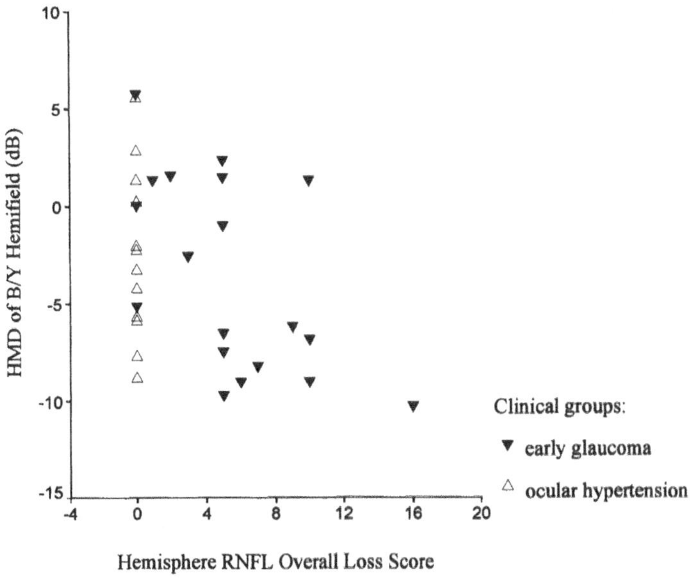

Fig. 2. The age- and lens-adjusted hemifield mean deviation (*HMD*) of blue-on-yellow (*B/Y*) visual fields obtained from "normal" (HMD better than −2 dB) white-on-white hemifields, plotted against the overall score of retinal nerve fiber layer loss from the respective hemisphere in patients with early glaucoma (Pearson's $R = -0.56$; $p = 0.012$) and ocular hypertension

obtained from "normal" W/W hemifields of ocular hypertensive patients (with zero RNFL loss score) and early glaucoma patients was not statistically significant (as determined using analysis of variances); but the respective B/Y hemifield data of normal subjects was statistically significantly different from that of patients with ocular hypertension and early glaucoma. However, the RNFL score was also abnormal in five hemispheres, corresponding to respective B/Y hemifields with an MD better than zero in patients with early glaucoma (Fig. 2). The results of our study suggest that, while the B/Y perimetry may in some cases reveal functional damage even before RNFL loss becomes clinically detectable, there are other patients in whom the glaucomatous RNFL abnormalities can be detected in spite of normal B/Y and W/W visual fields.

In summary, the B/Y perimetry MDs are well correlated with results of optic nerve head and RNFL assessment. B/Y visual field, optic nerve head and RNFL evaluation may reveal glaucomatous damage in a hemifield found to be normal on W/W perimetry.

Acknowledgements. Supported in part by a grant from the Silmäja Kudospankki Foundation.

References

Johnson CA (1996) Diagnostic value of short-wavelength automated perimetry. Curr Opin Ophthalmol 7:54–58

Quigley HA, Addicks EM (1982) Quantitative studies of the retinal nerve fiber layer defects. Arch Ophthalmol 100:807–814

Sommer A, Katz J, Quigley HA, et al. (1991) Clinically detectable nerve fiber atrophy precedes the onset of glaucomatous field loss. Arch Ophthalmol 109:77–83

Teesalu P, Airaksinen PJ, Tuulonen A, et al. (1997) Fluorometry of the crystalline lens for correcting blue-on-yellow perimetry results. Invest Ophthalmol Vis Sci 38:697–703

Tuulonen A, Lehtola J, Airaksinen PJ (1993) Nerve fiber layer defects with normal visual fields. Ophthalmology 100:587–598

CHAPTER 18

Comparison of Conventional and High-Pass Resolution Perimetry in a Prospective Study of Patients with Glaucoma and Normal Controls

B. C. Chauhan · P. H. House · T. A. McCormick · R. P. LeBlanc

Abstract. *Objective:* To determine whether high-pass resolution perimetry detected glaucomatous visual field progression earlier than conventional perimetry. *Methods:* In a prospective longitudinal study, we followed 113 open-angle glaucoma patients with early to moderate visual field damage and 119 normal controls. Each subject was tested at intervals of 6 months with both conventional and high-pass resolution perimetry using program 30-2 of the Humphrey Field Analyzer and the Ring program of the Ophthimus perimeter, respectively. Our predetermined criterion for progression with conventional perimetry was the presence of four or more overlapping non-edge locations outside the fifth percentile for test-retest variability of threshold deviations (defined by the STATPAC Glaucoma Change Probability Analysis) in two of three consecutive visual fields. We employed the identical criterion for progression with high-pass resolution perimetry using our own test-retest variability data. We repeated this procedure in the normal controls to measure the false positive rate of progression. *Results:* Patients were followed for a median of 4.5 years and 11 examinations with each technique: 57 (50.4 %) patients did not progress with either technique; 24 (21.2 %) patients showed progression with high-pass resolution perimetry; 6 (5.3 %) showed progression with conventional perimetry alone. Of the remaining, 26 (23.0 %) patients who showed progression with both techniques: 14 (53.8 %) showed progression with high-pass resolution perimetry first (median: 12 months earlier); 5 (19.2 %) showed progression with conventional perimetry first (median 6 months earlier); 7 (26.9 %) showed progression at the same time. Normal controls were followed for a median of 5 years and 11 examinations with each technique. One (0.8 %) showed progression with high-pass resolution perimetry. *Conclusions:* Our results suggest that high-pass resolution detects glaucomatous visual field progression earlier than conventional perimetry in the majority of patients with progression.

CHAPTER 19

Third Generation Rapid Algorithms for Static Computerised Perimetry, SITA. Development, Results and Observations

A. Heijl · B. Bengtsson

Introduction

This article is a follow-up to *Improved Test Algorithms for Automated Perimetry* previously published in *Glaucoma Update V* after the previous Quebec meeting of the Glaucoma Society of the International Congress of Ophthalmology in 1994 [1]. More than 10 years ago, we started a project to create better test procedures for computerised static-threshold perimetry. The new methods aimed at achieving a considerable reduction of test time without any decrease in test quality. This should be obtained by combining modern knowledge about visual field physiology in normal subjects and patients with glaucoma to model the visual field, and by modifying this model continuously during the perimetric test, using computer-intensive mathematical maximum-likelihood calculations in real time. Such an approach would permit continuous estimation not only of threshold values but also of threshold value errors.

Our new family of algorithms has developed considerably since the last article was written in 1994. The new algorithms have also been tested in simulations as well as in patients with glaucoma and in normal subjects, and the resulting Swedish interactive thresholding algorithms (SITA) have become available as standard tests on modern Humphrey field analyzer (HFA) II perimeters. The purpose of the current article is to summarise and describe these developments and results and to draw conclusions about the practical usage of the two different test programs we developed, SITA Standard and SITA Fast.

General Features of the New Algorithms

Some important features of the new algorithms are clear from the block diagram in Fig. 1. The perimeter has a priori knowledge of normal and abnormal visual field characteristics; this knowledge is already available prior to the test. The algorithms use conventional staircase testing, but threshold value estimates and estimates of threshold accuracy across the entire field are calculated and updated in real time continuously during the test. A so-called error-related factor is used to terminate the staircase when the measurement error at a point reaches a predetermined level of accuracy [2].

False-negative and false-positive frequencies are calculated with new time-saving techniques. False-positive errors are quantified without the use of any catch trials at all and thus without expenditure of test time [3].

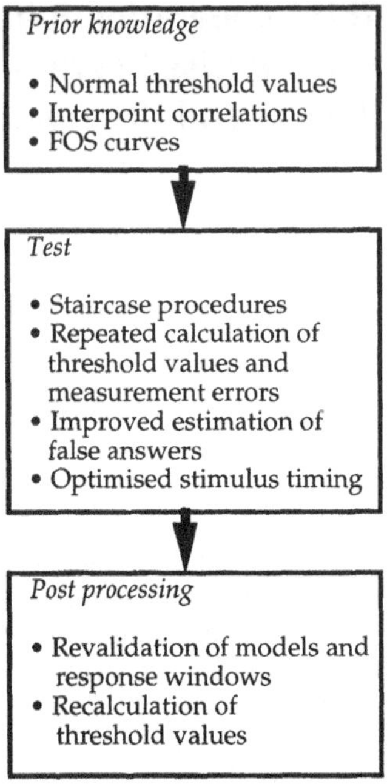

Fig. 1. Some Swedish interactive thresholding algorithm features

Stimulus timing has been optimised; stimulus pacing will follow the patient better than in previous programs and will change during the test, adapting both to very fast and very slow responders. This contributes to the high patient acceptance of the newer tests.

The final results are post processed when all results of the tests are collected. At that time, the patient's reaction times in response to stimuli and any changes in reaction time during the test are known and are used to recalculate response windows, i.e. the period of time during which legitimate responses typically are made after stimulus presentations. The patient's frequencies of false-positive and false-negative answers are also known. These frequencies are incorporated in the visual field models and will influence threshold estimations.

Development

Simulations

Simulations played a very important part in the development of the new algorithms. During recent years the simulator was improved, allowing different rules for early closing of testing at individual test-point locations. The similarity to physiological conditions was increased using defect depths instead of absolute sensitivity levels. With the new simulator, we could study perimetric behaviour in glaucomatous fields in detail. This helped us optimise levels for the error-related factor (see above). The simulator allowed us to analyse how varying this factor influenced accuracy at various eccentricities and defect depths, and the cost, in number of stimulus exposures, associated with higher accuracy.

Patient-Based Development

Our new family of algorithms was incorporated in the HFA II and made available to us in early 1996 for further clinical development. SITA produces response list files, detailed recordings of the perimetric test; every stimulus exposure, every patient response, fixation behaviour and exact time points are recorded. These response list files made it possible for us to make detailed studies of patient behaviour during perimetry. We found that re-opening of previously closed points did not lead to improved test results. Instead, test–retest variability was larger after the second sequence than after the first. Points subjected to such testing were almost always situated at the border of scotomata, where variability is inherently large. Re-opening of previously closed points was consequently abolished. The results of second-test staircases, initiated when estimated threshold values deviated much from initially expected values, were equally discouraging, and stricter criteria were introduced for initiation of such staircases.

SITA Fast

With access to response list files, we saw that test points in normal areas often had very small threshold error estimates and were closed by the error-related factor. This made us realise that there was a potential to develop an even faster test logic than that initially described, which was later called SITA Standard [2]. It seemed possible to develop a very fast algorithm that could give almost the same precision as SITA Standard and at least the same as Fastpac. We developed SITA Fast, which uses only one step size at regular points (4 dB) and only one staircase reversal [4] (Table 1). Criteria for early closing are less strict than in SITA Standard; a larger error-related factor is

Table 1. Procedures in Swedish interactive thresholding algorithm (SITA) Standard and SITA Fast

	SITA Standard	SITA Fast
No. of staircases at regular points	1–2	1–2
Step sizes at regular points (dB)	4–2	4–0
No. of stair cases at primary points	2	2
Step sizes at primary points	4–2, 4–2	4–0, 4–2
No. of reversals per staircase		
Maximum	2	1
Minimum	1*	0**
Error-related factor (lower values require higher accuracy)	0.69	0.89

* If error-related factor is <0.69.
** Is stimulus is seen and error-related factor is <0.89.

Table 2. Results from studies comparing SITA with traditional full-threshold and/or Fastpac

	Full threshold	Fastpac	SITA standard	SITA fast
Normal eyes (n = 20) [6]				
Test time (min)	12.3	7.3	6.1	-
Reproducability RMSE (dB)	1.1	1.2	1.0	-
Glaucoma and glaucoma suspect eyes (n = 32) [5]				
Test time (min)	14.5	9.2	7.8	-
Reproducability RMSE (dB)	1.7	1.8	1.7	-
Glaucoma and glaucoma suspect eyes (n = 30) [4]				
Test time (min)	14.6	9.4	5.0	-
Reproducability RMSE (dB)	2.0	2.0	1.8	-
Glaucoma eyes (n = 45) [7]				
Test time (min)	16.0	-	8.6	5.4
Reproducability RMSE (dB)	2.8	-	3.0	2.9

accepted, and it is possible to interrupt testing at a point after only one perceived stimulus if the error of the measurement is small.

Clinical Evaluations

SITA Fast and SITA Standard have undergone clinical evaluations in patients with suspect and manifest glaucoma and in normal subjects [4–8]. SITA Standard was designed to replace the Humphrey full threshold program, and SITA Fast to replace Fastpac. The designed test programs met our development goals. Thus, SITA Standard saves about half the test time of the Humphrey full threshold program, with at least the same precision measured as in test-re-test reproducibility. Similarly, SITA Fast saves about 50 % of the time used for Fastpac and actually has smaller variability than Fastpac (Table 2).

Visual Fatigue – Differences between Algorithms with Different Lengths

SITA Standard, full threshold, SITA Fast and Fastpac usually give very similar results when used to test the same eye. However, when using the various test logics, we noticed early on that the shorter test algorithms rather frequently result in smaller and/or shallower glaucomatous field defects than the more time-consuming, older programs (Fig. 2). The average differential light sensitivity was also higher with the shorter test algorithms, particularly with the fastest test. This is most probably due to visual fatigue [9]. The latter is a physiological phenomenon, not entirely understood, resulting in a decrease of differential light sensitivity during the test itself, i.e. the visual field deteriorates during the test. Visual fatigue is not homogeneous across the field and is larger in glaucomatous than in normal visual fields.

When using the different test algorithms, we noticed that differences between measured threshold values were larger in eyes where test-time differences were large, supporting the hypothesis that differences in visual fatigue account for the systematic differences between the test algorithms.

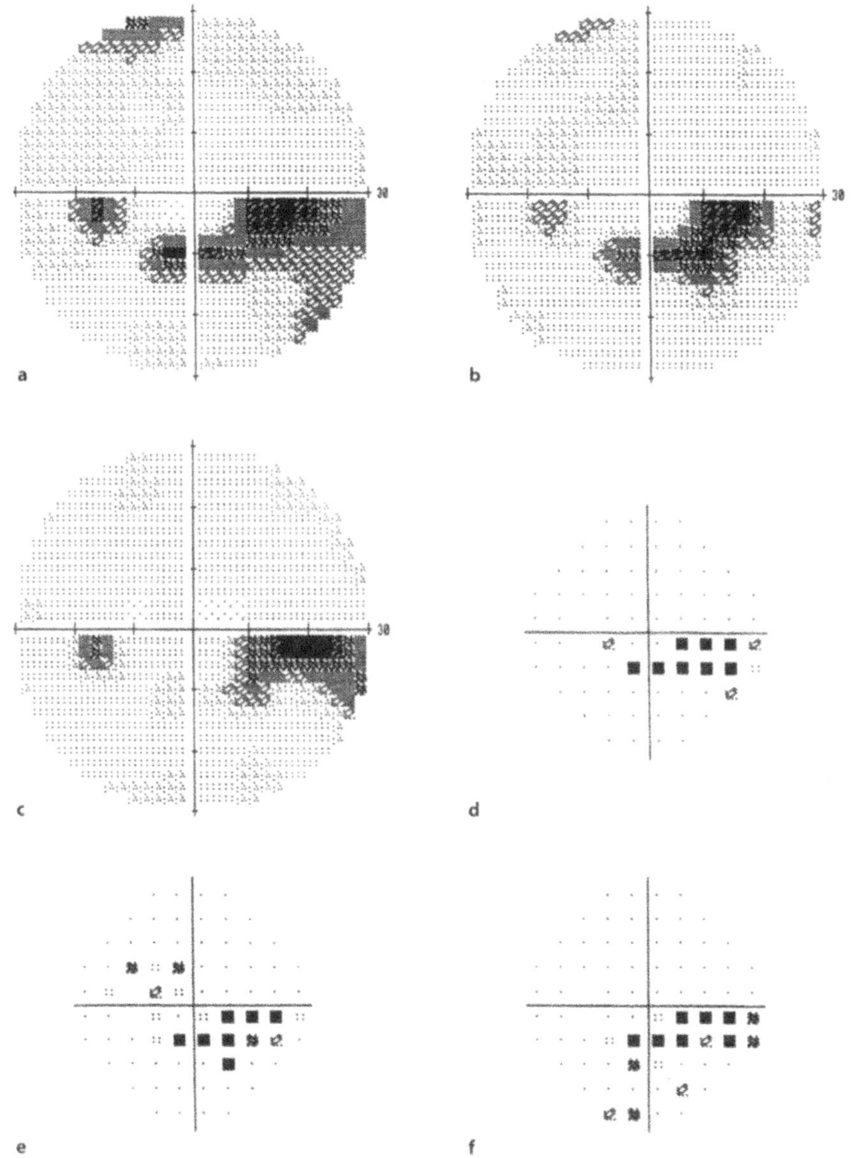

Fig. 2a–f. Grayscale printouts of test results obtained using three different strategies from the same glaucomatous eye. **a** Full threshold using 16 min, 1 s. **b** Swedish interactive thresholding algorithm (SITA) Standard requiring 8 min, 46 s. **c** SITA Fast with 4 min, 57 s. Defects appear larger/deeper with the long full-threshold program than in shorter tests. In corresponding pattern deviation-based probability maps, the number of significantly depressed points was somewhat smaller when using full threshold (**d**) than with both SITA Standard (**e**) and SITA Fast (**f**), indicating that the shorter tests give at least as much significant field loss as the longer full-threshold test

Normal Limits, Normal Variability

A large multi-centre trial has been conducted to establish normal limits for Statpac for SITA. The results show that the shorter and newer SITA programs have higher sensitivity and smaller inter-individual variability than the older ones. Normal individuals have smoother fields with SITA tests. This smaller variability is highly desirable, of course, leading to narrower normal limits for the newer tests. These narrow limits may be a result of the smaller visual fatigue of the shorter tests.

Sensitivity to Glaucomatous Field Loss

SITA's narrower limits mean that in order to reach significance, SITA Standard and SITA Fast defects do not have to be as deep as defects identified when using the older tests. This higher sensitivity compensates for the somewhat smaller/shallower defects in the SITA tests. In fact, the number of significantly depressed points in glaucomatous fields are as large with SITA as with, for example, full threshold. Even in cases when field defects appear smaller and/or shallower with the SITA algorithms than with their more time-consuming predecessors, the significance of field defects – as indicated, for example, in probability maps – are often as high with SITA as with the older algorithms (Fig. 2).

Practical Usage of SITA

SITA Standard and SITA Fast have been available as standard tests on the HFA II perimeters (Humphrey Instruments, San Leandro, Calif.) since 1997. Statpac for SITA was made available in spring 1998. The very high requirements on computer power and the need for fast changes of stimulus position make it impossible to adapt the older HFA I perimeters for SITA. SITA Standard is intended as a better replacement for the full-threshold algorithm, and SITA Fast can replace Fastpac. The existence of visual fatigue makes it non-optimal to compare visual field tests obtained with tests of different duration. While patients having normal fields, therefore, can be switched immediately from full-threshold or Fastpac to SITA, one must decide whether to continue to follow patients with established field loss with one of the old algorithms or whether to establish a new baseline for follow-up.

Summary

The new SITA algorithms represent a new generation of threshold algorithms for computerised static perimetry. They are faster than the older standard algorithms that they are intended to replace. They have higher patient acceptance and they are at least as reproducible as the older algorithms. Studies with the older and the newer algorithms confirm that visual fatigue is of importance in clinical perimetry and that shorter tests give somewhat smaller or shallower glaucomatous visual field defects than longer tests, and also that shorter tests have narrower normal limits. The narrower normal limits compensate for the smaller/shallower glaucomatous visual field defects, so that the shorter algorithms identify at least as much significant glaucomatous visual field loss as the older, more time-consuming ones. Patients with normal visual fields can be switched immediately to the newer, faster tests, while follow-up of patients with established field loss should continue with the older algorithms or be switched to SITA and a new baseline established.

It should be pointed out that SITA is a new set of algorithms for threshold perimetry; it is a more efficient way of collecting patient data. It is not a new test modality like, for example, short-wavelength automated perimetry or motion-detection perimetry. SITA can be adapted for all such new tests. Such adaptation requires considerable effort, however, since accurate visual field models are necessary for SITA to optimally increase test efficacy. Normal age-corrected values, inter-point correlations and frequency-of-seeing curves, for example, must be known.

References

1. Heijl A (1995) Improved test algorithms for automated perimetry. In: Krieglstein GK (ed) Glaucoma update, vol V. Kaden, Heidelberg, pp 168–173
2. Bengtsson B, Olsson J, Heijl A, Rootzén H (1997) A new generation of algorithms for computerized threshold perimetry, SITA. Acta Ophthamol 75:368–375
3. Olsson J, Bengtsson B, Heijl A, Rootzén H (1997) An improved method to estimate frequency of false positive answers in computerized perimetry. Acta Ophthalmol 75:181–183
4. Bengtsson B, Heijl A (1998) SITA Fast, a new rapid perimetric threshold test. Description of methods and evaluation in patients with manifest and suspect glaucoma. Acta Ophthalmol Scand 76:431–437
5. Bengtsson B, Heijl A (1998) Evaluation of a new threshold visual field strategy, SITA, in patients with suspect and manifest glaucoma. Acta Ophthalmol Scand 76:268–272
6. Bengtsson B, Heijl A, Olsson J (1998) Evaluation of a new threshold visual field strategy, SITA, in normal subjects. Acta Ophthalmol 76:165–169
7. Bengtsson B, Heijl A (1997) Test time with SITA and full threshold strategies in glaucoma patients (abstract). Final program of the 1997 Annual Meeting of the American Academy of Ophthalmology, San Francisco, California, p 171
8. Cunliffe IA, Pacey IE, Wild JM, Sedgewick G, O'Neill EC (1998) The validity and reproducibility of the SITA Standard and SITA Fast threshold algorithms in glaucoma. Invest Ophthalmol Vis Sci ARVO Suppl 39:26
9. Heijl A, Drance SM (1983) Changes in differential threshold in patients with glaucoma during prolonged perimetry. Br J Ophthalmol 67:512–516

CHAPTER 20

Frequency-Doubling Threshold Perimetry in Glaucoma, Glaucoma Suspect, and Normal Eyes

P. A. Sample · C. F. Bosworth · B. L. Lee · J. S. Perez · R. N. Weinreb

Abstract. *Purpose:* This study was undertaken in order to compare frequency-doubling threshold perimetry (FDT) results with standard achromatic automated perimetry (SAP) results in normal eyes, ocular-hypertensive (OHT) eyes, glaucoma-suspect eyes, and eyes with primary open-angle glaucoma (POAG) for detection of visual field loss and severity by location. *Methods:* Ninety patient eyes (29 OHT, 35 suspect, and 26 POAG) and 42 normal eyes were evaluated by FDT and SAP. Standard visual fields were done using the normal protocols. FDT thresholds were measured with 16 ten-degree targets, which covered most of the Humphrey-program 24-2 field area. Each target consisted of a 0.25-cycle per degree sinusoidal grating flickering at 25 Hz in counterphase. Abnormality for both tests was determined by comparison with the manufacturer's internal normative database. A variety of definitions of "abnormal on FDT" were evaluated. The results below used the criteria that two adjacent points outside the 95 % probability limits as abnormal. Thresholds for the two tests were also compared by visual-field location to determine whether defective areas overlapped. *Results:* Of the 61 suspect or POAG eyes, 75 % (46) were abnormal on FDT and 48 % (29) on SAP; 44 % (27) were abnormal on both tests, with results overlapping in at least one quadrant. FDT showed more abnormal quadrants (2.74 ± 1.26) than SAP (1.70 ± 0.91). There was a significant correlation between mean deviation for SAP and that for FDT in patient eyes ($p < 0.001$). *Conclusions:* Frequency-doubling perimetry had a sensitivity of 75 % when specificity was set to 90 %; however, a larger number of OHT eyes were identified as abnormal than would be expected to convert to glaucoma (48 %). Longitudinal follow-up of these eyes will help determine the predictive value of FDT for the development of glaucoma.

Introduction

Psychophysical tests of visual function that favor detection by one particular type of ganglion cell have been shown to be superior to standard visual fields for early detection of vision loss associated with glaucoma [1–23]. Frequency-doubling threshold perimetry (FDT) is a test which has been proposed to detect one type of ganglion cell.

FDT favors detection by the parasol ganglion cells, which project to the magnocellular layers of the lateral geniculate nucleus (LGN) in macaque and are therefore also called the M-ganglion cells. These ganglion cells make up about 10 % of the total population of ganglion cells. It has been suggested that the test may be evaluating a small subset of the M-ganglion cells, the My subset (see Discussion). The test is based on the frequency-doubling visual illusion [24], where the subject perceives the spatial frequency of a grating pattern with twice as many bars as are physically present. This illusion is thought to result from non-linear mechanisms in the visual-response pathway [25]. The test has been shown to differentiate normal from glaucomatous eyes [26] and to be useful as a screening test for glaucoma [27].

We compared the results of FDT in a large number of patient and normal eyes and showed that it has good sensitivity and specificity but may over-identify eyes with ocular hypertension (OHT).

Methods

Visual Fields

All eyes were tested using both standard automated perimetry (SAP) and FDT within a 3-month period. Standard visual fields were measured by means of a Humphrey field analyzer (HFA) I perimeter, using program 24–2. FDT was measured using the HFA Model 710 with Welch Allyn Frequency-Doubling Technology software version 1.20, program C-20. Abnormality for both tests was determined by comparison with the manufacturer's internal normative database. Visual-field results were evaluated to determine whether the defective areas for the two tests fell within the same quadrant of the visual field.

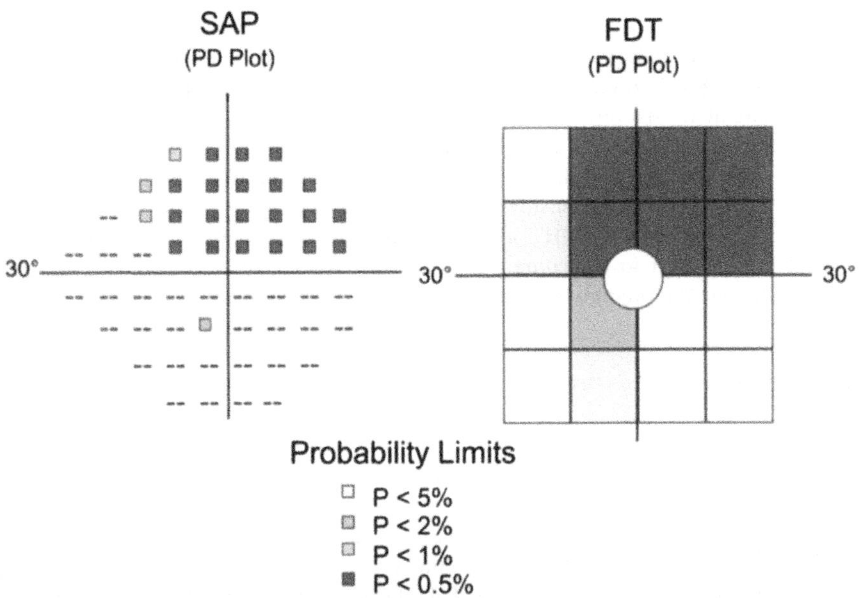

Fig. 1. The 16 test locations for frequency-doubling perimetry on the right. Each box covers an area of 10 × 10° of visual angle. The standard achromatic automated perimetry (*left*) and frequency-doubling threshold perimetry (*right*) pattern deviation results from a patient are also shown. In this case, there is good overlap between the defective areas found for each test

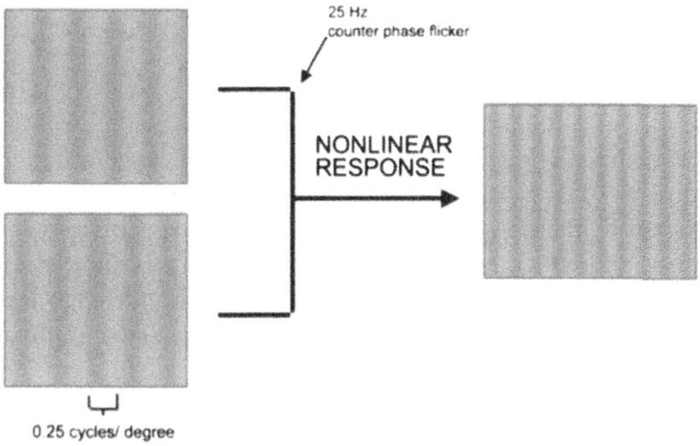

Fig. 2. A schematic representation of the frequency-doubling illusion. The two *boxes* on the *left* show time one (*top*) and time two (*bottom*) of the counterphase flicker of the 0.25-cycle-per-degree stimulus. These two alternate at a rate of 25 Hz. The *box* on the *left* shows the perceived doubling of the spatial frequency

Standard visual fields were classified as abnormal if the glaucoma hemifield test (GHT) was outside normal limits, the corrected-pattern standard deviation was triggered at the 5 % probability or worse, or the mean deviation (MD) was triggered at the 5 % probability or worse with no generalized depression on two consecutive visual fields. Quadrants were identified as abnormal by a cluster of more than three points at the 5 % probability limit or worse on the pattern-deviation plot. Frequency-doubling fields were abnormal when a cluster of two adjacent points reached the 5 % probability limit or worse. This gave a specificity for the normal controls of 90 %.

FDT consists of 16 targets, each 10×10° of visual angle covering the central 20° radius of the visual field (Fig. 1). The target consisted of a low spatial frequency sinusoidal grating (0.25 cycles/degree [c/d]), which undergoes a high temporal frequency counterphase flicker at 25 Hz. This produces an illusory perception of twice as many light and dark bars than are physically present; that is, the spatial frequency appears to be doubled to 0.50 c/d (Fig. 2). To obtain threshold, the contrast between the light and dark bars is varied until the stripes of the grating appear. The subject's task is to respond by pushing a button when the grating pattern can be seen, regardless of whether it is seen as doubled. A modified binary-search procedure is used to obtain the contrast threshold [27].

Subjects

All subjects had a complete ophthalmological exam, which included relevant medical history, best-corrected visual acuity, slit-lamp biomicroscopy (including gonioscopy), applanation tonometry, dilated fundoscopy, and stereoscopic ophthalmoscopy of the optic disc with a 78-D lens. Simultaneous stereophotographs were obtained on both eyes and graded in a masked fashion by a glaucoma expert. Photographs were graded abnormal when any one of the following was identified: a cup/disc asymmetry of more than 0.2 mm, rim thinning, notching, excavation, nerve-fiber-layer defect, or disc hemorrhage.

Inclusion Criteria

The criteria for inclusion were: open angles, a best corrected acuity of 20/40 or better, a spherical refraction within ± 5.0 D, cylinder within ± 3.0 D, and reliable standard Humphrey 30–2 or 24–2 visual fields (defined as less than 25 % false positives, 25 % false negatives, and 25 % fixation losses). A family history of glaucoma is allowed. In addition, normal controls were required to have intraocular pressures (IOPs) less than 22 mmHg on all known occasions, normal standard visual fields, and a grade of "normal" on stereophotograph review.

Exclusion Criteria

The criteria for exclusion were: a history of intraocular surgery in normals and suspect groups (except for uncomplicated cataract surgery), secondary causes of elevated IOP (exfoliation syndrome, pigment dispersion, corticosteroid use, iridocyclitis, trauma), other intraocular eye diseases, other diseases affecting the visual field (pituitary lesions, demyelinating diseases, human immunodeficiency virus or acquired immunodeficiency syndrome, or diabetes), generalized depression or "sensitivity too high" result on GHT, or problems (other than glaucoma) affecting color vision.

One eye was selected randomly from each subject after written consent was obtained according to protocols approved by the Human Subjects Committee of the University of California, San Diego. The 90 patient's eyes were divided into those with only OHT (defined as pressures greater than 23 mmHg) on two occasions (n = 29), those who had abnormal standard fields but normal stereophoto reviews (n = 3), those who had glaucomatous stereophoto reviews but normal standard fields (n = 32), and those with both abnormal standard fields and glaucomatous stereophotos (n = 26). No criteria for IOP was applied to the suspect or glaucoma groups. In addition, 42 normal control eyes were evaluated.

Results

Of the 61 glaucoma or suspect eyes, 75 % (46) were abnormal on FDT and 48 % (29) were abnormal on SAP (Table 1); 44 % (27) were abnormal on both tests. Of these 27 eyes, 93 % (25) had defective results that overlapped in at least one quadrant. An example is shown in Fig. 1. Greater areas of defect were found for FDT than SAP. The mean number (± SD) of abnormal quadrants in FDT was 2.72 ± 1.26, while SAP had 1.70 ± 0.91 ($p < 0.001$, paired t-test). There was a significant correlation between the MD for SAP and the MD for FDT in patient eyes ($p < 0.001$, $r^2 = 0.389$; Fig. 3).

FDT identified more OHT eyes as abnormal than would be expected to convert to glaucoma over a period of 10 years or more. Of the 29 OHT eyes, 48 % (14) were abnormal on FDT, while estimates usually place the expected number between 11 %

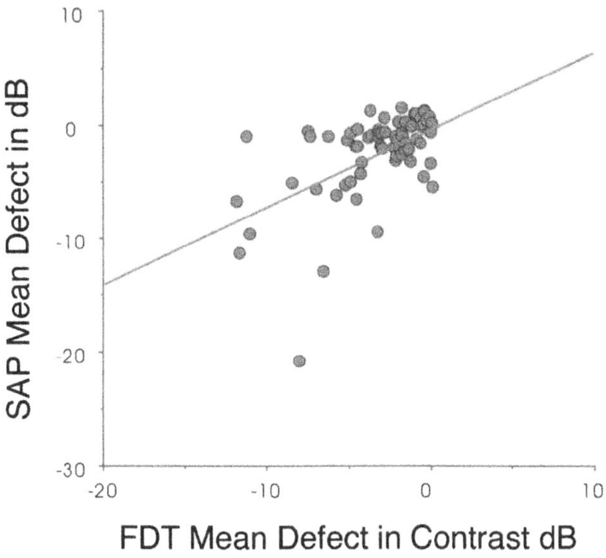

Fig. 3. The correlation in mean deviation between standard achromatic automated perimetry and frequency-doubling threshold perimetry

Table 1. Number of eyes (%) classified as normal or abnormal in each study group for both frequency-doubling threshold perimetry (FDT) and standard achromatic automated perimetry (SAP)

Field classification	POAG	Field only	Nerve only	OHT only
Abnormal on both	92 (24/26)	100 (3/3)	n/a	n/a
Abnormal on SAP only	8 (2/26)	0 (0/3)	n/a	n/a
Abnormal on FDT only	n/a	n/a	59 (19/32)	48 (14/29)
Normal on both	n/a	n/a	41 (13/32)	52 (15/29)
FDT abnormal		75 (46/61)		48 (14/29)
SAP abnormal		48 (29/61)		n/a by definition

POAG, primary open-angle glaucoma; OHT, ocular hypertension.

and 25% [28–31]. The stereophoto grades for the OHT eyes were all normal by definition; however, 29 of the 32 eyes were evaluated with the Heidelberg Retina Tomograph (HRT), a confocal scanning laser ophthalmoscope. Preliminary analysis of HRT results comparing the OHT eyes, which were abnormal on FDT, and those normal on FDT showed no significant differences for any measure (Table 2).

Discussion

Our results show that FDT has better sensitivity for detection of visual-field loss in eyes with abnormal optic discs on stereophoto review. Sensitivity was 75% when specificity was set to 90% on FDT. Standard fields using routine clinical criteria for

Table 2. Heidelberg Retina Tomograph (HRT) comparison in ocular hypertension (OHT): frequency-doubling threshold perimetry (FDT) normal versus FDT abnormal

Parameter	Normal FDT (n = 15)	Abnormal FDT (n = 14)	p value
Disc area (mm^2)	1.76±0.34	1.75±0.31	0.89
Rim area (mm^2)	1.23±0.18	1.24±0.14	0.99
Cup area (mm^2)	0.53±0.29	0.51±0.31	0.87
Rim volume (mm^3)	0.32±0.11	0.32±0.07	0.85
Cup volume (mm^3)	0.13±0.11	0.13±0.11	0.97
Height-variation contour (mm)	0.36±0.1	0.38±0.09	0.57
Maximum cup depth (mm)	0.61±0.19	0.59±0.22	0.76
Mean RNFL thickness (mm)	0.06±0.02	0.05±0.01	0.53
Cup shape measure	–0.18±0.07	–0.17±0.07	0.53
Linear discriminant function (% abnormal)	53 (8)	43 (6)	

RNFL, retinal nerve fiber layer.

abnormality identified only 48 %. This suggests that FDT may be useful for more than just screening for glaucoma. However, in the OHT group of patients, FDT was abnormal in 48 %, a percentage that is much higher than is expected to convert to glaucoma, and also much higher than the percentage shown for other ganglion-cell-specific tests. Short-wavelength automated perimetry (SWAP) and motion automated perimetry (MAP) usually identify between 20 % and 25 % of the OHT eyes, depending on the study [8, 10, 14, 18]. The reason that FDT is abnormal in so many OHT eyes needs to be evaluated further before it can be used as a diagnostic tool. Preliminary work in our laboratory showed that there were no significant differences in measures of optic-disc topographic parameters using HRT for OHT eyes identified as normal by FDT when compared with those identified as abnormal on FDT.

Another issue surrounding FDT that needs further study is the suggestion that FDT is processed by a small subset of the M-ganglion cells, called the My ganglion cells [26, 27]. This proposal is based on work by several physiologists who have identified cells at the level of the LGN which respond to pooled inputs from different parts of their receptive fields in a non-linear way; that is, the cell responds best to 2× the fundamental spatial frequency when there is a phase shift of 90° [32]. Others have not found evidence to support the existence of a distinct, non-linear class of magnocellular unit, and propose that the changes in temporal frequency leading to alterations in the spatial frequency contrast response could be found in both M and P units at retina and LGN [33, 34].

Attempts to relate the frequency-doubled perception to My- and M-type cells using a variety of techniques in human observers are in progress but are, as yet, inconclusive [35, 36]. At present, we can say that the combination of high temporal flicker (25 Hz) and low spatial frequency (0.25 c/d) used in FDT makes it likely that the test is at least utilizing the M cells, and is processed by no more than 10 % of the retinal-ganglion-cell population.

FDT has some advantages over standard visual fields. The test time is about 50 % of the time required for a full-threshold 24–2 field, primarily due to the smaller number of test locations used. The results are unaffected by blur, pupil-size differences if greater than 2 mm in diameter, or bifocal correction [27]. It is similar to standard visual fields in that statistical analysis packages can be developed to give global indices, such as MD and PSD, and pattern-deviation probability-style plots can be derived.

Although FDT shows promise for early detection of visual loss due to glaucoma, more work is needed. Prospective longitudinal studies with the device, especially studies addressing the over-identification of OHT eyes, will determine its predictive value and its usefulness for following the progress of visual loss.

Acknowledgements. This research was supported by a grant from the National Eye Institute, NEI EY 08208

References

1. Bosworth CF, Sample PA, Weinreb RN (1997) Motion perception thresholds in areas of glaucomatous visual field loss. Vis Res 37:355–364
2. Bosworth CF, Sample PA, Weinreb RN (1996) Perimetric motion thresholds are elevated in glaucoma suspects and glaucoma patients. Vis Res 37:1989–1997
3. Bullimore MA, Wood JM, Swenson K (1993) Motion perception in glaucoma. Invest Ophthalmol Vis Sci 34:3526–3533
4. Casson EJ, Johnson CA, Shapiro LR (1993) Longitudinal comparison of temporal-modulation perimetry with white-on-white and blue-on-yellow perimetry in ocular hypertension and early glaucoma. J Opt Soc Am A 10:1792–1806
5. deJong LAMS, Snepvangers CEJ, van den Berg CT (1990) Blue-yellow perimetry in the detection of early glaucomatous damage. Doc Ophthalmol 75:303–314
6. Demirel S, Johnson CA (1996) Short wavelength automated perimetry (SWAP) in ophthalmic practice. J Am Optom Assoc 67:451–456
7. Johnson CA, Adam AJ, Casson EJ, Brandt JD (1993) Progression of early glaucomatous visual field loss for blue-on-yellow and standard white-on-white automated perimetry. Arch Ophthalmol 111:651–656
8. Johnson CA, Adams AJ, Casson EJ, Bradnt J (1993) Blue-on-yellow perimetry can predict the development of glaucomatous visual field loss. Arch Ophthalmol 111:645–650
9. Johnson CA (1994) Selective versus nonselective losses in glaucoma. J Glaucoma 3:S32–S44
10. Johnson CA, Brandt JD, Khong AM, Adams AJ (1995) Short-wavelength automated perimetry in low-, medium-, and high-risk ocular hypertensive eyes. Arch Ophthalmol 113:70–76
11. Johnson CA (1996) Diagnostic value of short-wavelength automated perimetry. Curr Opin Ophthalmol 7:54–58
12. Sample PA, Weinreb RN (1990) Color perimetry for assessment of primary open-angle glaucoma. Invest Ophthalmol Vis Sci 31:1869–1875
13. Sample PA, Weinreb RN (1992) Progressive color visual field loss in glaucoma. Invest Ophthalmol Vis Sci 33:2068–2071
14. Sample PA, Taylor JDN, Martinez GA, Lusky M, Weinreb RN (1993) Short-wavelength color visual fields in glaucoma suspects at risk. Am J Ophthalmol 115:225–233
15. Sample PA, Martinez GA, Weinreb RN (1993) Color visual fields: A 5 year prospective study in eyes with primary open angle glaucoma. In: Mills R (ed) Perimetry update 1992/1993: proceedings of the Xth international perimetric society meeting. Kugler, Amsterdam, pp 473–476
16. Sample PA, Madrid ME, Weinreb RN (1994) Evidence for a variety of functional defects in glaucoma suspect eyes. J Glaucoma 3:S5–S18
17. Sample PA, Plummer DJ, Weinreb RN (1995) Standard achromatic perimetry vs. short-wavelength automated perimetry for following glaucoma. In: Kriglestein GK (ed) Glaucoma update V. Springer, Berlin Heidelberg New York, pp 197–204
18. Sample P, Bosworth C, Weinreb R (1997) Short-wavelength automated perimetry and motion automated perimetry in glaucoma. Arch Ophthalmol 115:1129–1133
19. Silverman SE, Trick GL, Hart WM Jr (1990) Motion perception is abnormal in primary open-angle glaucoma. Invest Ophthalmol Vis Sci 31:722–729
20. Trick GL, Steinman BS, Amyot M (1995) Motion perception deficits in glaucomatous optic neuropathy. Vis Res 25:2225–2233
21. Wall M, Kathryn M, Ketoff BS (1995) Random dot motion perimetry in patients with glaucoma and in normal controls. Am J Ophthalmol 120:587–596

22. Wild JM, Moss ID, Whitaker D, O'Neill EC (1995) The statistical interpretation of blue-on-yellow visual field loss. Invest Ophthalmol Vis Sci 36:1398–1410
23. Yamagishi N, Anton A, Sample PA, et al. (1997) Mapping structural damage of the optic disc to visual field defect in glaucoma. Am J Ophthalmol 123:667–676
24. Kelly D (1966) Frequency doubling in visual responses. J Opt Soc Am 56:1628–1633
25. Kelly DH (1981) Nonlinear visual responses to flickering sinusoidal gratings. J Opt Soc Am 71:1051–1055
26. Maddess T, Henry G (1992) Performance of nonlinear visual units in ocular hypertension and glaucoma. Clin Vis Sci 7:371–383
27. Johnson C, Samuels S (1997) Screening for glaucomatous visual field loss with frequency-doubling perimetry. Invest Ophthalmol Vis Sci 38:413–425
28. Lundberg L, Wettrell K, Linner E (1987) Ocular hypertension. A prospective twenty-year follow-up study. Acta Ophthalmol 55:705
29. Perkins ES (1973) The Bedford glaucoma survey. I: long-term follow-up of borderline cases. Br J Ophthalmol 57:179–185
30. Sorensen PN, Nielsen NV, Norskov K (1978) Ocular hypertension. A 15-year follow-up. Acta Ophthalmol 56:363
31. Quigley HA, Enger C, Katz J, et al. (1994) Risk factors for the development of glaucomatous visual field loss in ocular hypertension. Arch Ophthalmol 112:644–649
32. Kaplan E, Shapley RM (1982) X and Y cells in the lateral geniculate nucleus of macaque monkeys. J Physiol (Lond) 330:125–143
33. Lee BB, Kremers J, Yeh T (1998) Receptive fields of primate retinal ganglion cells studied with a novel approach. Vis Neurosci 15:161–175
34. Derrington AM, Lennie P (1984) Spatial and temporal contrast sensitivities of neurones in lateral geniculate nucleus of macaque. J Physiol (Lond) 357:219–240
35. Bedford S, Maddess T, Rose KA, James AC (1997) Correlations between observability of the spatial frequency doubled illusion and a multi-region pattern electroretinogram. Aust N Z J Ophthalmol 25:S91–S93
36. Maddess T, Bedford S, James A, Rose K (1997) A multiple-frequency, multiple-region pattern electroretinogram investigation of non-linear retinal signals. Aust N Z J Ophthalmol 25:S94–S97

CHAPTER 21

The Spatial Distribution and Severity of Visual Field Defects in Asians with Primary Open-Angle Glaucoma and Primary Angle-Closure Glaucoma

S. K. L. Seah · P. J Foster · J. G. Devereux · F. T. S. Oen · P. T. Khaw · P. T. K. Chew

Background

Descriptions of the characteristics of visual-field loss in primary angle-closure glaucoma (PACG) are scarce and contradictory. In Japan, a study of 110 subjects with acute angle-closure (42 subjects) and chronic PACG (68 subjects) using Goldmann kinetic perimetry concluded that the pattern of visual-field loss in PACG was similar to that in primary open-angle glaucoma (POAG) [1]. Another study of subjects with primary and secondary angle-closure found that most (9/11) subjects with chronic PACG had nerve-fibre-bundle pattern visual-field loss. Conversely, 11 of 18 subjects who had suffered an acute, symptomatic attack of angle-closure had no impairment of the visual field. The remaining 7 showed typical nerve-fibre-bundle visual-field loss [2]. However, a study of 25 cases of acute unilateral angle-closure described a "significant" field defect in over half of this group, usually characterised by constriction of the upper field (not felt to be typically "glaucomatous" in nature) [3]. In Singapore, a previous retrospective study of PACG (Goldmann perimetry, 50 subjects: 20 acute, 30 chronic), field loss was found to be more common in chronic than acute angle closure. Field loss was worse in eyes with higher intraocular pressure (IOP) [4].

Method

Subjects were enrolled prior to undergoing surgery for medically uncontrolled glaucoma. The inclusion criteria for this prospective study were: IOP over 21 mmHg on at least one occasion, reduction in width of part of the neuroretinal rim to under 0.1 of the cup/disc area ratio (alternatively, a "glaucomatous optic disc" in the opinion of a fellowship-trained glaucoma specialist), and a visual-field defect consisting of at least two points reduced by over 5 dB or one point reduced by over 10 dB below an age-specific threshold.

Data were collected from one eye only of each subject. Previous glaucoma therapy was recorded, and the number of "drop months" was calculated by summing the duration of treatment (in months) of all topical medications used since diagnosis. At enrolment, a detailed examination was carried out, including refraction, axial-length measurement and applanation tonometry. The degree of lens opacity was graded using standard photographs of the lens opacity classification system III scheme.

Visual-field examination was carried out using a static automated perimeter (model 750, Zeiss Humphrey). At least two visual-field tests were performed using the

24–2 program. If the field was classified as "low patient reliability" it was discarded. If the mean defect in these tests differed by more than 2 dB, further tests were carried out until this condition had been met. When pupil diameter was less than 3 mm, the pupil was dilated. Advanced Glaucoma Intervention Study (AGIS) scores were calculated from the total deviation matrix in the last test completed, using a spreadsheet program on a personal computer [5]. AGIS scores were compared in three clusters: nasal (scored 0–2), upper and lower (both scored 0–9), with 0 indicating no significant defect in each case. The scores in each of the three clusters were summed to produce a total score ranging from 0 (no defect) to 20 (all clusters deeply depressed).

Results

One hundred and seven subjects were examined. Of these subjects, 84 were ethnic Chinese (79 %), 13 were Malay (12 %) and 11 were Indian (9 %). Fifty-eight subjects with POAG were included (47 men, 11 women, mean age 60.8 years). Forty-nine subjects had PCAG (28 men, 21 women, mean age 63.3 years). There were 52 right eyes and 55 left eyes included in this study.

Table 1 summarises the demographic and ophthalmic characteristics of the POAG and PACG groups. The major differences between the two groups were the great excess of men in the POAG group and the mean axial length (POAG: 23.9 mm, PACG: 22.6 mm, $p < 0.001$). There was no significant difference between the groups in age, pre-operative IOP, pupil diameter during visual-field testing, "drop-months", spherical equivalent of refraction or lens opacity. The median time from diagnosis to listing for surgery was 12 months in the POAG group but only 7 months in the PACG group,

Table 1. Demographic and ophthalmic characteristics of subjects with primary open-angle glaucoma (POAG) and primary angle-closure glaucoma (PACG)

Parameter	P/NP[a]	POAG	PACG	Difference between POAG and PACG (p)
Age (years)	P	60.8 (10.7)	63.3 (9.0)	0.18
Sex (M:F)	–	47:11	28:21	–
IOP (mmHg)	P	22.4 (5.7)	22.6 (5.2)	0.88
Axial length (mm)	P	24.0 (1.3)	22.6 (0.8)	0.000
Pupil diameter (mm)	P	5.6 (1.3)	5.6 (1.5)	0.96
Time from diagnosis (months)	NP	12 (1 to 120)	7.0 (0 to 240)	0.24
"Drop months"	NP	17 (0 to 186)	15 (0 to 480)	0.70
Spherical equivalent (D)	NP	–0.5 (–8.25 to +3.00)	–0.19 (–5.13 to +2.00)	0.11
LOCS (NO)	NP	3 (2 to 5)	3 (1 to 5)	0.12
LOCS (NC)	NP	3 (2 to 5)	3 (1 to 5)	0.52
LOCS (C)	NP	1 (0 to 4)	0 (0 to 3)	0.22
LOCS (P)	NP	0 (0 to 3)	0 (0 to 3)	0.14

[a]P/NP indicates that data is distributed parametrically (P) or non-parametrically (NP). Parametric data is summarised with mean and standard deviation. Probability of the null hypothesis is derived from an independent sample *t*-test. Non-parametric data is summarised with median and range. Probability of the null hypothesis is derived from the Mann-Whitney U-test.
IOP, intraocular pressure; LOCS, Lens Opacity Classification System; NC, nuclear color; NO, nuclear opalescence; C, cortical cataract; P, posterior subcapsular cataract.

Table 2. Advanced Glaucoma Intervention Study (AGIS) score by category of severity and region. AGIS scores are categorised as follows: mild = 0–5, moderate = 6–11, severe = 12–17 and end-stage = 18–20

	POAG				PACG			
Mild	Moderate	Severe	End-stage	Mild	Moderate	Severe	End-stage	
n	25	15	10	8	12	10	12	15
AGIS	2.5±1.7	8.3±1.6	14.1±1.8	20±0.0	1.5±1.7	8.1±1.4	14.6±1.5	19.7±0.6
AGIS upper	1.1±1.4	4.9±2.4	7.1±2.6	9.0±0.0	1.1±1.4	4.0±2.2	6.7±2.4	8.9±0.4
AGIS lower	0.6±0.9	2.1±1.9	5.2±2.4	9.0±0.0	1.1±2.6	2.8±1.1	5.9±2.7	8.86±0.5
AGIS difference[a]	0.52±1.8	2.8±4.1	1.9±4.7	0.0±0.0	0.0±1.9	1.2±3.2	0.83±4.9	0.0±0.6

[a] AGIS difference represents upper hemifield cluster AGIS score minus lower hemifield cluster AGIS score. POAG, primary open-angle glaucoma; PACG, primary angle-closure glaucoma.

although this difference did not attain significance at the 5 % level ($p = 0.24$). Table 2 gives a summary of the AGIS score for upper- and lower-hemifield clusters in POAG and PACG patients sub-divided into mild, moderate, severe and end-stage glaucomatous field loss. The upper cluster has a higher AGIS score than the lower field in mild, moderate and severe POAG and moderate and severe PACG. Among the POAG group, 40 subjects had mild/moderate field loss, while 18 had severe/end-stage field loss. For the PACG group, 22 had mild/moderate field defects and 27 had severe/end-stage fields. This difference in severity between POAG and PACG groups was significant ($p = 0.012$).

Discussion

In POAG, there was significantly greater field loss in the upper field than in the lower at all stages of the disease except end stage. A similar pattern is seen in "moderate" and 66 "severe" PACG cases. It has been previously reported that the area of the visual field most often affected in the early stages of POAG is the Bjerrum area adjacent to the optic disc in the upper visual field [6]. In Europeans, early glaucoma (presumably POAG is described in this group) has a predilection for the inferio-temporal segment of the neuroretinal rim, producing an upper-field defect [7]. Only at a later stage does the supero-temporal rim become involved. Our findings suggest that, in Asians, POAG and PACG both have a similar propensity to cause loss of visual field in the upper-hemifield cluster in the early/intermediate stages. Evolution of a field defect in the lower-hemifield cluster lags behind until a relatively late stage in the disease.

There were significantly more subjects with severe and end-stage disease in the PACG group at a similar stage of hospital management. We believe this reflects a tendency for late presentation among this group, possibly reflecting a lower health awareness.

References

1. Horie T, Kitazawa Y, Nosé H (1975) Visual field changes in primary angle- closure glaucoma. Jpn J Ophthalmol 19:108–115
2. Douglas GR, Drance SM, Schulzer M (1975) The visual field and nerve head in angle-closure glaucoma. Arch Ophthalmol 93:409–411
3. McNaught EI, Rennie A, McClure E, Chisholm IA (1974) Pattern of visual damage after acute angle-closure glaucoma. Trans Ophthalmol Soc U K 94:406–415
4. Dhillon B, Chew PT, Lim ASM (1990) Field loss in primary angle-closure glaucoma. Asia Pac J Ophthalmol 2:85–87
5. The Advanced Glaucoma Intervention Study Investigators (1994) Advanced glaucoma intervention study. 2. Visual field test scoring and reliability. Ophthalmology 101:1445–1455
6. Hart WM, Becker B (1982) The onset and evolution of glaucomatous visual field defects. Ophthalmology 89:268–279
7. Jonas JB, Fernandez MC, Stunner J (1993) Pattern of glaucomatous neuroretinal rim loss. Ophthalmology 100:63–68

Normal Pressure Glaucoma

CHAPTER 22

Parapapillary Atrophy in the Chronic Open-Angle Glaucomas

J. B. Jonas · W. M. Budde · P. J. Lang

Introduction

The chronic open-angle glaucomas form a heterogeneous group of optic-nerve diseases, which can be differentiated from each other by their elevations of intraocular pressure (IOP), levels of IOP, the age of the patients, the refractive error, and the atrophic appearance of the posterior fundus [1–3]. The heterogeneity of the whole group of the chronic open-angle glaucomas is paralleled by a marked variability in the appearance of the intrapapillary region of the optic-nerve head [1–3]. The purpose of the present study was to evaluate the parapapillary region in the various chronic open-angle glaucomas.

Patients and Methods

The study included 631 patients with primary open-angle glaucoma (POAG), 123 patients with secondary open-angle glaucoma (pseudo-exfoliative glaucoma $n = 86$; pigmentary glaucoma $n = 37$), and 481 normal subjects. POAG was differentiated into non-highly myopic POAG ($n = 425$, no pronounced fundus tessellation), age-related atrophic POAG ($n = 89$, age greater than 50 years, marked fundus tessellation), highly myopic POAG ($n = 32$), juvenile-onset POAG (n = 33, age less than 40 years), and focal normal-pressure glaucoma ($n = 52$). Color stereo optic-disc photographs were morphometrically evaluated.

Results

The beta zone of parapapillary atrophy was significantly ($p< 0.0001$) larger in highly myopic POAG than in age-related atrophic POAG, in which the beta zone was significantly larger than in pseudo-exfoliative glaucoma ($p = 0.02$), pigmentary glaucoma ($p< 0.001$), and non-highly myopic POAG ($p< 0.001$). Compared with non-highly myopic POAG and age-related atrophic glaucoma, the beta zone was significantly smaller in focal normal-pressure glaucoma ($p = 0.02$) and juvenile-onset POAG ($p< 0.01$). The two latter groups did not vary significantly ($p = 0.27$) in the size of the beta zone. Compared with all glaucoma groups, the beta zone was significantly smaller in the normal eyes. Taking all glaucoma types except focal normal-pressure glaucoma, the beta zone increased significantly ($p = 0.01$) with decreasing mean IOP.

Discussion

The occurrence of parapapillary chorioretinal atrophy in glaucoma has been described by many authors during the last 30 years [1–4]. Ophthalmoscopically, parapapillary chorioretinal atrophy has been divided into a central beta zone with visible sclera, and a peripheral alpha zone with irregular hypopigmentation and hyperpigmentation [4]. Clinical histological studies revealed that the beta zone correlates with a complete loss of retinal pigment epithelium cells and a markedly diminished count of retinal photoreceptors, and that the alpha zone is the equivalent of pigmentary irregularities in the retinal pigment epithelium [4]. Correspondingly, the blind spot of the visual field is larger in eyes with pronounced parapapillary chorioretinal atrophy than in eyes with small parapapillary atrophy [4], due to an absolute scotoma in the beta zone and a relative scotoma in the alpha zone. In contrast to glaucomatous optic neuropathy, eyes with non-glaucomatous optic-nerve damage do not show a marked parapapillary atrophy which, among other variables, serves to differentiate between glaucomatous and non-glaucomatous optic-nerve atrophy [4].

As with many biological variables, including the size and shape of the optic disc and neuroretinal rim, parapapillary atrophy shows a pronounced interindividual variability [4], which sometimes led researchers to doubt the existence of an association between parapapillary atrophy and glaucomatous optic neuropathy. Previous cross-sectional and longitudinal studies, however, have shown that, at least in some eyes, glaucoma is associated with an unusually large parapapillary atrophy [4]. Correspondingly, a previous longitudinal optic-disc study on experimental high-pressure glaucoma in monkeys revealed an enlargement of parapapillary atrophy after elevation of IOP (SS Hayreh, unpublished data).

One of the reasons for the marked interindividual variability of parapapillary atrophy may be the inhomogeneity of the total glaucoma group. The present study shows that the amount of parapapillary atrophy varies considerably among the different chronic open-angle glaucomas. Parapapillary atrophy was the smallest in eyes with juvenile-onset POAG (Table 1). Parapapillary atrophy was medium sized in eyes with POAG without marked fundus tessellation, eyes with pseudo-exfoliative glaucoma and eyes with pigmentary glaucoma. Parapapillary atrophy was relatively large in age-related atrophic glaucoma, and it was largest in eyes with highly myopic primary open-angle glaucoma (Table 1). Taking all these glaucoma types into consideration, parapapillary atrophy increased significantly with decreasing mean minimal IOP readings. Correspondingly, parapapillary atrophy increased with decreasing mean IOP, calculated as the mean minimal IOP plus one-third of the difference between the mean maximal IOP minus the mean minimal IOP. The lower the mean IOP was, the larger the parapapillary atrophy.

However, this inverse correlation between the size of the parapapillary atrophy and level of IOP was not found in eyes with focal normal-pressure glaucoma. Eyes with focal normal-pressure glaucoma did not vary in parapapillary atrophy from eyes with juvenile-onset primary open-angle glaucoma, despite marked differences in IOP (Table 1). The question arises: which factors may be responsible for the discrepancy? One of the reasons could be that patients with focal normal-pressure glaucoma and patients with juvenile-onset POAG share some similarities in the pathogenesis of their optic-nerve damage. As a hypothesis, the trans-lamina cribrosa pressure gradi-

Table 1. Composition of the study groups and optic disc measurements (mean ± SD)

	Non-highly myopic POAG	Age-related atrophic glaucoma	Highly myopic POAG	Juvenile-onset POAG	Focal normal-pressure glaucoma	Pseudo-exfoliative glaucoma	Pigmentary glaucoma	POAG, matched for refractive error with pigmentary glaucoma	Normal subjects
n	425	89	32	33	52	86	37	148	481
Age (years)	62.91 ± 11.33	65.11 ± 8.79	55.94 ± 15.00	32.70 ± 5.49	50.52 ± 10.94	69.76 ± 9.21	42.43 ± 10.68	61.80 ± 12.46	45.37 ± 16.43
Refractive error (D)	−0.57 ± 2.50	−1.22 ± 2.39	−11.28 ± 4.34	−1.21 ± 2.27	−0.45±2.15	−0.03 ± 2.36	−2.47 ± 2.26	−2.69 ± 2.19	−0.25 ± 2.11
Refractive error range	−7.62 to +7.00	−6.75 to +2.50	−24.00 to −8.00	−5.50 to +4.87	−6.75 to +3.50	−7.85 to +6.50	−7.25 to +1.50	−7.62 to +0.5	−7.88 to +7.75
Neuroretinal rim (mm^2)	1.12 ± 0.50	0.93 ± 0.50	1.32 ± 1.02	1.18 ± 0.38	1.14 ± 0.39	0.99 ± 0.56	1.15 ± 0.40	1.12 ± 0.51	1.78 ± 0.38
Intraocular pressure (mmHg)									
Mean maximal IOP	20.89 ± 5.39	20.76 ± 4.91	20.19 ± 5.59	23.57 ± 8.34	16.13±2.16	24.09 ± 6.17	25.14 ± 8.76	20.76 ± 6.07	
Mean minimal IOP	12.84 ± 3.66	13.26 ± 2.93	11.62 ± 3.30	15.10 ± 3.82	12.70±2.27	13.62 ± 4.38	14.29 ± 3.32	13.03 ± 4.62	
Amplitude	8.05 ± 5.25	7.35 ± 4.97	8.29 ± 5.69	8.48 ± 7.84	3.29 ± 2.52	10.65 ± 5.52	10.86 ± 8.07	7.73 ± 5.31	
Parapapillary atrophy									
Beta zone (mm^2)	0.66 ± 1.06	1.00 ± 1.37	4.11 ± 3.42	0.33 ± 0.72	0.29 ± 0.38	0.65 ± 0.93	0.42 ± 0.58	0.87 ± 1.23	0.18 ± 0.57
Beta zone range (mm^2)	0.00–8.65	0.00–8.52	0.00–11.48	0.00–3.60	0.00–1.45	0.00–5.24	0.00–2.72	0.00–8.65	0.00–6.59
Alpha zone (mm^2)	0.78 ± 0.67	1.04 ± 0.92	0.96 ± 1.46	0.76 ± 0.72	0.92 ± 0.64	0.75 ± 0.72	0.95 ± 0.72	0.84 ± 0.80	0.57 ± 0.57
Alpha zone range (mm^2)	0.00–4.84	0.00–4.67	0.00–4.24	0.00–2.80	0.00–3.22	0.00–3.24	0.00–2.54	0.00–4.84	0.00–4.19

POAG, primary open-angle glaucoma.

ent, which is the difference between the pressure in the intraocular space and the pressure in the optic nerve sheaths, may be increased in both glaucoma types - in high-pressure glaucoma due to an abnormally high IOP, and in focal normal-pressure glaucoma due to an abnormally low cerebrospinal-fluid pressure. This theory, which has already been described in the literature [5], suggests a pressure-associated aspect in the pathogenesis of focal normal-pressure glaucoma. It could resolve the discrepancy between a small parapapillary atrophy in focal normal-pressure glaucoma and the inverse correlation between IOP and parapapillary atrophy. A structural weakness of the lamina cribrosa in the normal-pressure glaucoma patients would be another mechanism leading to similarities in the optic-disc morphology between focal normal-pressure glaucoma and high-pressure glaucoma. A normal trans-lamina cribrosa pressure gradient in combination with a weak lamina cribrosa might then be sufficient for a mechanical distortion of the lamina cribrosa, which may directly or indirectly damage the optic-nerve fibers.

The finding of the present study that focal normal-pressure glaucoma and high-pressure glaucoma do not vary markedly in parapapillary atrophy agrees with other investigations reported in the literature. Caprioli and Spaeth found no significant differences in optic-disc morphology between patients with high-pressure glaucoma and those with low-pressure glaucoma [2]. Park and coworkers reported that, in patients with normal-pressure glaucoma, parapapillary atrophy is significantly correlated with structural and functional damage. It agrees with the present study, in which parapapillary atrophy was slightly larger in focal normal-pressure glaucoma than in normal eyes (Table 1).

The results of our present investigation disagree with those of a previous study of ours. In the previous study, however, focal normal-pressure glaucoma had not been separated from other types of normal-pressure glaucoma. The inclusion of patients with age-related atrophic open-angle glaucoma, in which IOP is often normal and a pronounced parapapillary atrophy prevails [1-3], may explain the discrepancies between the studies. Despite similarities in the appearance of parapapillary atrophy in focal normal-pressure glaucoma and high-pressure glaucoma, one should not forget that both glaucoma types show characteristic differences in the morphology of the optic-nerve head, such as different frequencies of localized retinal nerve-fiber-layer defects, disc hemorrhages, and neuroretinal rim notches [1].

The variability of parapapillary atrophy in the whole study group suggests that it should be included in the panoply of optic-disc features used to differentiate the various types of open-angle glaucoma. To cite examples, eyes with the highly myopic type of POAG have secondary or acquired macrodiscs of an abnormal shape, and shallow and concentric disc cupping. Disc hemorrhages and localized retinal nerve-fiber-layer defects are relatively rare, and IOP measurements are often in the normal range [1-3]. In the juvenile-onset type of POAG, optic-disc cupping is steep and deep. Frequencies of disc hemorrhages, neuroretinal rim notches and localized retinal nerve-fiber-layer defects are low, and the minimal and maximal values of IOP measurements are high. Eyes with the age-related atrophic type of POAG show a shallow and concentric disc cupping. Disc hemorrhages, rim notches, and localized retinal nerve-fiber-layer defects are seldom found, and IOP readings are in the lower range. In focal normal-pressure glaucoma, as originally described in 1976 by Spaeth, Hitchings, and Sivalingam, IOP often is normal, and the optic disc shows focal emaciation of the neuroretinal rim, typically in the inferotemporal and superiotemporal disc sectors. Secondary open-angle glaucoma due to pseudo-exfoliation of the lens ("pseudo-exfoliative glaucoma") and secondary open-angle glaucoma due to primary melanin dispersion syndrome ("pigmentary glaucoma") do not show clinically significant peculiarities in the morphology of the optic disc.

The large parapapillary atrophy in highly myopic POAG is primarily associated with the myopic stretching of the globe and optic disc, leading to the acquired macrophthalmos and secondary macrodisc. A recent histomorphometric study has shown that non-highly myopic eyes with glaucoma and highly myopic glaucomatous eyes show qualitative differences in the parapapillary region. In the parapapillary region of highly myopic eyes, Bruch's membrane is absent, and the sclera is covered only by the retinal nerve-fiber layer or its remnants. In contrast, in non-highly myopic glaucomatous eyes with parapapillary atrophy, the parapapillary region is totally covered by Bruch's membrane which is devoid of retinal-pigment epithelium cells and retinal photoreceptors.

The association of a relatively large beta zone with marked fundus tessellation in eyes with age-related POAG raises the question of whether, in at least some eyes with this type of chronic open angle glaucoma, changes may occur in the deep retinal layers, including the retinal-pigment epithelium. It may lead to a higher ophthalmoscopic visibility of the vascular architecture of the choroid. The finding that the beta zone and alpha zone were significantly larger in the group with juvenile-onset POAG and the group with focal normal-pressure glaucoma than in the normal eyes shows that, even in these types of open-angle glaucoma, parapapillary atrophy is associated with the glaucomatous process. The finding that the various chronic open-angle glaucomas differ more in the beta zone than in the alpha zone corresponds to a more pronounced difference in the beta zone when normal eyes and eyes with glaucoma are compared (Table 1). It agrees with previous studies on patients with glaucoma that showed that measurement of the beta zone of parapapillary chorioretinal atrophy is more important than evaluation of the alpha zone.

Acknowledgement. Supported by the Deutsche Forschungsgemeinschaft (SFB 539).

References

1. Spaeth GL (1994) A new classification of glaucoma including focal glaucoma. Surv Ophthalmol 38:S9–S17
2. Caprioli J (1993) Correlation between disc appearance and type of glaucoma. In: Varma R, Spaeth GL (eds) The optic nerve in glaucoma. Lippincott, Philadelphia, pp 91–98
3. Nicolela MT, Drance SM (1996) Various glaucomatous optic nerve appearances: clinical correlations. Ophthalmology 103:640–649
4. Jonas JB, Fernández MC, Naumann GOH (1992) Glaucomatous parapapillary atrophy: occurrence and correlations. Arch Ophthalmol 110:214–222
5. Morgan WH, Dao-Yi Y, Cooper RL, et al. (1995) The influence of cerebrospinal fluid pressure on the lamina cribrosa tissue pressure gradient. Invest Ophthalmol Vis Sci 36:1163–1172

CHAPTER 23

Can Pulsatile Ocular Blood Flow Be a Predictor of Future Visual Field Loss in Normal-Tension Glaucoma?

R. A. Hitchings

Introduction

This presentation looks at the association between pulsatile ocular blood flow (pobf) and visual loss in normal-tension glaucoma (NTG). Progression in glaucoma is best recognised as change in visual function. This is usually seen as a reduction in static visual loss on white-on-white perimetry. It should be identified as a change in focal rather than global parameters, and this can either be by event analysis (as shown on STATPAC 2) or trend analysis (demonstrated by linear progression, e.g. the PROGRESSOR program) [1]. Studies using a significance level set at $p< 0.05$ have shown that both STATPAC 2 and PROGRESSOR identify the same progressing locations, but that PROGRESSOR will identify them sooner [2].

Because trend analysis will provide a measure of rate of change, we adopted trend analysis. Using trend analysis, we have defined progression as one or more locations with a slope significant at the $p< 0.01$ level, having a rate of change greater than or equal to 1 db per year (for the inner 20 °, 2 db per year for the outer 10 °) of a 30° field. With this definition, we have looked for the incidence of progression in patients with NTG.

At the NTG clinic at Moorfields Eye Hospital, we identified patients who had 5 years or more of continuous follow-up. These patients were divided into 'progressors' or 'non-progressors' on the basis of their visual-field change. Factors that could influence the development of progression at the outset, such as age, gender, severity of the visual-field defect and height of the intraocular pressure (IOP) were looked for. The pobf level, where available, was checked against these presenting features.

pobf Values have been obtained in several studies of patients with glaucoma. These demonstrated a general reduction compared with normal values [3, 4]. The extent of the reduction has bearing on the extent of the visual loss; Fontana et al. [4] showed that, in comparing pobf values in the two eyes of NTG patients with asymmetric disease, the eye with the lower mean deviation (MD) had the lower pobf value. With this observation in mind, it seemed worthwhile to see whether any relationship existed between the eye developing visual-field loss and pobf values.

Patients and Methods

The patient records from the Moorfields NTG clinic were reviewed. Features of those patients who had been followed for 5 years or more were checked for: starting age, starting MD, starting corrected-pattern standard deviation (CPSD), starting IOP, refraction, and gender. Treatment, when given, was noted. The time from presentation to the development of a visual-field defect was noted. The pobf values, where present, were noted.

Multiple-regression analysis was performed to assess the relationship, if any, among any of the starting variables and the progression of the visual-field loss. The association of the pobf values with progression or lack of it was noted.

Results

One hundred and ninety glaucomatous patients had been followed for 5 years or more. Progression occurred in at least one eye of 145 patients; 29 patients showed progression only in the right eye and 33 only in the left eye. Progression was not related to the gender or age of the patient at presentation. Progression was not seen in 'non-progressors', followed for more than 5 years. Progression was not related to the diurnal pressure curve or starting values of MD or CPSD.

Pobf Values were available for 100 patients. If the pobf was lower in the left eye, progression was more likely in that eye, and vice versa. A comparison was made of the interocular differences between patients with no progression in either eye (23 patients), patients with progression in both eyes (38 patients) and those with progression in only one eye (39 patients). The median interocular difference [interquartile (IQ)] in eyes with unilateral progression was 104 μl/min (53, 159) (A), bilateral non-progression was 68 μl/min (33, 105) (B), and unilateral progression was 64.5 μl/min (74, 109) (C). Comparisons between (B) and (A) and (B) and (C) gave significance values of $p < 0.05$ and $p = 0.07$, respectively (Mann Whitney U test). These results suggested that an eye with progressive glaucoma was more likely to have a lower pobf value, irrespective of the starting IOP or the extent of the visual-field defect.

Discussion

pobf Values vary greatly in the normal population. Several studies have demonstrated a reduction in pobf values from normal in glaucoma [3, 4]. This can be expected from the known reduction in choroidal vasculature that occurs in chronic glaucoma. The pobf represents total ocular blood flow, and approximately 1% supplies the optic nerve. This supply to the optic nerve and choroid is thought to be poorly autoregulated [5], so that any variations in IOP will have a direct affect on both. Surgical reduction in IOP has been shown to increase pobf values [6]. We have seen such an increase in eyes with NTG that have undergone trabeculectomy. In the absence of autoregulation redistributing the blood flow around the ocular structures, it can be assumed that this overall increase will result both in an increase in the choroid blood flow and in the optic nerve. This may well exert a beneficial effect on the course of visual-field loss in glaucomatous patients.

References

1. Fitzke PW, Hitchings RA, Poinoosawmy D, McNaught AI (1996) Analysis of visual field progression in glaucoma. Br J Ophthalmol 80:40–48
2. Viswanathan AC, Fitzke FW, Hitchings RA (1997) Early detection of visual field progression in glaucoma: a comparison of PROGRESSOR and STATPAC 2. Br J Ophthalmol 81:1037–1043
3. Yang YC, Hulbert MF, Batterbury M, Clearkin LG (1997) Pulsatile ocular blood flow measurements in healthy eyes: reproducibility and reference values. J Glaucoma 6:175–179
4. Fontana L, Poinoosawmy D, Bunce C, Hitchings RA (1998) Pulsatile ocular blood flow investigation in asymmetric normal tension glaucoma and normal subjects. Br J Ophthamol 82:731–736
5. Pillunat LE, Stodtmeister R (1989) Pressure compliance test of the optic nerve head: influence of different antiglaucoma drugs. Surv Ophthalmol 33[Suppl]:465–466
6. James CB (1994) Effect of trabeculectomy on pulsatile ocular blood flow. Br J Ophthalmol 78:818–822

CHAPTER 24

Changes in the Optic-Nerve Head over Time in Normal-Tension Glaucoma

G. Tomita · Y. Kitazawa · N. Hayashi

Introduction

Recently, various kinds of computer-assisted image-analysis systems and instruments have been developed in the field of glaucoma diagnosis [1–3]. It has been stressed that one of the advantages of using computerized image-analysis methods is the ability to detect changes over time in the optic-nerve head or nerve-fiber layer [4]. This is because computerized techniques are not influenced by bias, unlike clinicians' subjective evaluations based on ophthalmoscopic findings. However, to what extent such techniques can detect differences in the configuration of the optic-nerve head over time is not yet fully understood. The purpose of this study was to evaluate changes in the optic-nerve head over time by means of scanning laser tomography in patients with normal-tension glaucoma.

Subjects and Methods

Study-Subject Selection

Patients with normal-tension glaucoma (NTG) were selected for this study from the database in our Heidelberg Retina Tomograph (HRT, Heidelberg Engineering GmBH, Heidelberg, Germany) from August 1993 to November 1997. We enrolled 30 eyes from 30 patients who met the following criteria: (1) the first and last optic disc measurements were over 2 years apart, (2) the HRT image quality was acceptable for further analyses; that is, the mean standard deviation of three consecutive images was less than 35 μm, and (3) a diagnosis of NTG had been established. Our criteria for a diagnosis of NTG in this study were:

1. At least one eye met the following criteria for visual-field loss by Humphrey field analyzer (Zeiss-Humphrey, Inc., San Leandro, Calif.), using program central 30–2, standard, full-threshold strategy.
   a. Three or more adjacent points with $p < 0.05$ in a total-deviation probability map
   b. Two or more adjacent points with $p < 0.02$ in a total-deviation probability map
   c. A difference of greater than 10 dB across the nasal horizontal meridian at two or more adjacent points [5]
   d. Fixation loss less than 20 % and false positive and negative rates less than 15 %
2. Intraocular pressure (IOP) of 21 mmHg or less based on measurements obtained at 2-h intervals over 24 h in both eyes by Goldmann applanation tonometry.

3. Gonioscopically normal anterior chamber angles in both eyes.
4. Glaucomatous disc abnormalities corresponding to visual-field defects defined ophthalmoscopically by two of us (GT and YK).
5. Absence of a history of laser surgery or intraocular surgery in either eye.
6. Absence of a history of systemic β-blocker or systemic or topical corticosteroid therapy.
7. Absence of intracranial abnormalities or lesions demonstrated on otolaryngologic or neurological examination, including computerized tomographic scan.

All eyes had a corrected visual acuity better than 20/30. Perimetry was performed within 3 months of disc measurements. If both eyes of a patient met inclusion criteria, we selected one eye randomly.

Subjects' Characteristics

Of 30 NTG patients enrolled in this study, 14 were followed-up without systemic or topical medications in both eyes for glaucoma during the period between the initial (time 1) and final (time 2) measurements of optic disc [medication (–) group], and 16 were treated with either anti-glaucoma eye drops or oral calcium-channel blockers or both [medication (+) group].

In the medication (–) group, 3 patients were male and 11 female. The age of patients ranged from 27 years to 70 years (mean age ± SD 53.6±13.2 years). The enrolled eyes had a refractive error of –1.80 ± 3.39 D in spherical equivalent (mean refractive error±SD). The period between times 1 and 2 measurements, i.e., follow-up period, ranged from 26 months to 50 months (mean period ± SD 39.4 ± 7.8 months). In the medication (+) group, the patients were 6 males and 10 females ranging in age from 41 years to 77 years (mean age ± SD 59.3± 11.4 years). The enrolled eyes had a refractive error of –1.50 ± 4.00 D in spherical equivalent (mean refractive error ± SD). The period between times 1 and 2 measurements ranged from 24 months to 53 months (mean period±SD 38.6 ± 7.1 months). Of 16 eyes, 8 were treated with oral calcium-channel blockers, 3 with topical IOP-lowering eye drops, and 5 with both. There were no statistically significant differences between the two groups in the mean age, refraction, or follow-up period.

Optic-Disc Measurements

Configuration of the optic-nerve head was measured using a HRT (program version 2.01). Three consecutive HRT images in a field 10 × 10° were taken to obtain a mean image with an average deviation of less than 35 μm. This mean image was used to determine the optic-disc parameters. A contour line, best fitted to the inner margin of the peripapillary scleral ring, was drawn to calculate the optic-disc parameters in the whole disc and the six defined areas of the optic disc (temporal-superior 45–90°; nasal-superior 90–135°; nasal 135–225°; nasal-inferior 225–270°; temporal-inferior 270–315°; and temporal 315–45°). The same contour line determined during the time-1 image was used to obtain the parameters during the time-2 image. The parameters we used included: cup area (mm^2), mean height of contour (mm), cup volume (volume below reference), rim volume (volume above reference), maximum cup depth, and cup-shape measure (third moment).

Statistical Analysis

Statistical analysis of the optic-disc measurements and other clinical data was done using the Wilcoxon's signed-rank test to evaluate the difference between times 1 and 2, and the Mann-Whitney *U* test was used to evaluate the difference between the medication (-) and medication (+) groups. Statistical significance was a *p* value less than 0.05.

Results

There were no statistically significant differences between the medication (-) and (+) groups in the initial IOP (IOP measured at the same day of the initial HRT measurements), the mean deviation (MD) or the corrected-pattern standard deviation (CPSD) of the visual-field indices. The IOP at time 2 was statistically significantly higher than that at time 1 in the medication (-) group (Table 1) (Wilcoxon signed rank test, $p< 0.01$). The MD at time 2 in the medication (-) group was lower than that at time 1, with a borderline significance ($p< 0.1$). There were no statistically significant differences between the two groups or between times 1 and 2 in all of the disc parameters in the whole disc (Table 1).

On analyzing defined small areas in the optic disc, the cup area of the temporal-inferior region in the medication (-) group was statistically significantly larger at time 2 than at time 1 (Wilcoxon signed-rank test, $p< 0.05$). The rim volume of the

Table 1. Parameter changes between time 1 and time 2, measured using the Wilcoxon signed rank test. Mean±SD

Value measured	Medication (-) $n = 14$ Time 1	Time 2	*p* value	Medication (+) $n = 16$ Time 1	Time 2	*p* value
IOP (mmHg)	13.8±1.7	15.4±1.3	<0.05	14.1±1.5	14.6±1.6	NS
Visual field indices						
MD (dB)	-2.22±2.37	-3.44±3.23	<0.1	-2.16±2.86	-3.04±3.47	NS
CPSD (dB)	3.69±2.67	4.68±2.80	NS	4.82±3.01	5.27±3.49	NS
Disc parameters in whole disc						
Cup area (mm^2)	1.23±0.63	1.27±0.55	NS	1.15±0.44	1.16±0.46	NS
Mean height of contour (mm)	0.13±0.05	0.14±0.07	NS	0.13±0.05	0.14±0.04	NS
Cup volume (mm^3)	0.38±0.35	0.38±0.32	NS	0.38±0.22	0.36±0.22	NS
Rim volume (mm^3)	0.31±0.20	0.28±0.16	NS	0.23±0.11	0.27±0.15	NS
Max cup depth (mm)	0.75±0.17	0.75±0.16	NS	0.80±0.19	0.76±0.25	NS
Cup-shape measure	-0.09±0.08	-0.09±0.08	NS	-0.11±0.05	-0.11±0.07	NS

NS, not significant; IOP, intraocular pressure; MD, mean deviation; CPSD, corrected-pattern standard deviation; Max, maximum.

Table 2. Disc parameter changes in the defined small areas, measured using the Wilcoxon signed rank test. Mean ± SD

Value measured	Medication (-) n = 14 Time 1	Time 2	p value	Medication (+) n = 16 Time 1	Time 2	p value
Cup area (mm^2): temporal-inferior	0.19±0.08	0.21±0.08	<0.05	0.16±0.08	0.17±0.09	NS
Rim volume (mm^3): temporal	0.05±0.15	0.01±0.01	NS	0.01±0.01	0.02±0.02	<0.05
Max cup depth (mm): nasal–inferior	0.67±0.10	0.63±0.12	NS	0.68±0.20	0.62±0.22	<0.05

NS, not significant; Max, maximum.

temporal region in the medication (+) group was statistically significantly larger (Wilcoxon signed-rank test, $p < 0.05$), and the maximum cup depth of the nasal-inferior region was statistically significantly smaller (Wilcoxon signed-rank test, $p < 0.05$) at time 2 than at time 1 (Table 2).

In the medication (+) group, the maximum cup depth of the nasal-inferior region at time 2 (mean ± SD 0.55 ± 0.16 mm) was statistically significantly shallower than that at time 1 (mean ± SD 0.62 ± 0.13 mm) in the subgroup of patients who had been treated with topical anti-glaucoma eye drops with or without adjunct use of oral calcium-channel blockers (n = 8). However, in the subgroup of patients who had been treated with oral calcium-channel blockers only (n = 8), no such differences were observed (mean±SD at time 1, 0.74 ± 0.25 mm; at time 2, 0.68 ± 0.27 mm). The IOP at time 1 was statistically significantly higher in the subgroup treated with glaucoma eye drops with or without calcium-channel blockers (mean ± SD 15.0 ± 1.3 mmHg) than in the group treated with calcium-channel blockers only (mean ± SD 13.3 ± 1.0 mmHg) (Mann-Whitney U-test, $p < 0.05$). However, no significant differences were observed in IOP in either subgroup between times 1 and 2.

Discussion

In this study, we used scanning laser tomography to evaluate changes in the optic-nerve head configuration in 30 patients with NTG after the mean follow-up period of over 3 years. Of 30 patients, 14 were followed without any medication for glaucoma and 16 were treated with topical glaucoma medication or oral calcium-channel blockers or both. We found that in the medication (-) group, the IOP at time 2 was significantly higher than that at time 1. The MD of visual-field indices decreased with a borderline significance, and the cup area in the temporal-inferior region increased significantly, while, in the medication (+) group, there were no differences in IOP or visual-field indices between times 1 and 2. The rim volume in the temporal area increased significantly and the maximum cup depth in the nasal-inferior region decreased significantly.

Our findings suggest that, without medication, some of NTG patients may show deterioration in the optic-nerve head before significant changes are detected in the visual-field indices. However, medication has a favorable effect on the visual field as well as on the optic-nerve head in some NTG patients. Regarding topical anti-glaucoma eye drops and calcium-channel blockers, it is not yet clear which one has more preventive effect on the progression of the disease. In a series of patients enrolled in this study, morphometrical improvement was observed in eight patients who had been treated with topical glaucoma eye drops, with or without adjunct use of calcium-channel blockers. However, this should be confirmed by further investigation with a larger number of subjects. In conclusion, the effect of treatment on optic-nerve head topography is detectable by means of scanning laser tomography.

References

1. Tomita G (1996) Application of laser scanning ophthalmoscopy in the diagnosis of glaucoma. Folia Ophthalmol Jpn 47:637–644
2. Weinreb RN, Shakiba S, Zangwill L (1995) Scanning laser polarimetry to measure the nerve fiber layer of normal and glaucomatous eyes. Am J Ophthalmol 119:627–636
3. Schuman JS, Hee MR, Puliafito CA, Wong C, Pedut-Kloizman T, Lin CP, Hertzmark E, Izatt JA, Swanson EA, Fujimoto JG (1995) Quantification of nerve fiber layer thickness in normal and glaucomatous eyes using optical coherence tomography: a pilot study. Arch Ophthalmol 113:586–596
4. Caprioli J, Weinreb RN (1994) Measurements of the optic nerve head and retinal nerve fiber layer in glaucoma. In: Kaufman PL, Mittag TW (eds) Textbook of ophthalmology, vol 7: glaucoma. Mosby, London, pp 6.22–6.30
5. Caprioli J (1991) Automated perimetry in glaucoma. Am J Ophthalmol 111:235–239

Role of Trabeculectomy and Calcium-Channel Blockers in the Treatment of Normal-Tension Glaucoma

T. Yamamoto · Y. Kitazawa · K. Ishida · L. Daugeliene

Introduction

Normal-tension glaucoma (NTG) seems to develop on a multipathogenetic basis. Relatively high intraocular pressure (IOP) has a pathogenetic role, even in NTG eyes [1]. IOP-independent factors also seem to be involved in the development of glaucomatous optic neuropathy in at least some NTG eyes [2]. The purpose of the current study was to investigate the effect of two different therapeutic strategies, *i.e.*, trabeculectomy [3] and calcium-channel blockers [4], on the visual-field progression of NTG eyes and to find clinical factors associated with the progression of visual-field loss.

Effect of Trabeculectomy on the Visual-Field Progression of NTG

The subjects were selected according to the following enrollment criteria: the subjects were progressive NTG patients trabeculectomized with mitomycin C between 1991 and 1994; they were followed up at least 12 months preoperatively and at least 24 months postoperatively; they had no previous ocular surgeries; their visual acuity was at least 20/40 preoperatively; the preoperative mean deviation (MD) was better than –20.00 dB; they had reliable visual fields, as measured with the Humphrey Field Analyzer, and had no complications that could affect the visual field. Of 32 cases, 32 eyes were analyzed. The follow-up period ranged from 1.0 year to 15.0 years (mean 3.8 years) preoperatively, and from 2.0 years to 6.0 years (mean 4.5 years) postoperatively.

The progressive visual field was defined in three ways: (a) MD slope over –0.50 dB/year, (b) depression by at least 15 dB at two contiguous points developed outside of the central 5° area, and (c) depression by at least 15 dB confirmed twice in the central 5° area. These field changes were found in 19, 4 and 9 eyes, respectively.

Figure 1 shows the distribution of the change in the annual MD slope between the preoperative and postoperative periods. The annual MD deterioration slowed down in all of the 10 eyes with a pretreatment IOP of 15 mmHg or higher and in 13 of the 22 eyes with a pretreatment IOP less than 15 mmHg. The visual field, however, did not change or even worsened in 9 eyes with a pretreatment IOP less than 15 mmHg.

A stepwise regression analysis was performed to find prognostic factors. The dependent variable was the difference between preoperative and postoperative annual MD changes. The explanatory variables included several clinical factors, such as IOP

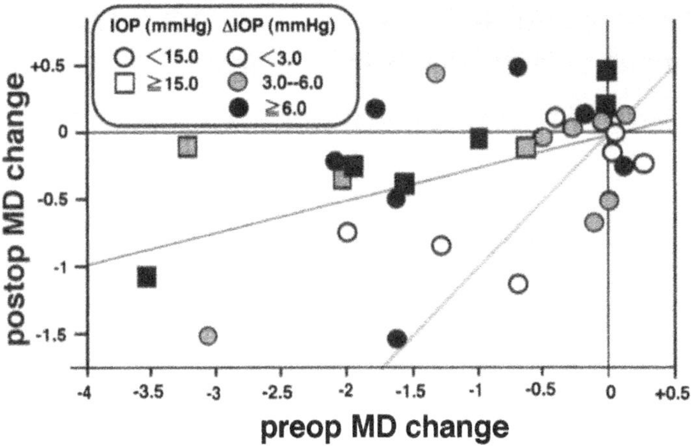

Fig. 1. Distribution of the change in the annual mean-deviation slope following mitomycin trabeculectomy

parameters, history of disc hemorrhage, and so on. The stepwise analysis revealed that better visual-field prognosis was associated with higher untreated mean diurnal IOP and the absence of diabetes mellitus.

Does the Calcium-Channel-Blocker Treatment Retard the Progression of NTG?

The subjects were selected according to the following selection criteria from our patient population consisting of 321 consecutive NTG cases: their follow-up period was at least 2 years; they had no previous intraocular surgeries; their pretreatment MD was better than −15.00 dB; their visual acuity was better than 20/40; and they had reliable perimetric results using the Humphrey Field Analyzer. Selected were 110 cases - 30 male, 80 female. The follow-up period ranged from 24 months to 112 months, with a mean of 51.5 months. The age ranged from 24 years to 75 years, with a mean of 56.9 years. Calcium-channel blockers prescribed were nifedipine in 8 cases, brovincamine in 26 cases, and nilvadipine in 2 cases.

The visual-field progression was defined in two ways: by MD deterioration over 3.00 dB detected twice and by point-by-point comparison, *i.e.*, threshold deteriorations greater than or equal to10 dB at two contiguous points, or greater than or equal to 5 dB at three contiguous points with one of them greater than or equal to 10 dB for two consecutive perimetric examinations. In either case, we defined the date when the change was detected for the first time as the endpoint.

The Kaplan-Meier life-table method and the Cox proportional-hazards model were used for analysis with PC-SAS software. The Kaplan-Meier life-table method revealed that the estimated probability (± standard error) of visual field non-progression was 91 ± 5 % for those treated with calcium-channel blockers and 68 ± 6 % for those treated without, when the MD definition was employed. The difference

Table 1. Clinical factors associated with visual-field progression by the mean-deviation definition. The number of cases that showed visual-field progression was 22 of 110 eyes

Clinical factor	Hazard ratio	95 % confidence	*p* value
Calcium-channel blocker			
Untreated	1		
Treated	0.14	0.04–0.49	0.002
Percent recovery at 1 min in a cold recovery test, by 1 % increase	0.96	0.83–0.99	0.005
Systolic blood pressure, by 1-mmHg rise	1.03	1.01–1.05	0.005
Disc hemorrhage			
Absent	1		
Present	3.62	1.40–9.32	0.008
Corrected pattern standard deviation, by 1-dB increase	1.13	1.01–1.28	0.039

was statistically significant ($p = 0.019$, Logrank test). When the visual-field defect was defined by the pointwise progression, the final probability was 65 ± 10 % and 39 ± 8 % for the treated and untreated groups, respectively. The difference was significant ($p = 0.009$, Logrank test).

The Cox proportional-hazards model demonstrated that the use of calcium-channel blockers, a parameter of cold recovery test, systolic blood pressure, disc hemorrhage and corrected pattern standard deviation, were associated with the visual-field outcome when the MD change was employed (Table 1). The favorable outcome was correlated with the use of calcium-channel blockers, better cold recovery test results, lower systolic blood pressure, no history of disc hemorrhage, and lower corrected-pattern standard deviation. When the pointwise definition was employed, the use of calcium-channel blockers, better initial MD, and smaller untreated IOP variation during a 24-h phasing were associated with the favorable outcome (data not shown).

Discussion

The current studies clearly demonstrate that both surgical reduction of IOP and use of systemic calcium-channel blockers help in preventing visual-field progression in NTG eyes. The effect of surgical IOP reduction was prominent in eyes with higher untreated IOP, *i.e.*, 15 mmHg or higher; however, this was not the case for eyes with lower IOP, which further forces us to believe that a mechanical factor is involved in the development and/or aggravation of optic neuropathy of NTG eyes with relatively high IOP. However, the results of administration of calcium-channel blockers conformed to those of the previous reports that demonstrated the favorable effect of several calcium-channel blockers on visual-field progression in NTG [5]. The favorable effect seems to provide further clinical evidence for the role that vascular insufficiency plays in the aggravation of glaucomatous optic neuropathy in some NTG eyes.

Taking into consideration the fact that both ocular hypotensive and calcium-channel-blocker treatments are effective in NTG, it would not be surprising if both

IOP-related and unrelated factors were associated with the visual-field prognosis. Of the associated factors identified using the Cox model, the recovery rate of a cold recovery test, systolic blood pressure, disc hemorrhage, and calcium-channel-blocker treatment have little to do with IOP.

The results of the current study confirm that clinical factors other than IOP are associated with the progression of NTG and that calcium-channel blockers may retard the glaucomatous visual-field progression, as does surgical IOP reduction. A practically important issue raised in clinical settings is the question of how to distinguish between the indications of the two totally different therapeutic modalities in an individual case based on the particular individual conditions.

References

1. Cartwright MJ, Anderson DR (1988) Correlation of asymmetric damage with asymmetric intraocular pressure in normal-tension glaucoma (low-tension glaucoma). Arch Ophthalmol 106:898–900
2. Geijssen HC (1991) Studies on normal pressure glaucoma. Kugler, New York
3. Daugeliene L, Yamamoto T, Kitazawa Y (1998) Effect of trabeculectomy on visual field in progressive normal-tension glaucoma. Jpn J Ophthalmol 42:286–292
4. Ishida K, Yamamoto T, Kitazawa Y (1998) Clinical factors associated with progression of normal-tension glaucoma. J Glaucoma 7:372–377
5. Netland PA, Chaturvedi N, Dreyer EB (1993) Calcium channel blockers in the management of low-tension and open-angle glaucoma. Am J Ophthalmol 115:608–613

Angle Closure Glaucoma

CHAPTER 26

Medical Therapy in Primary Angle-Closure Glaucoma: a Model for Evaluation of Its Efficacy

P. T. Hung · Y. C. Chen

Introduction

Primary angle-closure glaucoma (PACG) is the most common form of glaucoma in East Asia. The racial difference is well known, as prevalence is especially high among populations of Eskimos, Mongolians, and Chinese. The specific features of PACG in these populations include a high proportion of chronic-type PACG. In addition, in these populations, both acute and chronic PACG tend to show gradual progression even after elimination of the pupillary block mechanism by iridectomy. This type of glaucoma was called post-iridectomy glaucoma by Forbes and Becker in 1964 [1, 2], residual glaucoma by Chandler and Grant in 1965 [3], and late chronic glaucoma in 1973 by Lowe [1, 4]. The mechanisms of intraocular-pressure (IOP) elevation include diffuse peripheral anterior synechia, trabecular functional damage, or iris angle crowding from plateau iris-like mechanisms, lenticular factors or ciliary-block mechanisms. Such residual post-iridectomy glaucoma is important because of its insidious progression to severe visual impairment via optic-nerve atrophy. Argon-laser gonioplasty or trabeculoplasty can be used for short-term relief; however, after failure of laser therapy, medical treatment remains as an essential therapeutic approach prior to a surgical procedure.

The mechanisms of IOP elevation in PACG are probably more complicated and different from those in primary open-angle glaucoma (POAG). The mechanical force of angle closure is another important factor in PACG; therefore, optic-nerve evaluation or visual-function tests, which are commonly used to detect early POAG, are not appropriate for early detection of PACG.

Many provocative tests for detecting PACG have been introduced, including the dark-room test, prone-position test, and mydriatic test. In order to test the efficacy of the hypotensive effect and the prevention of angle closure by medical therapy, a non-pharmacological provocative procedure of combined dark prone-position tests was carried out while the patient was under the test medication [5]. We compared the efficacy of pilocarpine, timolol, and dorzolamide for IOP control in patients with PACG.

Materials and Methods

This study featured 60 patients (96 eyes) with acute or chronic PACG. Group A consisted of 36 patients (72 eyes) with previous laser iridectomy (7 men, 29 women, 42–68 years of age). Group B consisted of 24 PACG patients (24 eyes) prior to iridectomy (6 men, 18 women, 48–81 years old). Data from group A have been reported previously [5], although the result analysis was modified for the present report.

Diagnostic criteria for acute PACG were elevated IOP above 25 mmHg and associated with angle closure. For chronic PACG, a positive dark prone test associated with peripheral anterior synechia of slit-occludable angle and biometric evidence [6] were required. In group A, the fellow eye received the test regardless of whether or not it met the diagnostic criteria. However, all eyes with PACG were in quiet condition for at least 2 weeks, and the IOP was below 20 mmHg prior to the test. The washing-out period for the previous medications was at least 3 weeks for beta-blockers and 1 week for other medications.

The first dark prone test was performed without any pre-medication. For subsequent tests, 3 h prior to the test, two drops of 1 % pilocarpine, 0.25 % timolol, or 2 % dorzolamide were instilled in both eyes and the eyes were kept closed for 3 min. A modified dark prone test was then performed, the patients remaining in sitting position with their faces down on a desk for 1 h in a dark room; darkness was enhanced with opaque goggles. IOP was measured before and at the end of the test. Gonioscopic examination was performed soon after the IOP measurement in the first dark prone test for each patient. Thereafter, patients underwent a second or third dark prone test after the instillation of the various test medications. A positive test result was defined as an increase in IOP of at least 8 mmHg.

Results

In the iridectomized eyes of group A, a rise of IOP of more than 8 mmHg occurred in 31 of 72 eyes (43 %) during the first test without medication. After treatment with pilocarpine, only 6 (8 %) eyes had positive results, while 23 (32 %) had a positive test result after treatment with timolol (1 eye with a positive result after pilocarpine and 2 with a positive result after timolol treatment had negative results in the non-medication test.) Only eyes with positive non-medication tests were included in the subsequent analysis. As shown in Table 1, treatment with pilocarpine resulted in a significantly lower rate of positive test results than treatment with timolol (16 % vs 68 %, $p < 0.05$)

In group B, all eyes had IOP increases of more than 8 mmHg in the first test. The provocation test demonstrated that 1 % pilocarpine also showed significantly better prevention of IOP elevation than 2 % dorzolamine in this group. Only 3 (38 %) eyes had positive provocative tests after pilocarpine treatment, compared with 11 (46 %) after dorzolamide treatment (Table 2).

Table 1. Results of dark prone provocation in 31 iridectomized primary angle-closure glaucoma eyes

Medication	Total number of eyes	Number of eyes giving a positive test (%)
None	31	31 (100 %)
Under 1 % pilocarpine	31	5 (16 %)*
Under 0.25 % timolol	31	21 (68 %)*

* $p < 0.05$, chi-square test.

Table 2. Results of dark prone provocation in 24 primary angle-closure glaucoma eyes before laser iridectomy

Medication	Total number of eyes	Number of eyes giving a positive test (%)
None	24	24 (100 %)
Under dorzolamide	24	11 (46 %)*
Under 1 % pilocarpine	8	3 (38 %)*

* $p < 0.05$, chi-square test.

Discussion

Early detection of PACG can avoid severe acute attacks as well as chronic ocular damage by a simple laser-iridotomy procedure. However, the optic-nerve studies and visual-function tests, including field examinations emphasized for POAG detection, are not suitable for PACG early detection. In recent decades, intensive biometric studies have been carried out for PACG and, in the future, image analysis of the chamber angle may be another promising technique for early diagnosis of PACG.

Provocative tests for detecting angle-closure glaucoma have been advocated since the beginning of this century. The positive rates have ranged from 63 % to 90 %. Hung et al. [7] used prone-position tests performed in a dark room to study iridectomized PACG [8]. Such tests, when repeated twice, obtained a positive rate of 78 % in the fellow eye of 32 patients with PACG. There are also several pharmacological tests for PACG. Hyams considered that provocative tests that closely mimic physiologic status yield a low rate of positive results but are highly specific for PACG.

An important characteristic feature of PACG in Asia is the slow progression of angle closure even after the pupillary-block mechanism has been eliminated by successful iridectomy. Many other mechanisms were proposed, and argon-laser peripheral iridoplasty or gonioplasty was introduced for therapy. However, such iridoplasty procedures do not provide a long-lasting effect, and repeated laser iridoplasty or filtering surgery may be necessary. Following failure of laser therapy, medical therapy to control IOP and subsequent surgical procedures are therefore of practical importance.

The dark prone-position test model described in this report is useful for evaluating the hypotensive effect of PACG medications. In PACG therapy, however, prevention of angle-closure is also essential. Our finding strongly indicates that pilocarpine shows excellent protective effects for angle closure both before and after laser iridectomy. Because pilocarpine decreased the frequency of positive provocative tests in iridectomized and pre-iridectomized eyes, this drug appears to be effective for both pupillary block and non-pupillary block mechanisms of PACG.

It is well known that long-term use of pilocarpine for glaucoma has some unfavorable side effects, which include miosis, iritis, cataract formation, visual field change, and retinal detachment. Other adverse effects include increased pupillary block leading to IOP elevation, forward movement of the lens-iris diaphragm and shallowing of the anterior chamber. Our Scheimpflug video image studies [6] showed that pilocarpine drops caused shallowing of the anterior chamber angle and depth in healthy eyes, and such narrowing preceded the hypotensive effect of pilocarpine by about 150 min. However, no significant change of angle width after placing topical pilocarpine in eyes with PACG was noted, probably because of the elimination of iris bombé. Therefore, pilocarpine may be considered as a safe medical therapy for PACG patients.

Conclusions

1. The mechanisms of IOP elevation in primary angle-closure glaucoma involve many different factors. It is therefore important to consider etiological factors involved when treating PACG.
2. Residual PACG after an iridotomy is an important issue in this form of glaucoma. Monitoring and treatment of residual glaucoma are essential.
3. The dark prone-position test provides an excellent tool for evaluation of the efficacy of medical treatment of PACG. The present experiment demonstrated that 1 % pilocarpine is most effective for treatment of angle-closure glaucoma.

Acknowledgement. Supported in part by National Science Council, Executive Yuan, ROC. NSC88-2314-B002-369.

References

1. Hung PT (1991) Treatment of post-iridectomy glaucoma. In: Koo CY (ed) Frontiers in ophthalmology. Elsevier Science, Amsterdam, pp 199–202
2. Forbes M, Becher B (1962) Iridectomy in advanced angle-closure glaucoma. Am J Ophthalmol 57:57–62
3. Chandler PA, Grand WM (1965) Angle-closure of glaucoma. In: Chandler PA, Grand WM (eds) Lectures on glaucoma. Lea and Febiger, Philadelphia, pp 183–184
4. Lowe RF (1973) Primary angle-closure glaucoma: a review 5 years after bilateral surgery. Br J Ophthalmol 57:457–463
5. Hung PT (1990) Provocation and medical treatment in post-iridectomy glaucoma. J Ocular Pharmacol 6:279–283
6. Congdon NC, Quigley HA, Hung PT, et al. (1996) Screening techniques for angle-closure glaucoma in rural Taiwan. Acta Ophthalmol Scand 74:113–119
7. Hyams SW, Friedman Z, Neumann E (1968) Elevated pressure in the prone position. A new provocative test for angle-closure glaucoma. Am J Ophthalmol 66:661–672
8. Hung PT, Chou LH (1979) Provocation and mechanism of angle-closure after iridectomy. Arch Ophthalmol 97:1862–1864
9. Yang CC, Chou SC, Hung PT, et al. (1997) Anterior chamber angles shallowing and intraocular pressure after topical pilocarpine. J Ocular Pharmacol 13:219–224

CHAPTER 27

Quantitative Ultrasound Biomicroscopy

H. Ishikawa · J. M. Liebmann · R. Ritch

Introduction

New imaging technologies are providing important information regarding disease pathophysiology, diagnosis, progression, and treatment. High-frequency ultrasound biomicroscopy (UBM, Paradigm Medical Industries, Inc., Salt Lake City, UT) provides high resolution *in vivo* imaging of the anterior segment. The structures surrounding the posterior chamber, previously hidden from clinical observation, can be imaged and their anatomic relationships assessed. The role of abnormal anterior segment architecture in disease states can be evaluated. Although an extensive literature on qualitative UBM findings now exists, quantitative analysis largely remains to be developed.

Equipment and Technique

UBM technology is based on 50- to 100-MHz transducers incorporated into a B-mode clinical scanner [1]. Higher frequency transducers provide fine resolution of more superficial structures and lower frequency transducers provide greater depth of penetration. The commercially available unit operates at 50 MHz and provides lateral and axial physical resolution of approximately 50 μm and 25 μm, respectively. Lateral distortion is minimized by a linear scan format. Tissue penetration is approximately 4–5 mm. The scanner produces a 5×5-mm field with 256 vertical image lines (or A-scans) at a scan rate of 8 frames/sec. (Fig. 1). Each A-scan is mapped into 1024 sampling points, and the number of points is downsized to 432 pixels, which have 256 gray-scale levels, to fit on the UBM monitor [2]. The real-time image is displayed on a video monitor and can be stored on videotape for later analysis. Acquisition of highly reproducible distance measurements are strongly dependent on the examiner's technique and experience [3]. The relative proportions of structures in images depend on the plane of the section and the degree of tilt of the scanning probe. Room illumination, fixation, and accommodative effort affect anterior-segment anatomy and should be held constant, particularly when quantitative information is being gathered.

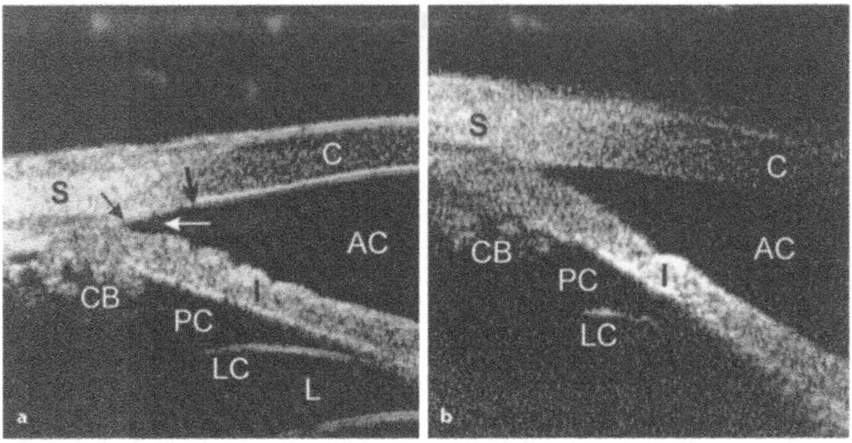

Fig. 1. a Normal eye. The cornea (*C*), anterior chamber (*AC*), iris (*I*), lens (*L*), lens capsule (*LC*), posterior chamber (*PC*), angle (*white arrow*), scleral spur (*thin black arrow*), Schwalbe's line (*thick black arrow*), sclera (*S*), and ciliary body (*CB*) are visible. The angle between the probe and the corneal surface affects the quality of the images. Two *bright white lines* are visible on the epithelial and endothelial surface of the center of the cornea. The approach of the probe to the corneal surface is ideal. **b** There is no reflecting line on either the epithelial or endothelial surface of the cornea. The observer needs to adjust the approach of the probe perpendicular to the corneal surface

Instrument Resolution and Measurement Precision

Understanding the difference between instrument axial resolution (the smallest object detectable along the axis of the beam and also how close two objects can be along the axis of the beam and still be detected as two distinct entities) and measurement precision (the width and height of a single pixel on the screen that can be identified by the operator using a screen cursor) is important [4]. The measurement software calculates distance by counting the number of pixels along the measured line and multiplies that number by the width or height of a single pixel. Thus, the result of the calculation always equals the width or height of a single pixel multiplied by some integer in a measurement along the vertical or horizontal line. However, it is possible for measurement precision to have a smaller value than the instrument axial resolution.

The commercially available instrument provides lateral and axial resolution of approximately 50 μm and 25 μm, respectively. The theoretical axial measurement precision on the monitor is about 12 μm (UBM cannot distinguish two small objects closer than 25 μm), though it is still possible to measure the distance between two objects far enough apart (> 50 μm) with 12 μm precision.

Sugimoto et al. [2] showed the usefulness of utilizing the internal raw data. Comparing the measurement on the UBM screen and the measurement based on the raw data, which has 1024 pixels vertically instead of 432 pixels, on-screen measurement allows only one digit after the decimal point because of the relatively low precision. However, measurements on raw data allow two digits after the decimal point (measurement precision is approximately 5 μm) in addition to better reproducibility.

Quantitative Measurement Methods

Corneal Thickness and Anterior-Chamber Depth

Both corneal thickness and anterior-chamber depth can be measured when images are taken with great care to produce sections perpendicular to the cornea and lens interfaces [4]. To determine the center plane of the anterior chamber, maximize the pupil diameter and the brightness of the signals from the epithelial and endothelial surfaces on the screen.

Anterior-Chamber Angle

Figure 1 shows a cross-sectional image of the anterior chamber angle produced by orienting the probe radially above the limbal region. One can consistently distinguish the scleral spur, a useful landmark presenting a constant reference point for measurement in the anterior-chamber-angle region. The angle-opening distance (AOD) has been defined by taking a point on the endothelial surface 500 μm anterior to the scleral spur and extending a line from this point perpendicular to the plane of the trabecular meshwork to the iris (Fig. 2a) [5]. Angular measurement in degrees ("trabecular-iris angle", ϑ_1) is determined by measuring the angle formed with the apex at the iris recess and the arms passing through (a) the point on the meshwork 500 μm from the scleral spur and (b) the point on the iris perpendicularly opposite [5].

Iris

Pavlin et al. [5] proposed several parameters to measure the iris.

1. Trabecular-ciliary process distance (TCPD) is defined as the distance between a point 500 μm from the scleral spur and the ciliary process on the line which is perpendicular through the iris (Fig. 2b).
2. The iris thickness (ID1) is defined along this line, as is the iris-ciliary process distance (ICPD).
3. Iris thickness can also be measured 2 mm from the iris root (ID2) and at its thickest point near the margin (ID3).
4. Iris-zonule distance (IZD) is defined a part of TCPD at a point just clearing the ciliary process.
5. The length of iris–lens contact (ILCD) and the angle at which the iris leaves the lens surface (ϑ_2) are easily measured.

Other Measurement Methods

Potash et al. [6] introduced a parameter for iris concavity in order to observe dynamic configurational changes. A line is first created from the most peripheral point to the most central point of iris-pigment epithelium. A perpendicular is extended from this line to the iris-pigment epithelium at the point of greatest concavity or convexity.

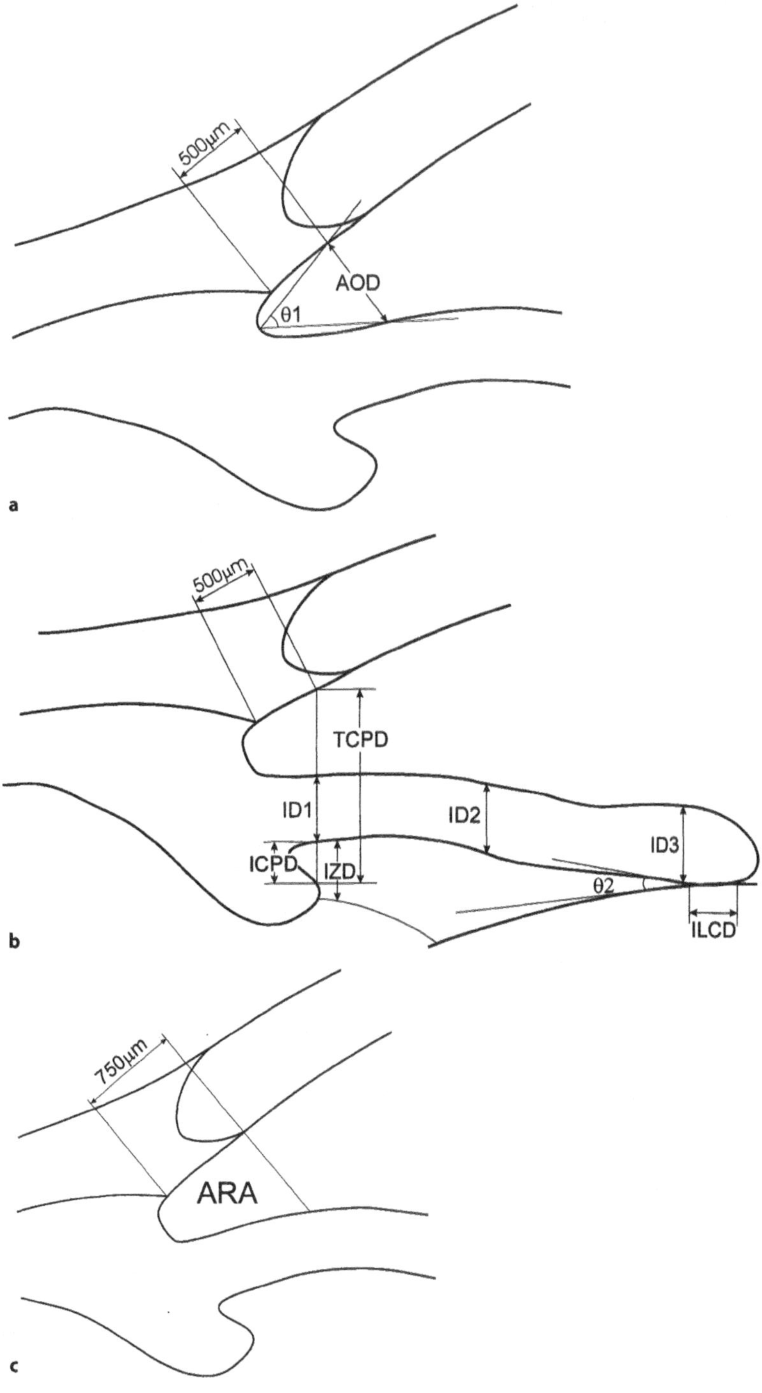
500μm
AOD
θ1
a
500μm
TCPD
ID1
ID2
ID3
ICPD
IZD
θ2
ILCD
b
750μm
ARA
c

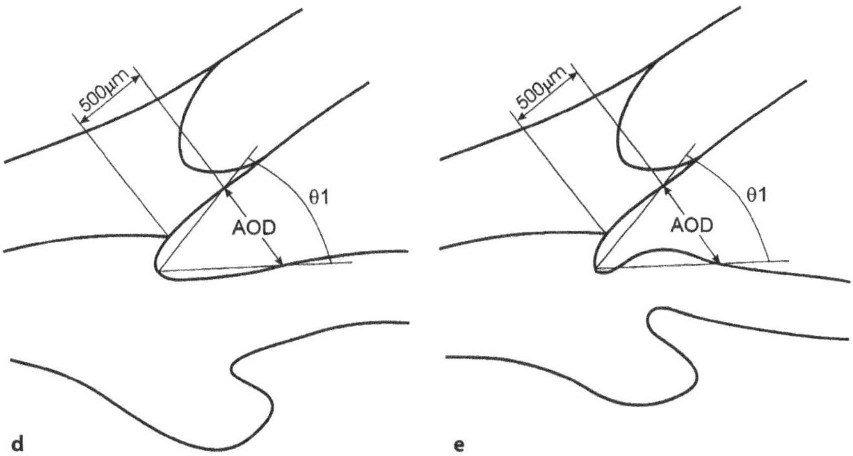

Fig. 2. **d, e** Limitation of AOD measurement. **d** and **e** have exactly the same value for the AOD and angle ϑ_1. However, it is evident that the angle in **e** is gonioscopically narrower and is more likely to be occludable than the normal-appearing angle in **d**.

Sakuma et al. [7] proposed subtypes of angle-closure glaucoma, "type S" being defined as appositional closure starting in the vicinity of Schwalbe's line and "type B" as appositional angle closure starting at the apex of the angle. They then introduced parameters capable of distinguishing subtypes of angle-closure [8]. Line X was defined as the distance between the scleral spur and the iris insertion, line Y as the iris thickness measured at the root, and line Z as the distance between the iris root and the cornea along the line perpendicular to the endothelial surface of the cornea.

Reproducibility of Measurements

Tello et al. [3] reported on the reproducibility of measurement of the above parameters. Intraobserver reproducibility is reasonably good, except for AOD, but interobserver reproducibility is not. Image acquisition is the major cause of this variability.

Fig. 2. **a** The angle-opening distance (AOD) is defined as the length of the line drawn from the point on the endothelial surface 500 μm anterior to the scleral spur to the iris surface perpendicular to the corneal endothelial surface. Angle ϑ_1 is defined as an angle formed with its apex at the iris recess and the arms passing through the point on the meshwork 500 μm from the scleral spur and the point on the iris perpendicularly opposite. **b** The trabecular-ciliary process distance (TCPD) is defined as the distance between a point 500 μm from the scleral spur and the ciliary process on the line which is perpendicular through the iris. The iris thickness (ID1) is defined along this line, as is the iris-ciliary process distance (ICPD). Iris thickness can also be measured 2 mm from the iris root (ID2) and at its thickest point near the margin (ID3). The iris-zonule distance (IZD) is defined as a part of TCPD at a point just clearing the ciliary process. The length of the iris-lens contact (ILCD) and the angle at which the iris leaves the lens surface (ϑ_2) are easily measured. **c** The angle-recess area (ARA). ARA is defined as a triangular area bordered by the anterior iris surface, corneal endothelium and a line perpendicular to the corneal endothelium drawn from a point 750 μm anterior to the scleral spur to the iris surface.

To minimize observer effects, automated selection of reference points is ideal. With current technology, it is difficult for software to detect the location of the scleral spur. Allowing the software program to perform a measurement calculation after the observer defines the location of the scleral spur is presently the most practical method. Ishikawa et al. [9] developed an automated software program capable of measuring consecutive AOD from the scleral spur to 750 μm anterior to the scleral spur. This improved intra- and interobserver reproducibility dramatically.

Improved Quantification Methods

AOD treats the iris surface as a straight line. Irregularities of iris contour and curvature are important considerations in angle-closure glaucoma. Ishikawa et al. [9] defined the angle-recess area (ARA) as the triangular area bordered by the anterior iris surface, corneal endothelium, and a line perpendicular to the corneal endothelium drawn to the iris surface from a point 750 μm anterior to the scleral spur (Fig. 2c). Figure 2d, e shows two schematics of the angle, demonstrating the same value for AOD and angle ϑ_1. However, it is evident that the angle on the right is gonioscopically narrower and is more likely to be occludable than the one on the left.

We developed a software program to calculate the ARA. After the observer selects the scleral spur, the program draws a border, processes the image, and calculates the ARA. The program plots consecutive AODs from the base of the angle recess to 750 μm anterior to the scleral spur and performs linear-regression analysis of consecutive AODs. This produces two figures: the acceleration and the y-intercept [10]. The equation for the linear regression is as follows:

$$y = ax+b$$

where a is the acceleration and b is the y-intercept.

Acceleration tells us how rapidly the angle is getting wider, using the tangent of the angle instead of degrees as the unit. Acceleration is an estimated value used to describe the angle opening, taking the irregular curvature of the iris surface into account. The y-intercept refers to the distance between the scleral spur and the iris surface along the perpendicular to the plane of the trabecular meshwork. In spite of these similarities, the acceleration and the y-intercept have unique characteristics. Since these values are calculated for linear-regression analysis, they can be negative numbers, which is impossible for routine on-screen measurements. A negative number for acceleration means that the angle has an almost-normal configuration at its peripheral part and becomes very shallow or is apposed to the cornea at its central part (e.g., appositional closure starting at Schwalbe's line with space remaining in the angle recess) (Fig. 3a). A negative y-intercept means that the angle recess is very shallow or is attached to the cornea at its periphery, while it is relatively wide centrally (Fig. 3b).

We have also developed software for measuring iris volume (Fig. 4) [11]. Since this calculation is based on a single UBM image, the calculated volume is not the precise volume. However, it is useful for purposes of comparing iris volumes in the same eye under different circumstances.

Quantitative analysis of UBM images is still in its infancy. Advances in software design will improve our theoretical understanding of the pathophysiology of

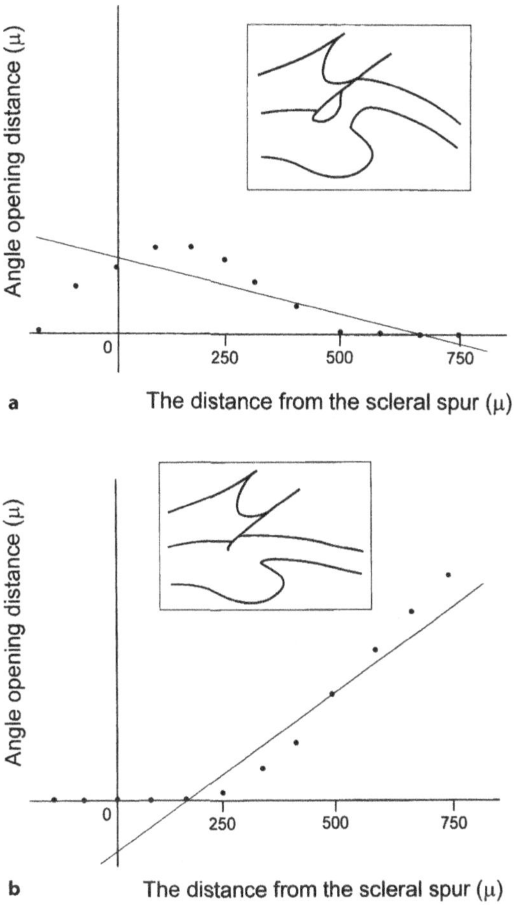

Fig. 3. a Linear regression analysis on the plot graph of angle opening distance versus distance from the scleral spur. The line of the linear regression shows negative acceleration, meaning that the angle almost has a normal configuration at its peripheral part and becomes very shallow or is apposed to the cornea at its central part, i.e., the appositional angle closure began at the level of Schwalbe's line. **b** A negative y-intercept means that the angle recess is very shallow or is attached to the cornea at its periphery, while it has a relatively wide angle recess centrally

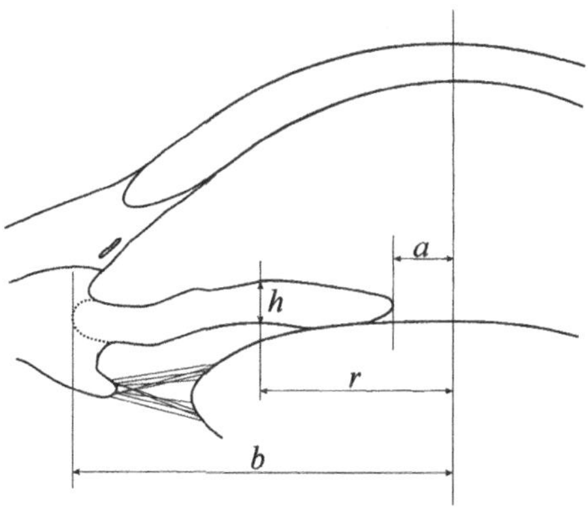

Fig. 4. Iris volume calculation: *a* is the distance between the optical axis and the pupillary edge; *b* is the distance between the optical axis and the point on the iris furthest away from the axis; *h* is the thickness of the iris at distance v from the optical axis. The equation for this calculation is as follows:

$$\int_a^b 2\pi v \cdot h \cdot dv$$

anterior-segment disorders. Future applications of quantitative techniques will yield important information regarding mechanisms of appositional angle closure, understanding of the dynamic functions of iris and other components of the anterior segment, and development of an automated diagnosing software program that will be used for telemedicine.

Acknowledgements. Supported in part by the Rudolph Robinson Research Fund of the New York Glaucoma Research Institute, New York, NY, and the David Warfield Fellowship program in Ophthalmology of the New York Community Trust and the New York Academy of Medicine (Dr. Ishikawa).

References

1. Foster FS et al. ■ (1993) Principles and applications of ultrasound backscatter microscopy. IEEE Trans Ultrason Ferroelectr Freq Contr 40:608
2. Sugimoto M, Ishikawa H, Esaki K, et al. (1998) The hidden information within ultrasound biomicroscopy (UBM) images. Invest Ophthalmol Vis Sci 39[Suppl]:S1032
3. Tello C, Liebmann J, Potash SD, et al. (1994) Measurement of ultrasound biomicroscopy images: intraobserver and interobserver reliaility. Invest Ophthalmol Vis Sci 35:3549–3553
4. Pavlin CJ, Foster FS (1995) Ultrasound biomicroscopy of the eye. Springer, Berlin Heidelberg New York
5. Pavlin CJ, Harasiewicz K, Eng P, Foster FS (1992) Ultrasound biomicroscopy of anterior segment structures in normal and glaucomatous eyes. Am J Ophthalmol 113:381–389
6. Potash SD, Tello C, Liebmann J, Ritch R (1994) Ultrasound biomicroscopy in pigment dispersion syndrome. Ophthalmology 101:332–339
7. Sakuma T, Yamamoto T, Kitazawa Y (1995) Observation of the chamber angle in primary angle-closure glaucoma with an ultrasound biomicroscope. Nippon Ganka Gakka Zasshi 99:806–810
8. Sakuma T, Sawada A, Yamamoto T, et al. (1997) Appositional angle closure in eyes with narrow angles: an ultrasound biomicroscopic study. J Glaucoma 6:165–169
9. Ishikawa H, Esaki K, Liebmann JM, et al. (1996) A new method of quantifying the anterior chamber angle with ultrasound biomicroscopy. Invest Ophthalmol Vis Sci 37[Suppl]:S820
10. Esaki K, Ishikawa H, Liebmann JM, et al. (1998) Factors associated with positive dark room provocation using ultrasound biomicroscopy (UBM). Invest Ophthalmol Vis Sci 39[Suppl]:S251
11. Ishikawa H, Ritch R, Hoh ST, et al. (1997) Iris volume before and after pupillary dilation using ultrasound biomicroscopy. Invest Ophthalmol Vis Sci 38[Suppl]:S166

Medical Therapy

Occurrence of Cystoid Macular Edema in Eyes Treated with Latanoprost: Preliminary Analysis

R. A. Schumer · C. B. Camras · A. Mandahl

Introduction

Prostaglandin (PG) analogues have recently been introduced for the pharmacological reduction of intraocular pressure (IOP) in the treatment of glaucoma (Alm et al. 1995; Mishima et al. 1996; Camras et al. 1996a, b; Watson et al. 1996, 1998). One such agent, latanoprost (13,14-dihydro-17-phenyl-18,19,20-trinor-$PGF_{2\alpha}$-isopropyl ester), has been available commercially in the United States since September 1996 and in numerous other regions worldwide soon thereafter.

Latanoprost, an analogue of the naturally occurring $PGF_{2\alpha}$, differs from $PGF_{2\alpha}$ by addition of an isopropyl ester group and by 17-phenyl substitution. It is a lipophilic prodrug, hydrolyzed to the active free acid in the cornea. Although many of the PGs are vasoactive, important interspecies differences exist, and latanoprost appears to have minimal vascular activity in humans. Pharmacokinetic studies demonstrate that little, if any, latanoprost is expected to accumulate in the posterior segment after topical application to normal, phakic eyes. Nevertheless, several clinical case reports (Moroi et al. 1997; Rowe et al. 1997; Avakian et al. 1998; Gaddie and Bennett 1998; Heier et al. 1998; Warwar et al. 1998) have shown that cystoid macular edema (CME) may occur in some eyes treated with latanoprost.

In a small study designed to investigate the potential of latanoprost to induce CME, 24 pseudophakic patients with posterior chamber lenses and with intact posterior capsules were treated unilaterally for 4 weeks. Sixteen received latanoprost 0.006 % twice daily (twice the clinical dose) and eight received placebo. They were examined by means of biomicroscopy and fluorescein angiography (FA) before and after treatment. There was no indication of macular edema in the latanoprost-treated eyes; one of the placebo-treated eyes had mild angiographic CME (Hoyng et al. 1997). For the present study, all cases of CME occurring in eyes treated with latanoprost that were known to the manufacturer (Pharmacia & Upjohn Co., Kalamazoo, Mich.) by 5 December 1997 or that were published in the literature have been analyzed.

Methods

Clinical information was extracted from reports of the co-occurrence of CME and latanoprost use arising from three general sources: clinical trials, the compassionate-use program, and post-market release spontaneous reports, including published reports of cases not independently reported to the manufacturer. The clinical trials included relatively short-term phase-I and -II trials and long-term, pre-approval safety and efficacy phase-III studies performed simultaneously in the United States, the United Kingdom, Scandinavia, and Japan from 1992 to 1994 (Alm et al. 1995; Camras et al. 1996a,b; Mishima et al. 1996; Watson et al. 1996, 1998), as well as separate, ongoing, long-term post-market approval safety studies (data on file).

In the compassionate-use protocol, carried out from May 1995 through September 1996, some 3500 patients were enrolled. Nomination for inclusion was at the discretion of designated physician participants. Patients receiving maximally tolerated medical therapy and in need of additional IOP reduction were included. No exclusions were made on the basis of concurrent ocular diagnoses or history, but all patients were required to have glaucomatous visual-field defects. Patients were treated once daily with 0.005 % latanoprost in addition to their other ocular medications.

The final, largest source of cases derives from all patients worldwide who had been treated with latanoprost following market introduction in their country. Spontaneous reports of occurrences of CME that were received by the manufacturer by 5 December 1997 are included in the present analysis. Since clinical information about these patients derives solely from spontaneous reports, great variation in the quality and comprehensiveness of available clinical information was encountered. Extensive efforts were made to contact submitting physicians to obtain detailed clinical information, but such efforts were not always successful, due to various factors, such as a physician's ability to cooperate, adequacy of patient records, and/or loss of patient to follow-up.

Twelve cases of CME in association with latanoprost use have been reported in recently published literature, including abstracts (Moroi et al. 1997; Rowe et al. 1997; Avakian et al. 1998; Gaddie and Bennett 1998; Heier et al. 1998; Warwar et al. 1998). Of these 12 cases, 6 had been reported to the manufacturer. We gathered information from the published descriptions of the other six cases for inclusion in the present analysis.

For each occurrence of CME, an attempt was made to identify all risk factors (RFs) for the development of CME. Candidate RFs were compiled from major, accepted causes of CME (Rocha and Deschenes 1996). Each RF was counted once for each occurrence in an individual eye to give a crude estimation of the relative risk for CME.

Other known clinical data of interest were compiled and tabulated to assess variables pertinent to the observations of CME. Insofar as the data were highly inhomogeneous and non-normative, and since there were no controls available in this post-hoc analysis, only descriptive statistics were generated. No attempt was made to perform tests of statistical significance.

Results

Putative CME arising in 72 eyes of 65 patients were collected (Table 1). The sources of these cases were: 3 eyes in 2 patients in clinical trials, 1 eye in 1 patient in the compassionate program, 62 eyes in 56 patients in spontaneous reports, and 6 eyes in 6 patients in published cases not already included in the spontaneous reports.

Table 1. Known risk factors for cystoid macular edema during latanoprost treatment

Patient number	Eye number	Source	Known risk factors*	Number of known risk factors
1	1	CT	1	1
2	2	CT	1, 2, 5, 11, 11, 11 OD	6 OD
2	3	CT	1, 2, 5 OS	3 OS
3	4	Comp	1, 4, 6, 7, 11	5
4	5	SR	1, 4, 13	3
5	6	SR + Gaddie + Bennett (1998)	1, 5	2
6	7	SR	9	1
7	8	SR	14	1
8	9	SR	1, 2, 4	3
9	10	SR	1, 2, 4	3
10	11	SR	1, 5, 8, 11	4
11	12	SR	?	?
12	13	SR	1, 5, 11	3
13	14	SR	1, 4	2
14	15	SR	1	1
15	16	SR	1, 3	2
16	17	SR	1, 4, 6, 6, 15	5
17	18	SR	1	1
18	19	SR	1, 4	2
19	20	SR	1, 4, 5	3
20	21	SR	1, 7, 7, 7	4
21	22	SR	1, 4	2
22	23	SR	1, 2, 4, 5 OD	4 OD
22	24	SR	1, 2, 4, 5 OS	4 OS
23	25	SR	1, 3 OD	2 OD
23	26	SR	1, 3 OS	2 OS
24	27	SR	1, 9, 14	3
25	28	SR	1, 3	2
26	29	SR	1, 7, 10, 14 OD	4 OD
26	30	SR	1, 14 OS	2 OS
27	31	SR	1, 5, 6, 14	4
28	32	SR	1, 11	2
29	33	SR	1, 9, 14	3
30	34	SR	1, 9	2
31	35	SR	1, 7, 9	3
32	36	SR	1, 11	2
33	37	SR	1, 4, 5, 6, 15, 20	6
34	38	SR	1	1
35	39	SR	1, 2, 4, 6, 22	5
36	40	SR	1, 9	2
37	41	SR	1, 2, 3, 5	4
38	42	SR	?	?
39	43	SR + Moroi et al. (1997)	8	1
40	44	SR + Moroi et al. (1997)	10	1
41	45	SR + Moroi et al. (1997)	1, 3	2
42	46	SR + Moroi et al. (1997)	8	1
43	47	SR	1	1
44	48	SR	1, 5, 14 OD	3 OD
44	49	SR	1, 5, 14 OS	3 OS
45	50	SR	1	1
46	51	SR	1, 11	2
47	52	SR	?	?
48	53	SR	?	?
49	54	SR	?	?
50	55	SR	1, 2, 7	3
51	56	SR	10 OD	1 OD

Table 1. (Continued)

Patient number	Eye number	Source	Known risk factors*	Number of known risk factors
51	57	SR	None	0 OS
52	58	SR	?	?
53	59	SR	1, 9 OD	2 OD
53	60	SR	1, 9 OS	2 OS
54	61	SR	1, 10	2
55	62	SR + Rowe et al. (1997)	1, 11	2
56	63	SR	?	?
57	64	SR	7	1
58	65	SR	7	1
59	66	SR	7	1
60	67	Heier et al. (1998)	1, 4, 5, 20	4
61	68	Warwar et al. (1998)	1, 4, 5, 11	4
62	69	Warwar et al. (1998)	1, 8	2
63	70	Avakian et al. (1998)	1, 4, 5, 6, 14	5
64	71	Avakian et al. (1998)	1, 15	2
65	72	Gaddie + Bennett (1998)	1, 4, 5, 8, 16, 22	6

CT, clinical trials; Comp, compassionate program; SR, spontaneous reports; OD, right eye; OS, left eye; ?, no clinical information available.
* Numbers indicate categories of risk factors as specified in Table 2.

Cases arising during clinical trials all derived from phase-III clinical trials, in which approximately 1300 patients were treated with latanoprost, over 90% for over 6 months, some for as many as 24 months. Prior phase-I and -II clinical trials, involving more than 360 eyes, some treated for as long as 3 months, gave rise to no episodes of CME. In the compassionate program, approximately 3500 eyes were treated with latanoprost in the United States. Following market approval of latanoprost and up to the database closure date of 5 December 1997, an estimated 600,000 patients with glaucoma or ocular hypertension were treated with latanoprost.

In seven cases of CME (all arising from spontaneous reports to the manufacturer), no clinical detail other than the apparent occurrence of CME was available because the submitting physicians either did not remember or did not have access to medical records, or did not respond to repeated inquiries from the investigators. Therefore, clinical information regarding 65 eyes from 58 patients was analyzed.

Table 2 shows the frequency of occurrence of each RF for the 65 eyes. The number of RFs may be underestimated because complete clinical information may have been lacking. Eyes that developed CME had an average of 2.6 RFs. Of these 65 eyes, 98 % had 1 or more RFs, 75 % had 2 or more, 43 % had 3 or more, and 25 % had 4–6 RFs. Of the 65 eyes, 55 (85 %) had undergone cataract surgery. Of these 55 aphakic or pseudophakic eyes, 49 (89 %) had other RFs for CME as well. Seventeen of these 55 eyes (31 %), had anterior-chamber intraocular lenses (AC IOLs) and 17 (31 %) had disrupted posterior capsules. One eye, not confirmed by FA, had no known risk factors. This eye had age-related macular degeneration.

Lens status was known in 1, 116 of the approxentely 3500 patients in the compassionate program, which included 138 aphakic eyes, 39 eyes with AC IOLs, and 344 eyes with posterior chamber IOLs. Although cataract surgery, aphakia, and AC IOLs are all major recognized RFs for CME, only one (0.2 %) of these eyes developed CME

Table 2. Frequency of occurrence of risk factors for cystoid macular edema (CME) during latanoprost therapy (total of 167 occurrences in 65 eyes)

Risk factor	Number of occurrences
1. Cataract surgery	55
2. Intracapsular cataract surgery	9
3. Aphakia	6
4. Anterior chamber intraocular lens implant	17
5. Absent posterior capsule (secondary to surgery or to Nd:YAG laser capsulotomy)	17
6. Anterior vitrectomy	7
7. Retinal or vitreoretinal surgery	10
8. History of uveitis	5
9. Concurrent uveitis	8
10. Premacular fibrosis	4
11. History of prior CME	11
12. Diabetic retinopathy	0
13. Retinal vein occlusion	1
14. Considerable intraocular pressure (IOP) reduction, low IOP	9
15. Filtering or other intraocular surgery (other than cataract surgery) within one year before CME	3
16. Concurrent treatment with epinephrine compounds	1
17. Subretinal neovascularization	0
18. Retinitis pigmentosa	0
19. Retinal detachment	0
20. Penetrating keratoplasty	2
21. Pan-retinal photocoagulation	0
22. Retinal inflammatory disease (e.g., pars planitis, birdshot, toxoplasmosis, others)	2
23. Radiation vasculopathy	0

Nd:YAG, neodymium-doped yttrium/aluminum garnet.

while treated with latanoprost. Such a rate is far lower than the spontaneous rate reported in most studies of the natural history of CME-susceptible eyes.

The duration of treatment with latanoprost until onset of CME was known for 56 of the 65 eyes. For these eyes, the mean duration of treatment prior to the diagnosis of CME was 9.5 weeks (range 1 day to 11 months; median 3.3 weeks).

Information regarding recovery following the diagnosis of CME was available in 54 of the 65 eyes. Latanoprost was discontinued in all but one eye following diagnosis of CME. By the time of follow-up reporting, 42 eyes experienced full recovery (including the eye in which latanoprost treatment was continued), and 11 additional eyes were reported to have partially recovered. One of two eyes in a bilateral case of CME with a complicated surgical history (eye # 29) had not improved after 7 months of follow-up. This eye had four RFs. Of 33 eyes for which information was available regarding duration of recovery or partial recovery, visual acuity recovered at an average of 2.2 months after discontinuation of latanoprost (range 2 days to 8 months; median 5.3 weeks).

Three cases are of special interest. One patient (# 22) with bilateral AC IOLs, who developed bilateral CME after being treated with latanoprost, was unilaterally re-challenged with latanoprost at an unknown number of weeks after bilateral resolution of the CME. CME subsequently recurred in the non-treated fellow eye, but not in the re-challenged eye. Another case of CME, not analyzed here but observed during the phase-III clinical trials, occurred contralateral to the eye being treated with latanoprost. In a third case (eye # 1), CME resolved despite the fact that latanoprost treatment was continued. These occurrences demonstrate the difficulties inherent in ascribing CME to latanoprost use in eyes that are otherwise at high risk for developing CME.

Discussion

Our analysis depends heavily on spontaneous reports by physicians. With few exceptions, these reported eyes were at high risk for the development of CME, independent of the latanoprost treatment. Necessarily, the analysis may be biased by factors that influence the frequency of reporting. Under-reporting of cases may be due to several factors, including the physicians' possible presumptions that well-known RFs caused the CME instead of latanoprost. Over-reporting may have occurred because latanoprost is a PG analogue and, as such, has been thought of as a causal factor in the development of CME, particularly since CME information was not yet included in the product insert. In addition, reporting physicians may be influenced by unsubstantiated claims of market competitors that a causal association between latanoprost and CME exists.

Aggregate analysis of all known cases of CME in conjunction with latanoprost use indicates that latanoprost is unlikely to cause CME in phakic eyes or in pseudophakic eyes with intact posterior capsules and without other RFs. With few exceptions, there were multiple other RFs for the development of CME. Our results, thus, neither support nor disprove that CME in these eyes was caused by latanoprost usage. Nevertheless, there appears to be an intriguing temporal association between the onset of latanoprost usage and the development of CME in some eyes. Latanoprost should be used with caution in eyes with multiple RFs for the development of CME. Long-term, randomized, placebo-controlled studies would be required to determine whether a causal relationship between latanoprost and CME exists in eyes with multiple RFs. However, such studies would be very difficult to undertake in view of the large numbers of patients required to provide an adequate sample size for evaluation of this rare potential side effect.

Acknowledgement. Supported in part by an unrestricted departmental grant from Research to Prevent Blindness, Inc., New York, NY (CBC).

References

Alm A, Stjernschantz J, Scandinavian Latanoprost Study Group (1995) Effects on intraocular pressure and side-effects of 0.005% latanoprost applied once daily, evening or morning. A comparison with timolol. Ophthalmology 102:1743–1752

Avakian A, Renier SA, Butler PJ (1998) Adverse effects of latanoprost on patients with medically resistant glaucoma. Arch Ophthalmol 116:679–680

Camras CB, Alm A, Watson PG, Stjernschantz J, Latanoprost Study Groups (1996a) Latanoprost, a prostaglandin analog, for glaucoma therapy: efficacy and safety after 1 year of treatment in 198 patients. Ophthalmology 103:1916–1924

Camras CB, US Latanoprost Study Group (1996b) Comparison of latanoprost and timolol in patients with ocular hypertension and glaucoma. A six-month, masked, multicenter trial in the United States. Ophthalmology 103:138–147

Gaddie IB, Bennett DW (1998) Cystoid macular edema associated with the use of latanoprost. J Am Optom Assoc 69:122–128

Heier JS, Steinert RF, Frederick AR (1998) Cystoid macular edema associated with latanoprost use. Arch Ophthalmol 116:680–682

Hoyng PFJ, Rulo A, Greve EL, Watson PG, Alm A (1997) Fluorescein angiographic evaluation of the effect of latanoprost treatment on blood-retinal barrier integrity: a review of studies conducted on pseudophakic glaucoma patients and on phakic and aphakic monkeys. Surv Ophthalmol 41[Suppl 2]:S83–S88

Mishima HK, Masuda K, Kitazawa Y, Azuma I, Araie M (1996) A comparison of latanoprost and timolol in primary open-angle glaucoma and ocular hypertension. A 12 week study. Arch Ophthalmol 114:929–932

Moroi SE, Gottfredsdottir MS, Johnson MW, Schteingart MT, Elner SG, Schertzer RM, Abrams GW (1997) Anterior uveitis and cystoid macular edema associated with latanoprost. Final program of the Proceedings of the American Academy of Ophthalmology Annual Meeting, San Francisco, CA, p 172

Rocha G, Deshcenes J (1996) Pathophysiology and treatment of cystoid macular edema. Can J Ophthalmol 31:282–288

Rowe JA, Hattenhauer MG, Herman DC (1997) Adverse side effects associated with latanoprost. Am J Ophthalmol 124:683–685

Warwar RE, Bullock JD, Ballal D (1998) Cystoid macular edema and anterior uveitis associated with latanoprost use. Ophthalmology 105:263–268

Watson PG, Stjernschantz J, Latanoprost Study Group (1996) A six-month, randomized, double-masked study comparing latanoprost with timolol in open-angle glaucoma and ocular hypertension. Ophthalmology 103:126–137

Watson PG, the Latanoprost Study Group (1998) Latanoprost. Two years' experience of its use in the United Kingdom. Ophthalmology 105:82–87

CHAPTER 29

Cytoskeletal and Cell-Junctional Modulation of Aqueous Outflow

P. L. Kaufman · J. A. Peterson · B. Tian · B. T. Gabelt · B. Geiger

Abstract. Cell-cell (C–C) and cell-extracellular matrix (C–ECM) adhesions in the trabecular meshwork (TM) contribute to overall TM geometry and thereby to flow resistance. Actin-disrupting agents (cytochalasins, latrunculins) and protein-kinase inhibitors, which inhibit actomyosin contractility (H-7, staurosporine), dramatically increase outflow facility in monkeys by causing separation of cells in the juxtacanalicular meshwork and inner canal wall, and distention of the TM. Interference with the cellular actin filament network functionally alters junctional complexes in the TM and Schlemm's canal, leading to easier fluid flow across the meshwork and washout of resistance-relevant ECM material. Resistance reduction is partially dependent on perfusion flow rates and pressure gradients across the TM, suggesting a looser, more "relaxed", more easily distensible tissue architecture. Although downregulation of C–C and C–ECM adhesions can be accomplished pharmacologically, as described, recent advances in molecular genetics and gene-transfer technology may allow long-term re-setting of these control mechanisms to therapeutic advantage in glaucoma.

Introduction

Epithelial and endothelial cell–cell (C–C) and cell–extracellular matrix (C-ECM) adherens junctions (AJs) are dynamic structures which vary in number, location and "adhesiveness" with the ambient physical and chemical milieu. AJs are complex molecular entities comprising structural and signal-transduction proteins, with the latter providing regulatory control over the former in response to intra- and extracellular conditions. In the trabecular meshwork (TM), AJs contribute to overall TM geometry and thereby to flow resistance. Compounds that affect AJs and the contractile proteins that interact with them can alter the shapes of cells in the juxtacanalicular meshwork and inner wall of Schlemm's canal, and can thereby change the overall geometry and stability of the TM so as to facilitate aqueous outflow and promote washout of resistance-producing ECM [1]. Actin microfilaments (MFs) are a major component of the cytoskeleton. They are attached to the submembrane plaque of AJs in many cell types. MFs are abundantly present in the cells of the corneoscleral and juxtacanalicular portions of meshwork and the inner wall of Schlemm's canal in cynomolgus and rhesus monkeys and in humans [2]. MFs are potential targets for TM-modulating compounds. We therefore studied the effects of the "direct" MF-disrupting agents cytochalasins and latrunculins and the protein kinase inhibitors H-7 and staurosporine (Fig. 1) on outflow facility in monkeys.

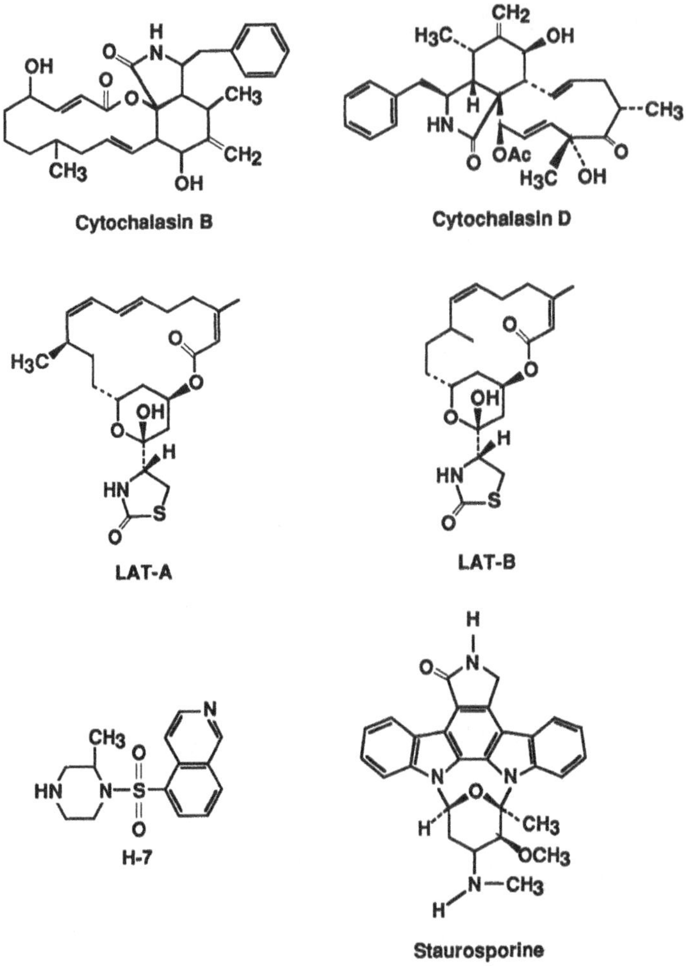

Fig. 1. Chemical structures of cytochalasin B, cytochalasin D, latrunculin A, latrunculin B, H-7 and staurosporine

Actin-Disrupting Agents

Cytochalasins are fungal metabolites which cap MF by mechanisms that are not entirely clear [3]. In cultured cells, exposure to the cytochalasins causes concentration-dependent changes in cell shape and actin organization. Latrunculins, a family of marine macrolides derived from Red-Sea sponges, destroy microfilaments by binding to G-actin and blocking filament nucleation and elongation [4]. Exposure of cultured cells to latrunculins induces cell shape and junction disruption (mainly C–C junctions, but to a lesser extent C–ECM junctions also).

In living monkeys, outflow facility was measured by two-level constant pressure perfusion of the anterior chamber (AC). Bolus injection of 0.1–10 μg cytochalasin B

(CB) or 0.1–5 μg cytochalasin D (CD) caused up to a sixfold increase in outflow facility (data not shown), unrelated to ciliary muscle contraction but accompanied by distention of the TM, cell separation, ruptures in the inner wall and washout of ECM. CD can relax carbachol-precontracted ciliary muscle and trabecular strips in vitro. Intracameral exchange infusion of 0.5–5 μM latrunculin A (LAT-A) or 0.02–2 μM LAT-B, or topical administration of 21–42 μg LAT-A or 3.95 μg LAT-B causes a dose- and time-dependent facility increase of up to fivefold (data not shown). While LAT-A is more potent in cell culture than LAT-B, the relative potency is reversed in vivo for reasons that are unclear. Although the increases in outflow facility are completely reversible, a residual perfusion-time-dependent effect still persists even 24 h after a single topical LAT-A dose, as will be discussed later.

Protein-Kinase Inhibitors Affecting Actomyosin Contractility

H-7 (1-(5-isoquinolinyl-sulfonyl)-2-methylpiperazine), a broad-spectrum serine-threonine kinase inhibitor, blocks the phosphorylation activity of diverse protein kinases, including protein kinase C, myosin light-chain kinase (MLCK) and rho kinase [5]. Exposure of cultured cells to H-7 inhibits acto-myosin contractility, leading to deterioration of the actin MF system and perturbation of its membrane anchorage, which in turn weakens C–ECM and to a lesser degree C–C contacts in various cell types. Staurosporine, another broad-spectrum serine-threonine kinase inhibitor, depletes actin MF bundles in cultured rat astrocytes [6], inhibits contraction of guinea-pig airway smooth muscle cells induced by the protein kinase C activator phorbol myristate acetate, and inhibits intracellular Ca^{2+}-dependent contractions induced by various agonists in rabbit aortic strips, all presumably as a result of the blocking of acto-myosin contractility in a manner analogous to acto-myosin blockage by H-7.

In living monkeys, AC-exchange perfusion with 10–300 μM H-7 increased outflow facility in a dose-dependent fashion (Fig. 2). In monkeys, staurosporine (0.1–10 μM) produced a facility effect similar to that of H-7 (data not shown). The dose ranges (100–300 μM H-7 or 1–10 μM staurosporine) producing a facility effect were identical or close to those inducing actin filament and AJ alterations in cultured cells, suggesting that H-7 and staurosporine increased facility by a cytoskeletal-cell junctional mechanism similar to that proposed for the cytochalasins and latrunculins.

Discussion

Perturbation of cell contractility and consequent cytoskeletal alterations and weakening of cell adhesions in the TM might lead to elevated outflow facility if fluid flow across a TM structure "loosened" by any of these four agents caused further loosening and separation of TM layers and cells, enhancing intercellular-flow pathways and washout of resistance-relevant ECM. Our facility data support this hypothesis. Following bolus injection (cytochalasins) or AC-exchange infusion (H-7, staurosporine, latrunculins), initial facility values were slightly but dose-dependently elevated (Fig. 2). Substantial facility elevation required continued perfusion, suggesting that

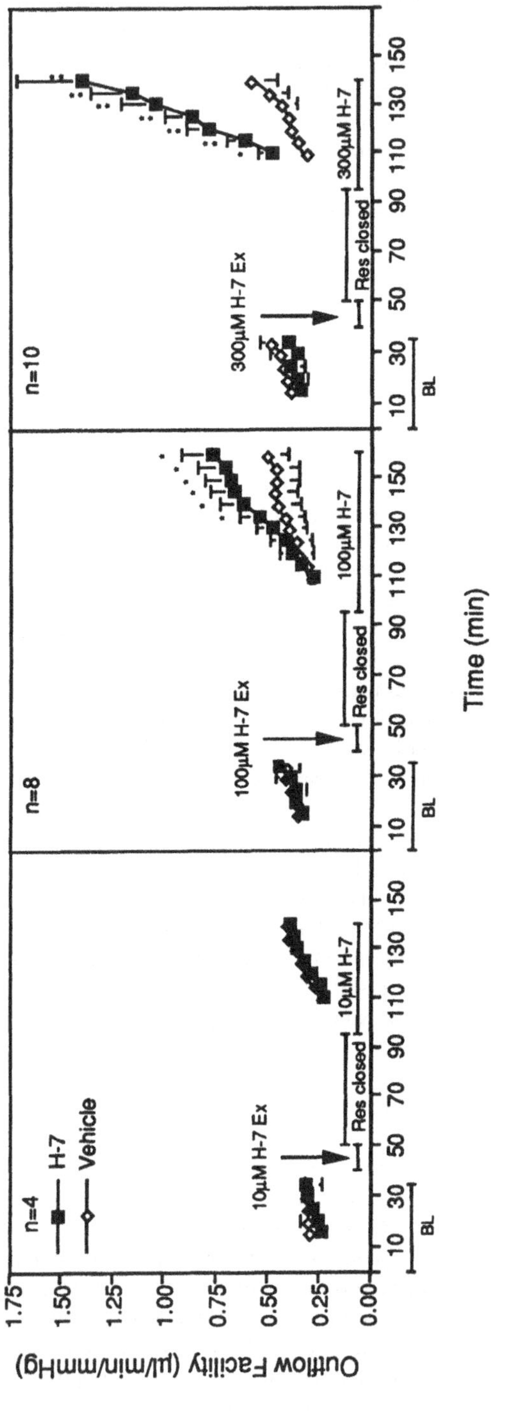

Fig. 2. Effect of intracameral exchange (*Ex*) infusion with 10–300 µM H-7 on outflow facility in monkeys. *BL*, baseline; *Res*, reservoir. Data are mean ± SEM µl/min/mmHg for *n* animals, each contributing one H-7- and one vehicle-treated eye. Difference between eyes ≠ 0.0 by the two-tailed paired *t*-test. $^{*}p < 0.05$, $^{**}p < 0.01$

the deterioration of the MF network destabilizes cell junctions within the TM and produces slight resistance washout at low trans-trabecular pressure gradients and flow rates. However, at higher pressure gradients or flow rates, e.g., during perfusion, the destabilized TM architecture is further disrupted, substantially reducing flow resistance. Under this scenario, these MF-disrupting agents may be effective in glaucoma patients with elevated IOP, especially if they are not receiving secretory suppressants, and digital ocular pressure may enhance the effect. A recent study has confirmed that the facility-increasing effect is a consequence of direct drug action on the TM rather than on other structures in the living eye [7].

A better understanding of the mechanisms responsible for these effects is crucial for the development of a clinically relevant therapy. Nonetheless, our data suggest that MF disruption by either pharmacologic or genetic means [8, 9] may allow long-term re-setting of these control mechanisms to increase outflow facility and reduce IOP to therapeutic advantage in the treatment of glaucoma.

Acknowledgements. This study was supported by the National Institutes of Health, Bethesda, MD [grant EY02698 (PLK)]; the Glaucoma Research Foundation, San Francisco, CA [Catalyst Program Award (PLK & BG)]; Research to Prevent Blindness, New York, NY [Senior Scientific Investigator Award & Unrestricted Departmental grant (PLK)]; the Ocular Physiology Research & Education Foundation, Madison, WI (BT); Yeda Research & Development, Ltd.; the Ruth Belilos Foundation, and the E. Neter Chair in Cell and Tumor Biology (BG).

References

1. Tian B, Kaufman PL, Volberg T, Gabelt BT, Geiger B (1998) H-7 disrupts the actin cytoskeleton and increases outflow facility. Arch Ophthalmol 116:633–643
2. Gipson IK, Anderson RA (1979) Actin filaments in cells of human trabecular meshwork and Schlemm's canal. Invest Ophthalmol Vis Sci 18:547–561
3. Godman GC, Miranda AF (1978) Cellular contractility and the visible effects of cytochalasin. In: Tannenbaum SW (ed) Cytochalasins: biochemical and cell biological aspects. North Holland, Amsterdam pp 277–429
4. Coué M, Brenner SL, Spector I, Korn ED (1987) Inhibition of actin polymerization by latrunculin A. FEBS Lett 213:316–318
5. Hidaka H, Inagaki M, Kawamoto S, Sasaki Y (1984) Isoquinolinesulfonamides, novel and potent inhibitors of cyclic nucleotide dependent protein kinase and protein kinase C. Biochemistry 23:5036–5041
6. Mobley PL, Hedberg K, Bonin L, Chen B, Griffith OH (1994) Decreased phosphorylation of four 20-kDa proteins precedes staurosporine-induced disruption of the actin/myosin cytoskeleton in rat astrocytes. Exp Cell Res 214:55–66
7. Tian B, Gabelt BT, Peterson JA, Kiland JA, Kaufman PL (1999) H-7 increases trabecular facility and facility after ciliary muscle disinsertion in monkeys. Invest Ophthalmol Vis Sci 40:239–242
8. Borras T, Tamm ER, Zigler JS (1996) Ocular adenovirus gene transfer varies in efficiency and inflammatory response. Invest Ophthalmol Vis Sci 37:1282–1293
9. Kaufman PL, Jia WW-G, Tan J, Chen Z, Gabelt BT, Booth V, Tufaro F, Cynader M (1999) A perspective of gene therapy in glaucomas. Surv Ophthalmol (in press)

CHAPTER 30

Prostaglandin Effects on the Uveoscleral-Outflow Pathway

R. N. Weinreb · J. D. Lindsey · K. Kashiwagi · T. Sagara · D. D. Gaton

Introduction

Prostaglandins (PGs) have been developed as a topical therapy used to lower intraocular pressure (IOP) in glaucoma [1–3]. Unlike other IOP-lowering treatments that primarily target conventional aqueous-humor outflow through Schlemm's canal, these drugs act primarily to enhance aqueous outflow through the ciliary muscle and into the suprachoroidal space (the uveoscleral pathway) [4, 5]. This review summarizes our recent studies supporting the view that the cellular basis of the PG-mediated increase of aqueous outflow through the ciliary muscle fibers reflects reduction of the density of ciliary-muscle collagens and other extracellular molecules. These studies show that PGs can act directly on ciliary-muscle cells to induce their secretion of matrix metalloproteinases (MMPs), a family of secreted enzymes that initiate extracellular-matrix degradation.

Background

When considered together, several independent investigations are consistent with the possibility that PGs induce extracellular-matrix changes in the ciliary smooth-muscle cells, which may explain increased uveoscleral outflow. First, early electron-microscopic analysis of the ciliary muscle confirmed that ciliary muscle cells are organized into long bundles that are separated from each other by extracellular spaces containing fibrillar collagen [6]. Second, subsequent experiments showed that tracer molecules injected into the anterior chamber moved into these spaces among the ciliary-muscle cell bundles at rates that far exceeded what could be explained by diffusion [7–10]. This suggests that these spaces correspond to the uveoscleral-outflow pathway. Third, repeated topical treatment of monkey eyes with PGF2α or PGF2α-isopropyl ester (a PGF2α analog) reduces extracellular matrix in the spaces between ciliary smooth-muscle fibers [11, 12]. Therefore, it seems plausible that PGF2α could induce ciliary smooth-muscle cells to degrade adjacent extracellular matrix, thereby reducing the hydraulic resistance around the fibers and facilitating aqueous flow through the muscle. In addition to having implications for uveoscleral-flow changes following topical administration of PGs, this response also might be important for IOP regulation. PGs are produced by cultured human trabecular-meshwork cells [13, 14], intact trabecular meshwork tissue [15], and within perfused human anterior segments in vitro [16]. Therefore, trabecular-meshwork PG, besides having local effects, may also alter the adjacent ciliary muscle.

Ciliary-Muscle Cells In Vitro

Initially, we investigated extracellular-matrix changes in human ciliary smooth-muscle cells in vitro [17]. We found that exposure of these cells to PGF2α, 17phenyltrinor-PGF2α, or 11-deoxy-PGE1 induced marked changes in the structure of collagen types I, III, and IV [18]. In addition, these PGs can induce increased concentrations of MMP-1, MMP-2, MMP-3, and MMP-9 in the culture medium of treated cells [19, 20]. These results supported the view that PGs induce increased turnover and remodeling of extracellular matrix adjacent to ciliary muscle cells.

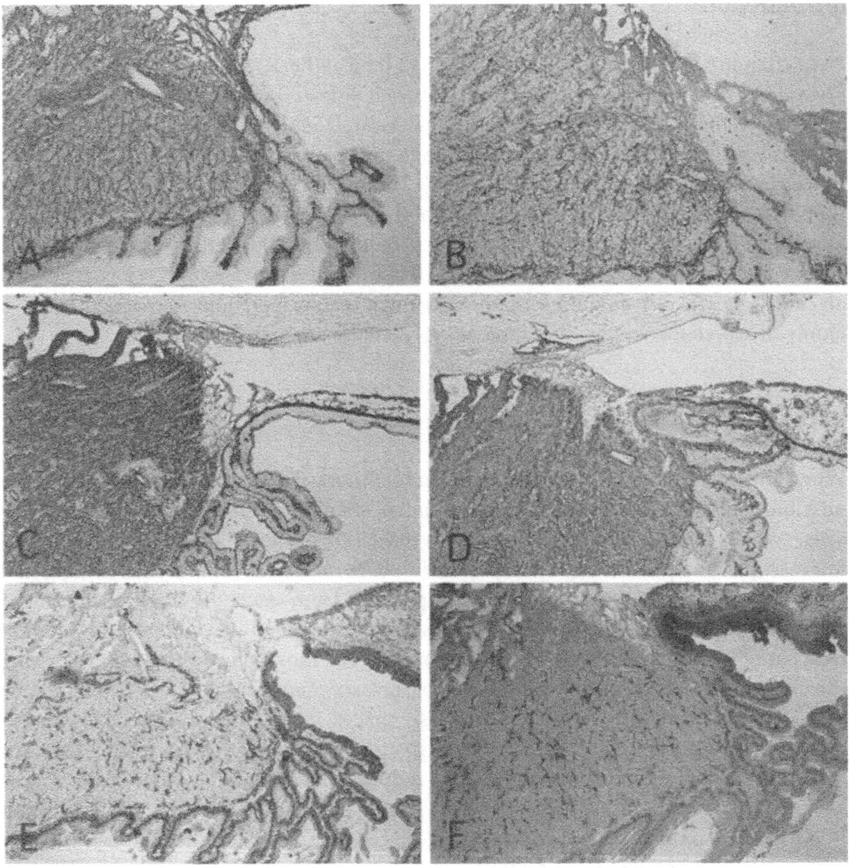

Fig. 1. Immunoreactivity for collagens III (**A, B**), and IV (**C, D**) as well as matrix metalloproteinase (MMP)-1 (**e,f**) in vehicle-treated cynomolgus monkey ciliary muscle (**A, D, E**), or following daily treatment with topical prostaglandin F2α-IE (**B, D, F**) for 5 days. Note reduced immunoreactivity for collagen types III and IV, and increased immunoreactivity for MMP-1. Collagen type-I immunostaining was similar to collagen type III. MMP-2 and MMP-3 were similar to MMP-1. Magnification × 50

Ciliary-Muscle Cells In Situ

Recently, we examined these responses in situ. Opposite eyes of four cynomolgus monkeys were treated with 2 μg PGF2α-IE or vehicle twice daily for 5 days. IOP reduction was 5 mmHg or more on day 4 in all monkeys. Sections from the anterior segments of these eyes were immunostained by means of standardized protocols using antibodies to collagen types I, III, and IV, as well as to MMPs-1, -2, and -3. We noted decreased collagen levels and increased MMP levels in the treated eyes (Fig. 1). To quantify these changes, average optical densities (ODs) of anterior-segment tissues were determined using two-dimensional imaging densitometry (Fig. 2). As shown in Table 1, these treatments induced significant reductions in the amount of collagen types I, III, and IV in the ciliary muscle and iris root. In the sclera, there is substantial collagen of types I and III, but very little collagen type IV. Here, we observed significant reductions in collagen types I and III in the PG-treated eyes. When we examined MMPs-1, -2, and -3 using this method, we found increases of OD scores for all three MMPs in the ciliary body, iris root, and sclera overlying the ciliary muscle (Table 2). These observations show that the decreases in ciliary-muscle collagens following PG treatment are mirrored by increases in MMP levels. In view of the ability of MMPs to initiate collagen degradation, these events are likely to be linked.

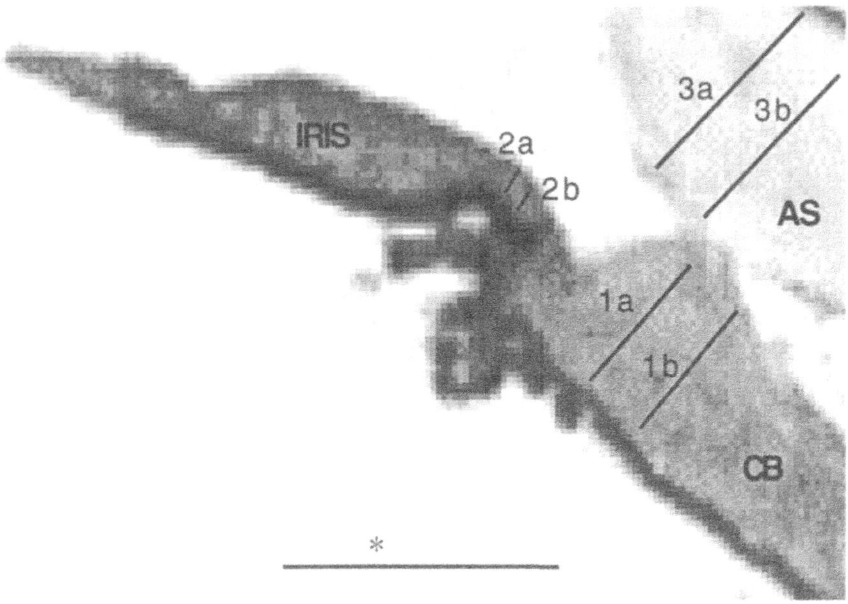

Fig. 2. Optical density was measured along two lines positioned over the structure of interest in each section. Here, lines *1a* and *1b* are over the ciliary body (CB), lines *2a* and *2b* are over the iris root, and lines *3a* and *3b* are over the adjacent sclera (AS). Background optical density in the optics of the densitometer and slide were measured using a line not over any structure (*asterisk*) and subtracted from the scores. Mean optical density was calculated from all corrected scan scores for each eye

Table 1. Reduction (expressed as a %) of collagen immunoreactivity in prostaglandin $F_{2\alpha}$: treated eyes versus vehicle-treated eyes [mean optical density ± standard deviation (*p* value, t-test)]

	Collagen I	Collagen III	Collagen IV
Ciliary muscle	52.0±6.8 (0.0004)	45.4±6.7 (0.0006)	34.1±10.6 (0.002)
Iris root	43.4±4.4 (0.01)	38.3±30.2 (0.008)	44.8±6.1 (0.003)
Sclera	43.0±31.6 (0.04)	44.6±13.2 (0.02)	6.3±31.4 (0.37)

Table 2. Increase (expressed as %) of matrix metalloproteinase (MMP) immunoreactivity: treated eyes versus untreated eyes [mean optical density ± standard deviation (*p* value, *t*-test)]

	MMP-1	MMP-2	MMP-3
Ciliary muscle	61±8 (0.002)	82±27 (0.003)	83±49 (0.007)
Iris root	89±16 (0.003)	129±53 (0.009)	207±84 (0.006)
Sclera	66±57 (0.01)	267±210 (0.005)	726±500 (0.02)

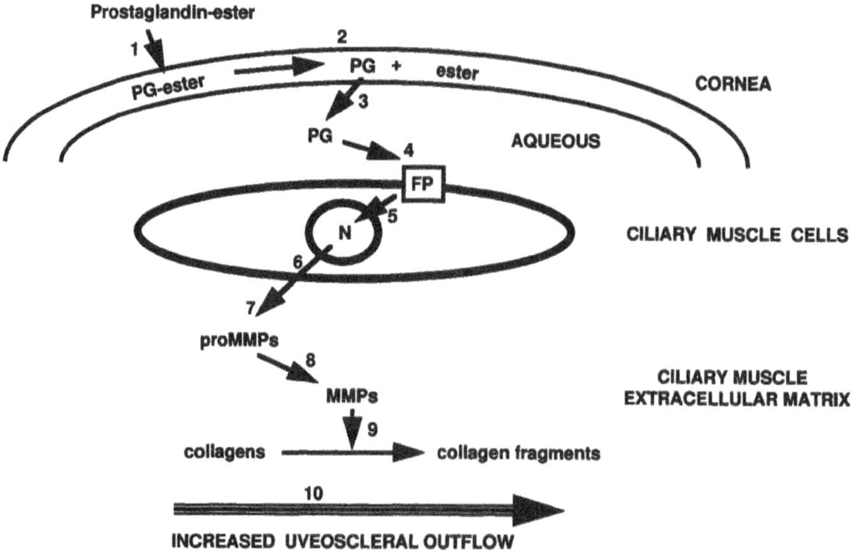

Fig. 3. Effect of prostaglandins (PGs) on uveoscleral outflow. Topical PG-ester is absorbed into the cornea (*1*) where it is converted to free PG (*2*). The free PG passes into the aqueous (*3*) and is carried into the ciliary muscle and binds to the FP receptor on the ciliary muscle cell surface (*4*). This binding initiates a signal cascade leading to AP1-transcription-factor formation (*5*) in the cell nucleus (*N*) that induces the transcription of matrix metalloproteinase (MMP) genes (*6*). The gene products are translated into proMMPs that are secreted into the extracellular space around the ciliary-muscle fibers (*7*). Proteolytic truncation induces activation of the MMPs (*8*), which initiates the degradation of extracellular matrix components, such as collagens (*9*). The reduction of collagens within the uveoscleral-outflow pathway reduces hydraulic resistance and facilitates uveoscleral outflow (*10*)

Conclusions

PGs can induce substantial remodeling of ciliary-muscle extracellular matrix in situ that reflects MMP-mediated collagen reduction. The sequence of cellular events underlying this response includes PG transduction at PG receptors on the surface of ciliary smooth-muscle cells, induction of MMP gene transcription, translation and secretion of proMMPs, activation of MMPs by proteolytic truncation, and MMP-mediated initiation of collagen degradation in the ciliary-muscle extracellular space (Fig. 3). In view of the evidence supporting passage of uveoscleral outflow through the ciliary-muscle extracellular spaces in situ, these findings support the view that extracellular-matrix remodeling may contribute to PG-induced increases in uveoscleral-outflow facility. Further studies are underway to evaluate the relationship of these changes to other PG-induced cellular responses.

Acknowledgements. Supported in part by National Eye Institute grant EY 05990 (RNW). The authors thank Paul L. Kaufman, M.D. and B'Ann True Gabelt of the University of Wisconsin, Madison, for their collaboration in our monkey studies.

References

1. Stjernschantz J, Selén G, Sjöquist B, Resul B (1995) Preclinical pharmacology of latanoprost, a phenyl-substituted $PGF_{2\alpha}$ analog. Adv Prostaglandin Thromboxane Leukot Res 23:513–518
2. Alm A, Camras CB, Watson PG (1997) Phase III latanoprost studies in Scandinavia, the United Kingdom and the United States. Surv Ophthalmol 41[Suppl 2]:S105–110
3. Watson PG, the latanoprost Study Group (1998) Latanoprost: two years' experience of its use in the United Kingdom. Ophthalmology 105:82–87
4. Toris CB, Camras CB, Yablonski ME (1993) Effects of PhXA41, a new prostaglandin F2α analog, on aqueous humor dynamics in human eyes. Ophthalmology 100:1297–1304
5. Toris CB, Camras CB, Yablonski ME, Brubaker RF (1997) Effects of exogenous prostaglandins on aqueous humor dynamics and blood-aqueous barrier function. Surv Ophthalmol 41[Suppl 2]: S69–75
6. Ishikawa T (1962) Fine structure of the human ciliary muscle. Invest Ophthalmol Vis Sci 1:587–608
7. Inomata H, Bill A, Smelser GK (1972) Unconventional routes of aqueous humor outflow in cynomolgus monkey (Macaca irus). Am J Ophthalmol 73:893–907
8. Inomata H, Bill A (1977) Exit sites of uveoscleral flow of aqueous humor in cynomolgus monkey eyes. Exp Eye Res 25:113–118
9. Wood RL, Koseki T, Kelly DE (1992) Uveoscleral permeability to intracamerally infused ferritin in eyes of rabbits and monkeys. Cell Tissue Res 270:559–567
10. Pederson JE, Toris CB (1987) Uveoscleral outflow: diffusion or flow? Invest Ophthalmol Vis Sci 28:1022–1024
11. Lutjen-Drecoll E, Tamm E (1988) Morphological study of the anterior segment of cynomolgus monkey eyes following treatment with prostaglandin $F_{2\alpha}$. Exp Eye Res 47:761–769
12. Tamm E, Lutjen-Drecoll E, Rohen JW (1990) Age-related changes of the ciliary muscle in comparison with changes induced by treatment with prostaglandin $F_{2\alpha}$. An ultrastructural study in rhesus and cynomolgus monkeys. Mech Ageing Dev 51:101–120
13. Weinreb RN, Polansky JR, Alvarado JA, Mitchell MD (1988) Arachidonic acid metabolism in human trabecular meshwork cells. Invest Ophthalmol Vis Sci 29:1708–1712
14. Weinreb RN, Mitchell MD (1989) Prostaglandin production by cultured cynomolgus monkey trabecular meshwork cells. Prostaglandins Leukot Essent Fatty Acids 36:97–100
15. Polansky JR, Weinreb RN (1990) Anterior segment inflammation and trabecular meshwork cell response. New Trends Lipid Mediators Res 5:56–64
16. Shaw BR, Lindsey JD, Weinreb RN (1993) Prostaglandin release in a perfused human anterior segment model. J Glaucoma 2:39–43

17. Lindsey J, Kashiwagi K, Kashiwagi F, Weinreb R (1997) Prostaglandin action on ciliary smooth muscle extracellular matrix metabolism: implications for uveoscleral outflow. Surv Ophthalmol 42[Suppl 2]:S53–59
18. Lindsey J, Kashiwagi K, Kashiwagi F, Weinreb R (1997) Prostaglandins alter extracellular matrix adjacent to human ciliary muscle cells in vitro. Invest Ophthalmol Vis Sci 38:2214–2223
19. Lindsey JD, Kashiwagi K, Boyle D, Kashiwagi F, Firestein GS, Weinreb RN (1996) Prostaglandins increase proMMP-1 and proMMP-3 secretion by human ciliary smooth muscle cells. Curr Eye Res 15:869–875
20. Weinreb RN, Kashiwagi K, Kashiwagi F, Lindsey JD (1997) Prostaglandins increase metalloproteinase activity in medium of human ciliary smooth muscle cells in vitro. Invest Ophthalmol Vis Sci 38:2772–2780

CHAPTER 31

A Comparison of the Ocular Hypotensive Efficacy, Safety and Acceptability of Brimonidine 0.2 % Twice Daily Versus Pilocarpine 2.0 % Thrice Daily as Adjunct Therapy with Beta-Blockers

S. Nagasubramanian

Abstract. The additivity, safety and acceptability of brimonidine (0.2 % b.i.d.) versus pilocarpine (2.0 % t.i.d.) were compared in 141 patients whose intraocular pressure (IOP) was inadequately controlled on beta-blocker monotherapy. Brimonidine and pilocarpine demonstrated equivalent additive ocular-hypotensive efficacy at peak and trough drug effect at every study visit. The overall mean additive IOP-lowering effects were 5.0 mmHg and 3.7 mmHg at peak and trough for brimonidine, respectively, and 4.5 mmHg and 2.9 mmHg at peak and trough for pilocarpine, respectively. Significantly more patients reported visual disturbance, headache and had worsening of far visual acuity in the pilocarpine group, while significantly more patients reported dry mouth in the brimonidine group. Thus, in addition to a highly favourable clinical safety and efficacy profile as monotherapy for ocular hypertension and open-angle glaucoma, brimonidine (0.2 % b.i.d.) is also safe and effective when used adjunctively with a beta-blocker, producing an additive IOP lowering effect equivalent to that of pilocarpine but with fewer adverse ocular effects and better patient acceptability.

Introduction

Although beta-blockers are commonly used as first-line therapy, approximately 50 % of glaucoma patients show an inadequate lowering of intraocular pressure (IOP) or efficacy is lost over time, leading to adjunctive therapy with other agents [1]. Pilocarpine is commonly used as an effective additive agent to beta-blocker therapy. Use of pilocarpine, however, is not always well tolerated and is often limited by serious ocular side effects [2].

Brimonidine is a highly selective and potent α_2-adrenoceptor agonist with a dual IOP-lowering mechanism of action [3]. Given twice daily (b.i.d), brimonidine produces an IOP lowering comparable with that of timolol [4] and superior to that of betaxolol [5]. Unlike nonselective beta-blockers, brimonidine is not contraindicated in patients who have or are at high risk for cardiopulmonary disease. In addition, in other clinical trials [4, 5], brimonidine produced relatively few of the ocular side effects that frequently preclude pilocarpine treatment [2]. Thus, brimonidine is a good candidate for use as an alternative to pilocarpine in adjunctive therapy of patients whose IOP is insufficiently controlled by beta-blockers. This study was designed to assess the ocular hypotensive efficacy, safety, and impact on quality of life of brimonidine and pilocarpine as additive therapies in patients uncontrolled by beta-blocker monotherapy.

Patients and Methods

A total of 141 patients aged 50 years or more with uncontrolled hypertension or open-angle glaucoma on beta-blocker monotherapy, but otherwise healthy, were enrolled in this open-label, randomised, parallel-group comparison trial conducted at 21 sites in Europe. All patients participated in a 2- to 4-week run-in treatment period with a beta-blocker b.i.d. Standard exclusion and inclusion criteria [4, 5] were used. The study consisted of a screening visit and four follow-up visits: visit 2 (day 1), visit 3 (day 10), visit 4 (day 40) and visit 5 (day 90). At visit 2 (baseline), patients were randomised to receive treatment for 90 days with either brimonidine tartrate (0.2 % b.i.d.) or pilocarpine hydrochloride [2.0 % t.i.d. (thrice daily)], in addition to their beta-blockers.

The primary efficacy variable was IOP, which was measured at baseline and at peak (2 h after morning dosing) and trough drug effects (approximately 12 h after the evening instillation) at every study visit. Patients were monitored throughout the study for signs and symptoms of systemic or ocular adverse events. Adverse events were assessed for severity, relationship to treatment and event resolution, and the investigator determined whether the subject should continue in the study based on both efficacy and safety considerations. Other variables included were resting blood pressures and heart rate, visual acuity and biomicroscopy. Ophthalmoscopy and visual-field assessments were performed at the screening visit. Patients completed a quality-of-life questionnaire consisting of a subset of seven questions from the Glaucoma Disability Index and the entire Visual Function-14 questionnaire. Patients were also asked to assess the acceptability of the study drug-dosing regimen. Data analyses were performed using standard statistical methods [4, 5].

Results

Of 141 patients enrolled, 118 patients (66 randomised to brimonidine and 52 to pilocarpine) met the protocol entry criteria and were included in the per protocol analysis of efficacy. All patients who received study treatment (brimonidine $n = 75$, pilocarpine $n = 66$) were included in the intent-to-treat analysis of safety. Due to protocol violations and/or failure to meet eligibility requirements, 23 patients were excluded from the per protocol analysis. No significant between-group differences were noted with regard to demographic parameters. The most commonly used beta-blockers, in descending order of frequency, were timolol, levobunolol, carteolol and metipranolol.

Treatment with either the combination of brimonidine or pilocarpine in addition to a beta-blocker significantly decreased the mean IOP from the baseline at peak (Fig. 1) and trough (Fig. 2) drug effect at every study visit ($p < 0.001$). The overall mean decrease from baseline IOP at peak effect was 5.0 mmHg (23 %) and at trough was 3.7 mmHg (15.7 %) in the brimonidine group and 4.5 mmHg (20.3 %) at peak and 2.9 mmHg (12.4 %) at trough in the pilocarpine group. The between-group difference in overall additive IOP lowering approached statistical significance favouring brimonidine ($p = 0.052$).

The significant side effects reported by patients treated with pilocarpine were visual disturbances (4/66, 6 %; $p = 0.046$) and headache (16/66, 24 %; $p < 0.001$)

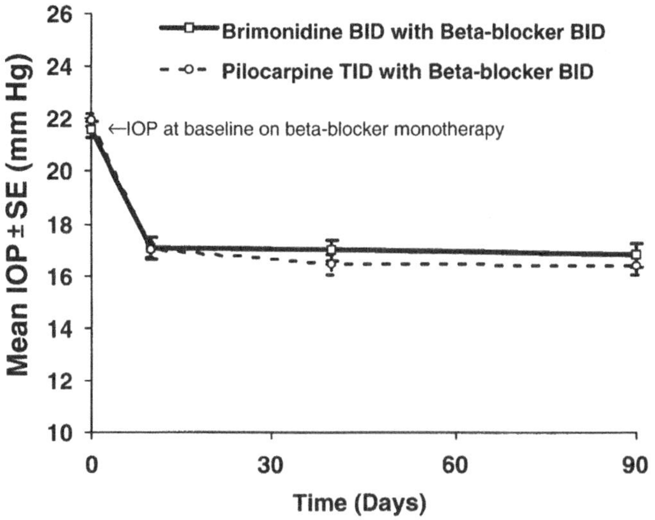

Fig. 1. Mean intraocular pressure (IOP) at peak drug effect. Comparison of the mean IOP±standard error at peak drug effect (2 h post-a.m. dosing) of brimonidine (0.2 % b.i.d.) or pilocarpine (2 % t.i.d.) plus beta-blocker b.i.d. Brimonidine (0.2 %) plus beta-blocker or pilocarpine plus beta-blocker significantly reduced the mean IOP from baseline at all follow-up visits ($p < 0.001$)

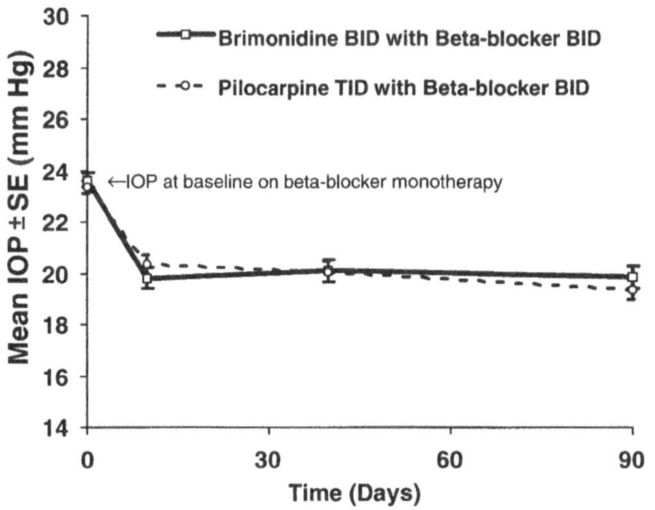

Fig. 2. Mean intraocular pressure (IOP) at trough drug effect. Comparison of the mean IOP±standard error at trough drug effect (approximately 12 h post-p.m. dosing) of brimonidine (0.2 % b.i.d.) or pilocarpine (2 % t.i.d.) plus beta-blocker b.i.d. Brimonidine (0.2 %) plus beta-blocker or pilocarpine plus beta-blocker significantly reduced the mean IOP from baseline at all follow-up visits ($p < 0.001$)

Table 1. Most frequently reported drug-related adverse events by treatment group

Adverse event	Brimonidine (0.2 %) and beta-blocker % (n = 75)	Pilocarpine (2 %) and beta-blocker % (n = 66)	p value
Oral dryness	8.0	0.0	0.030
Headache	0.0	24.2	<0.001
Visual disturbance	0.0	6.1	0.046

Table 2. Far visual acuity at exit visit, by treatment group

Change from baseline	Brimonidine (0.2 %) and beta-blocker % (n = 74)	Pilocarpine (2 %) and beta-blocker % (n = 65)	p value
Worse	1.4	7.7	0.016
No change	94.6	92.3	
Better	4.1	0.0	

(Table 1), and oral dryness was the significant side effect experienced by patients treated with brimonidine (6/75, 8 %; $p = 0.030$). Three patients treated with brimonidine (4 %) and four patients treated with pilocarpine (6 %) discontinued due to a treatment-related ocular or systemic adverse events.

At the exit visit, far visual acuity was significantly worse in patients treated with pilocarpine than those treated with brimonidine ($p = 0.016$). A total of five patients treated with pilocarpine (7.7 %) had a worsening of far visual acuity of two lines or more compared with one (1.4 %) of those randomised to brimonidine (Table 2). Three patients (4.1 %) treated with brimonidine experienced an improvement of far visual acuity at the final visit compared with baseline.

There were no clinically significant within-group or between-group differences in the mean heart rate and systolic and diastolic blood pressure measurements at peak or trough drug effect at any study visit. No significant between-group changes were detected from patient answers to the subset of seven representative questions from the 31-item Glaucoma Disability Index.

Patient responses to the Visual Function-14 questions indicated that a greater number of patients in the pilocarpine group (27.2 %) had difficulty with vision – specifically, difficulty driving during the day – than those randomised to brimonidine (8.4 %). Significantly more patients in the brimonidine group (81.3 %) reported taking all of their doses, compared with those in the pilocarpine group (64.4 %, $p = 0.001$).

Discussion

The data collected in this multi-centre, randomised clinical trial show that brimonidine (0.2 % b.i.d.) has a sustained additive ocular hypotensive efficacy at peak and trough drug effects that is equivalent to that of pilocarpine (2 % t.i.d.) in patients with insufficient IOP control on beta-blocker monotherapy. The combination of brimonidine and beta-blocker therapy was well tolerated and was associated with fewer ocular and systemic adverse events, better patient quality of life, and better patient compliance than the pilocarpine combination therapy.

Well-known ocular side effects frequently associated with pilocarpine treatment, some of which were encountered in this study, include brow ache and vision disturbances which reduce visual acuity, such as myopia and miosis. In addition, less common but more severe ocular side effects associated with pilocarpine treatment include retinal holes, retinal detachment and iris cysts [2]. Thus, despite the long-standing use of pilocarpine, it is no longer preferred as a first-line therapy and is used mainly as an adjunct therapy.

Brimonidine has been shown to be safe and effective as a first-line therapy with a favourable patient tolerability and few systemic or ocular side effects [3–5]. Brimonidine demonstrates ocular hypotensive efficacy comparable with that of timolol [4] and superior to that of betaxolol [5], and has not been documented to cause any significant visual disturbances.

When considering the established clinical profile of brimonidine as monotherapy along with the results of the present study, we conclude that brimonidine (0.2 % b.i.d.) is a safe and effective therapy for the treatment of ocular hypertension and open-angle glaucoma whether used as a monotherapy or as an adjunct therapy with beta-blockers.

Acknowledgements. This study was supported by a grant from Allergan, Inc., Irvine, California, USA. The investigators and centres involved in the Brimonidine Additivity Study Group I are Mr. S. Nagasubramanian, Moorfields Eye Hospital, London, United Kingdom; Dr. Arabela Futre Coelho, Instituto Gama Pinto, Lisbon, Portugal; Dr. Med. Joachim Zeisberg, Berlin, Germany; Dr. Med. Jörg Koch, St. Franziskus Hospital, Münster, Germany; Dr. Med. Joachim Preuss, Städtisches Krankenhaus, Hildesheim, Germany; OA Dr. Med. Detlev Spiegel, Klinikum d. Universität Regensburg, Regensburg, Germany; Dr. Med. Rüdiger Korff, Waldshut-Tiengen, Germany; Prof. Knorz, Munich, Germany; Prof. Dr. Julian Garcia Sanchez, Universidad Conplutense, Madrid, Spain; Dra Mercedes Vaquero Ruano, Clinical Puerta de Hierro, Madrid, Spain; Prof. Dr. Antonio Pinero Bustamante, Hospital Universitario Virgen de Valme, Sevilla, Spain; Prof. Dr. J.C. Pastor Jimeno, Hospital Universitario de Valladolid, Valladolid, Spain; Prof. Dr. Juan A. Duran de la Colina, Hospital de Cruces, Cruces (Vizcaya), Spain; Prof. Dr. Francisco Honrubia Lopez, Hospital Miguel Servet, Zaragoza, Spain; Professeur Gérard Brasseur, Chru Charles Nicolle, Rouen Cedex, France; Docteur Serge Zaluski, Perpignan, France; Docteur Jean-Claude Dascotte, Loos-les-Lille, France; Professeur Alain Bron, Hôpital Général, Dijon Cedex, France; Prof. Bruno Boles Carenini, Universita di Torino, Torino, Italy; Prof. Massimo Bucci, Universita di Tor Vergata, Roma, Italy; Prof. Mario Zingirian, Universita di Genova, Genova, Italy; Dr. Stefano Gandolfi, Universita de Parma, Parma, Italy.

References

1. Kass MA (1983) Efficacy of combining timolol with other antiglaucoma medications. Surv Ophthalmol 28:274–279
2. Nardin GF, Zimmerman TJ (1996) Ocular cholinergic agents. In: Ritch R, Shields MB, Krupin T (eds) The glaucomas, 2nd edn. Mosby, St. Louis, pp 1399–1407
3. Cantor BL, Burke J (1997) Drug evaluation: brimonidine. Exp Opin Invest Drugs :1063–1083
4. Schuman JS, Horwitz B, Choplin NT, David R, Albracht D, Chen K (1997) A 1-year study of brimonidine twice daily in glaucoma and ocular hypertension. A controlled, randomized, multicenter clinical trial. Arch Ophthalmol 115:847–852
5. Serle JB (1996) A comparison of the safety and efficacy of twice daily brimonidine 0.2 % versus betaxolol 0.25 % in subjects with elevated intraocular pressure. Surv Ophthalmol 41[Suppl 1]: S39–S47

Surgery I

CHAPTER 32

Classification of Developing Filtering Blebs after Trabeculectomy

F. Grehn · G. Picht

Abstract. The development of the filtering blebs after trabeculectomy of 55 eyes was followed to establish a classification of filtering blebs with a score system. The number of microcysts, the amount of vascularization, the appearance of "corkscrew vessels", encapsulation, and the height of the filtering bleb were evaluated semi-quantitatively. Two groups were defined: (1) eyes with a spontaneous favorable clinical outcome, and (2) eyes that needed further postoperative interventions (5-fluorouracil injections, needling, or revision). In group I, microcysts were frequent, excessive vascularization and the presence of "corkscrew vessels" were rare, encapsulation was infrequent, and the bleb was moderately elevated. In contrast, in group II, microcysts were generally absent, vascularization, "corkscrew vessels" and encapsulation were frequent, and the bleb was usually highly elevated. This behavior parallels the different activities of wound healing of the subconjunctival connective tissue. Observation of the developing filtering bleb after trabeculectomy according to standardized slit-lamp criteria may help to predict the outcome and may provide clues for the necessity of further treatment independent from post-operative intraocular pressure.

Introduction

The long-term success of filtering surgery depends on the development of adequate aqueous humor outflow into the subconjunctival drainage area. The wound-healing processes involved exhibit several phases that determine the amount of fibrosis at the site of filtration; consequently, the short-term development of the filtering bleb determines the later functional outcome. Most of the processes of fibrosis occur in the subconjunctival connective tissue. The scleral site is rarely involved in the initial process of scarring of the filtering bleb. In the subconjunctival connective tissue, the process of wound healing can be followed by means of slit-lamp biomicroscopy.

Many ophthalmologists evaluate the postoperative development of filtering surgery according only to the intraocular pressure (IOP). However, IOP values can be low despite ongoing scar formation during the first 2–3 weeks after filtering surgery. The biomicroscopical signs of the developing filtering bleb must be taken into consideration and may have a higher predictive value in early phases of bleb development than the IOP itself. For example, if choroidal detachment is present, the IOP is low due to increased uveoscleral outflow or ciliary muscle detachment, while the filtering site is not perfused and may obliterate despite low IOP.

The following classification of filtering blebs was established to improve our understanding and evaluation of early signs of favorable and unfavorable filtering-bleb development. The necessity of therapeutic measures, such as enhanced steroid treatment, needling of the filtering bleb, and/or 5-fluorouracil (5-FU) injections, can be deduced from morphologic follow-up of the filtering bleb.

Patients and Methods

Fifty-five eyes of 53 patients underwent filtering surgery. Trabeculectomy with a fornix-based conjunctival flap was performed by one surgeon. A 4 × 3-mm scleral flap was dissected and a trabeculectomy of 2 × 0.8-mm was performed (Grehn 1990). Of the 55 eyes, 42 had standard trabeculectomy, 6 had primary trabeculectomy with mitomycin-C (MMC), 4 had trabeculectomy with MMC after previous filtering surgery, and 3 had primary trabeculectomy with topical 5-FU. Mitomycin was given in a dose of approximately 100 µl of a 0.2 mg/ml solution soaked into a flat sponge of 8 × 8-mm. The sponge was applied between subconjunctiva and sclera for 5 min. The sclera was rinsed thereafter with 30 ml of balanced salt solution (BSS). Topical 5-FU was applied using the same procedure at a concentration of 40 mg/ml. Postoperative slit-lamp examination and applanation tonometry were both performed at 5 days, 3 weeks, and 3 months.

Standardized morphologic criteria were developed to classify the postoperative filtering bleb. The following criteria were used to establish a semiquantitative classification:

1. Presence or absence of microcysts at three sectors of the filtering bleb (0 = no microcysts, 1 = one sector, 2 = two sectors, 3 = three sectors). One sector was defined as the area overlying the scleral flap. The two other sectors were the areas adjacent to the temporal or nasal border of the scleral flap.
2. Quantity of conjunctival vessels compared with standard photographs (0, 1+, 2+, 3+).
3. Quantity of "corkscrew vessels" compared with standard photographs (0, 1+, 2+, 3+).
4. Presence or absence of encapsulation of the filtering bleb (no = 0; yes = 3).
5. Height of the filtering bleb compared with standard photographs (0, 1+, 2+, 3+).

Different filtering blebs are shown in Fig. 1. Microcysts are tiny spaces of aqueous humor directly underneath the conjunctival epithelium and can best be recognized by means of the narrow slit of the slit lamp (Fig. 1a). "Corkscrew vessels" probably develop due to contraction of fibrous subconjunctival tissue (Fig. 1b). Encapsulation occurs when the Tenon forms an impermeable monocyst while scleral passage of aqueous humor is patent (Fig. 1c).

In those eyes that needed further therapy to obtain favorable bleb function, 5-FU injections or needling in combination with subsequent subconjunctival 5-FU injections were performed. For needling, a 14-gauge cannula was mounted on a 5-ml syringe filled with BSS. Usually, the Tenon cyst was perforated by multiple punctures or cut tangentially, when possible, from the nasal, superior, and temporal directions. 5-FU was given as 5-mg doses (0.4 ml) by means of subconjunctival injections. The total dose varied between 15 mg and 65 mg.

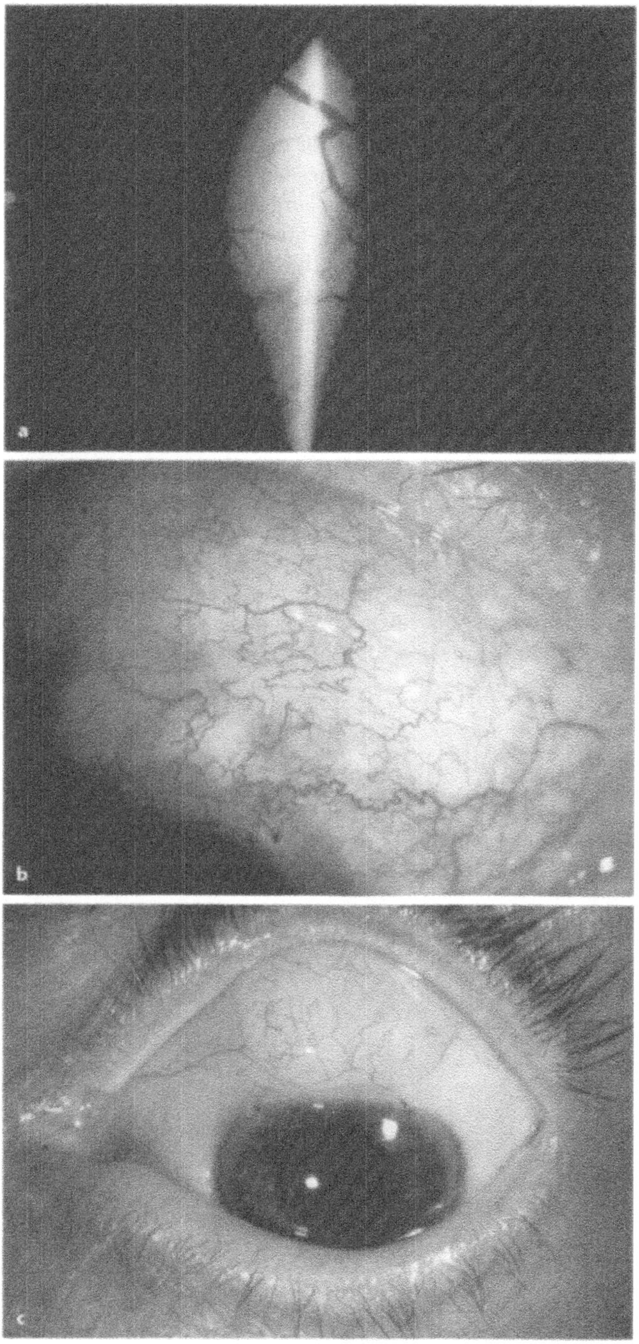

Fig. 1a–c. Different types of filtering blebs: **a** filtering bleb with microcysts; **b** filtering bleb with "cork screw vessels"; **c** encapsulated filtering bleb

Results

Thirty-eight eyes (71.7 %) showed a favorable outcome with controlled IOP (less than or equal to 18 mmHg) on no medication after 3 months (mean IOP 12 mmHg; range 7–18 mmHg). Due to signs of incipient scarring and/or uncontrolled IOP (mean IOP 16.1 mmHg, range 11–31 mmHg), 17 eyes (32.1 %) needed further treatment during the 3-months follow-up. Of these, one eye underwent surgical revision of the filtering site using topical 5-FU (IOP 31 mmHg prior to intervention), and six eyes underwent needling of the filtering bleb followed by subconjunctival 5-FU injections (mean IOP 17 mmHg prior to needling; range 14–24 mmHg). Ten eyes received subconjunctival 5-FU injections alone (mean IOP 14.1 mmHg prior to 5-FU injections; range 11–22 mmHg).

The score for each of the above-mentioned semiquantitative criteria was calculated for two cohorts of filtering blebs: (1) 38 eyes that had no further intervention postoperatively (group I), and (2) 17 eyes that needed further intervention postoperatively (group II). Microcysts were frequent in group I (mean score 1.8) and infrequent in group II (mean score 0.3). The quantity of conjunctival vessels was lower in group I (mean score 0.9) and higher in group II (mean score 2.0). The quantity of "corkscrew vessels" was lower in group I (mean score 0.1) and higher in group II (mean score 1.1). Encapsulation was infrequent in group I (mean score 0.3) and frequent in group II (mean score 2.7). The height of the filtering bleb was moderate in group I (mean score 1.2) and increased in group II (mean score 2.0). These results are summarized in Fig. 2.

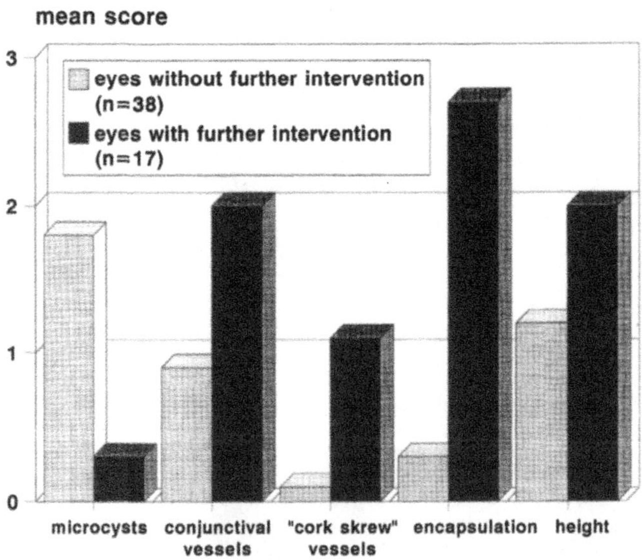

Fig. 2. Mean score values of slit-lamp criteria of filtering blebs comparing group I (eyes without further intervention during follow-up) and group II (eyes with further intervention during follow-up)

Discussion

The present investigation shows differences in the slit-lamp appearance of the filtering bleb between eyes that needed further interventions to develop a patent filtering bleb, and eyes with spontaneous favorable outcome. The scoring system mentioned in the section *Patients and Methods* was used to semiquantitatively describe the filtering bleb. The data for filtering-bleb scoring was obtained independently of the clinical decision for further treatment.

It was found that the presence and quantity of microcysts was a sign of favorable development, whereas increased vascularization, the presence and quantity of "corkscrew vessels", encapsulation, and increased height of the filtering bleb were signs of impending fibrosis. Although these signs are generally thought to be important by most glaucoma surgeons, a classification of developing filtering blebs using a score system seems helpful in facilitating decisions for further interventions such as needling, 5-FU injection, or bleb revision. In contrast to bleb morphology, IOP is a weak indicator of filtering-bleb development, especially within the early postoperative period (2–3 weeks).

A generally accepted classification of filtering blebs has not yet been established. Criteria for postoperative filtering blebs have been described by Vesti (1993) and Shingelton (1996). The above-mentioned score classification of filtering blebs was recently discussed by Picht and Grehn (1998) in the context of wound healing and histopathology. The different slit-lamp criteria of unfavorable bleb development are paralleled in the different phases of wound healing, namely cellular and vessel proliferation, formation of granulation tissue, and collagen secretion (Skuta and Parrish 1987; Miller et al. 1989; Costa et al. 1993; Khaw and Cordeiro 1998).

Some factors that predispose to failure are well known, i.e., inflammation, previous glaucoma medication, previous extra- or intraocular surgery, neovascular types of glaucoma, etc. (Sherwood et al. 1989; Broadway et al. 1993, 1994). Other intrinsic factors, however, cannot be evaluated in an individual patient prior to surgery, but may play an equally important role.

The aqueous humor contains a number of growth factors that may influence wound healing of the filtering site after glaucoma surgery. In particular, transforming growth factor β-2 (TGFβ-2) seems to play a major role (Herschler et al. 1980; Tripathi et al. 1994; Khaw and Cordeiro 1998). We have recently found a correlation between the TGFβ-2 concentration of aqueous humor collected prior to glaucoma operations and the outcome of filtering surgery measured by bleb score and the need of further intervention. Eyes that later showed impaired bleb development and needed additional measures to maintain bleb function showed increased levels of TGFβ-2. Primary open-angle glaucoma and juvenile-glaucoma eyes generally showed higher levels of TGFβ-2 than cataract eyes used as controls, whereas pseudo-exfoliative glaucoma eyes had normal TGFβ-2 levels in the aqueous humor prior to surgery (Picht et al. 1999). Thus, preoperative extrinsic and intrinsic factors as well as signs of postoperative filtering-bleb development can probably be used as predictors and guidelines for further treatment in order to obtain successful glaucoma surgery.

References

Broadway DC, Grierson I, Hitchings R (1993) The effect of topical antiglaucomatous medications on the conjunctiva. Br J Ophthalmol 77:590–596

Broadway DC, Grierson I, O'Brien C, Hitchings R (1994) Adverse effects of topical antiglaucoma medication, I: the conjunctival cell profile. Arch Ophthalmol 112:1437–1445

Costa VP, Spaeth GL, Eiferman RA, Orengo-Nania S (1993) Wound healing modulation in glaucoma filtration surgery. Ophthalmic Surg Lasers 24:152–170

Grehn F (1990) Chirurgische Glaukomtherapie. Fortschr Ophthalmol 87[Suppl]:S175–S186

Herschler J, Clafin AJ, Fiorentina G (1980) The effect of aqueous humor on the growth of subconjunctival fibroblasts in tissue culture and its implications for glaucoma surgery. Am J Ophthalmol 89:245–249

Khaw PT, Cordeiro MF (1998) Neutralizing effects of new recombinant human TGF-β2 monoclonal antibody on in vitro human conjunctival fibroblast-mediated scarring response (ARVO abstract). Invest Ophthalmol Vis Sci 39:S1107 (no 5115)

Miller MH, Grierson I, Unger WI, Hitchings RA (1989) Wound healing in an animal model of glaucoma fistulizing surgery in the rabbit. Ophthalmic Surg 20:350–357

Picht G, Grehn F (1998) Classification of filtering blebs in trabeculectomy: biomicroscopy and functionality. Curr Opin Ophthalmol 9:2–8

Picht G, Welge-Luessen U, Grehn F, Lütjen-Drecoll E (1999) Aqueous humor TGFβ-2 content and total protein versus postoperative filtering bleb development in different types of glaucoma. J Glaucoma (submitted)

Sherwood MB, Grierson I, Millar L, Hitchings RA (1989) Long-term morphological effects of antiglaucoma drugs on the conjunctiva and Tenon's capsule in glaucomatous eyes. Ophthalmology 96:327–335

Shingelton BJ (1996) Management of the failing glaucoma filter. Surg Rev 27:445–451

Skuta GL, Parrish RK II (1987) Wound healing in glaucoma filtering surgery. Surv Ophthalmol 32:149–170

Tripathi RC (1994) Aqueous humor in glaucomatous eyes contains an increased level of TGF-β2. Exp Eye Res 59:723–727

Vesti E (1993) Filtering blebs: follow-up of trabeculectomy. Ophthalmic Surg Lasers 24:249–255

Surgery II

CHAPTER 33

Effects of Irrigation on Mitomycin-C Concentration and Pharmacokinetics Parameters in Rabbit's Eyes

C. G. Machado · R. Susanna Jr.

Introduction

Mitomycin-C (MMC) has been used as an adjunctive therapy to glaucoma filtration surgery, increasing the success rate of the surgery. Excessive inhibition of wound healing results in hyperfiltration and its consequences [1–3]. In attempts to reduce the incidence of these complications, several parameters have been varied: drug concentration, duration of exposure, the site of application and the irrigation of tissues after drug exposure. Irrigation is the least-studied parameter [4, 5]. This experiment was designed to determine the influence of external irrigation on the pharmacokinetic parameters of MMC and its concentration in sclera and aqueous humor.

Materials and Methods

The MMC application was exactly the same in all animals. Using identical 5 × 5 × 2-mm dry cellulose sponges (Weck cel Surgical Spears, Weck Ophthalmics, Research Triangle Park, N.C., USA) uniformly soaked with 0.2 ml of the MMC solution, 5 min scleral application of MMC (0.5 mg/ml) was performed in 100 rabbit eyes. The sponges were placed over a 5 × 5-mm previously delineated scleral flap and left in place for 5 min, with the conjunctiva draped over them. The eyes were divided into three groups: eyes irrigated with 0 ml (35 eyes), 10 ml (35 eyes) and 50 ml (30 eyes). The irrigation rate was 10 ml/min. The saline solution was dripped on the center of the delineated area from 3 cm above.

The scleral flap was dissected as thick as possible and removed. A volume of 0.1–0.2 ml of aqueous humor was obtained by aspiration using a 30-gauge needle. Following sampling, the animals were killed with an overdose of sodium pentobarbital.

High-performance liquid chromatography (HPLC) was used to determine the MMC concentration in scleral and aqueous samples obtained at 0, 5, 15, 30, 60, 90 and 120 min for the non-irrigated eyes, 1, 5, 15, 30, 60, 90 and 120 min for the 10-ml-irrigated eyes, and 5, 15, 30, 60, 90 and 120 min for the 50-ml-irrigated eyes after sponge removal. For each period of time, the mean concentration of MMC in the sclera and aqueous humor of five eyes was calculated.

Sclera samples were homogenized (Polytron, Kinematica GmbH, Suiss) at 25,000 cycles/min. The scleral and aqueous-humor samples were immediately frozen at −80 °C. The MMC concentration was determined by means of HPLC. The equipment used was a Shimadzu LC-10AS, with injector SIL 10B and detector UV-VIS230 model SPD 10AV. The validated method was linear over a concentration range of 2.5–300 ng/ml, with a minimum detected concentration in the aqueous humor of 2.5 ng/ml and of 0.02 μg/g in the sclera.

Results

Increasing irrigation volume resulted in decreased amounts of MMC absorbed in the scleral and aqueous-humor, as calculated via AUC (area under the curve). The AUC and EBA (extension of bioavailability) for scleral exposed sites was, respectively, 36.05 μg/h/g and 100 % in nonirrigated eyes, 27.23 μg/h/g and 76 % for eyes irrigated with 10 ml, and 9.75 μg/h/g and 27 % for eyes irrigated with 50 ml of saline. The AUC and EBA for aqueous humor was, respectively, 334.00 ng/ml and 100 % in nonirrigated eyes, 103.10 ng/ml and 31 % for eyes irrigated with 10 ml, and 18.20 ng/ml and 5 % for eyes irrigated with 50 ml of saline. The aqueous-humor concentration of MMC peaked at 30 min. Increasing irrigation volume resulted in decreased mean residence time of MMC in aqueous humor. The residence time for nonirrigated eyes was 90 min, for eyes irrigated with 10 ml it was 30 min, and for eyes irrigated with 50 ml it was 15 min.

MMC half-life for the sclera did not change with external irrigation, (range 0.25–0.28 h), although the rate of distribution, alpha (in units of h^{-1}), of MMC from sclera decreased as the irrigation volume increased. It was 24.75 for the nonirrigated eyes, 9.24 for eyes irrigated with 10 ml, and 6.93 for eyes irrigated with 50 ml.

Figure 1 shows the concentration of MMC in the sclera as a function of time for the three groups. Figure 2 shows the concentration of MMC in the aqueous humor as a function of time for the three groups.

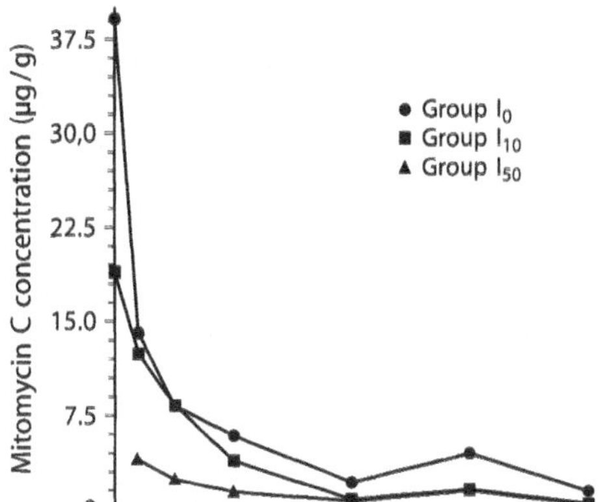

Fig. 1. Concentration of mitomycin-C (*MMC*) in the sclera as a function of time

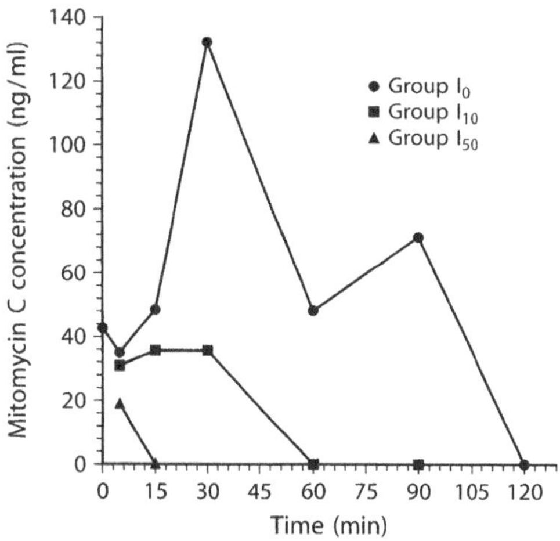

Fig. 2. Concentration of mitomycin-C (*MMC*) in the aqueous humor as a function of time. I_0 (*line with circles*), group eyes without rinsing; I_{10} (*with squares*), group eyes with 10 ml rinsing; I_{50} (*with triangles*), group eyes with 50 ml rinsing

Discussion

Our results reconfirm that MMC rapidly reaches the anterior chamber after topical application. Aqueous-humor concentrations of MMC in the nonirrigated eyes are much higher than those in the irrigated eyes, and this suggests that a significant amount of MMC remains on the ocular surface after the removal of the sponge. In the early phase in nonirrigated eyes, there is a correlation between the decrease of the concentration of MMC in the sclera and the increase of MMC in the aqueous humor, suggesting that there is a high transference of MMC from the sclera to the aqueous humor. Also, increasing irrigation volume decreased the mean residence time of MMC in the aqueous humor and the rate of distribution in sclera.

This study suggests that it is possible to decrease the amount and time of residence of MMC in the anterior chamber where it is not desirable, and yet have high concentrations of this drug on the target tissue. Many studies have been done to determine the best concentration and time of application of MMC in order to increase the success rate and minimize the complications of surgery. The volume of irrigation after the removal of the sponge is an important parameter that has not received the attention that it deserves.

References

1. Zacharia PT, Deppermann SR, Schuman JS (1993) Ocular hypotony after trabeculectomy with mitomycin C. Am J Ophthalmol 116:314–326
2. Greenfield DS, Suner IJ, Miller MP, Kangas TA, Palberg PF, Flynn HWJR (1996) Endophthalmitis after filtering surgery with mitomycin. Arch Ophthalmol 114:943–949
3. Jampel HD, Paquale LR, Dibernardo C (1992) Hypotony maculopathy following trabecutomy with mitomycin C. Arch Ophthalmol 110:1049–1050
4. Kawase K, Nishimura K, Matsushita H, Yamamoto T, Kitazawa Y (1992) Mitomycin concentration in rabbit and human ocular tissue after topical administration. Ophthalmology 99:203–207
5. Prata JÁ, Mincler DS, Koda RT (1995) Effects of external irrigation on mitomycin C concentration in rabbit aqueous and vitreous humor. J Glaucoma 4:32–35

Investigation of the Lectin from the Edible Mushroom Agaricus bisporus as an Inhibitory Modulator of Healing after Trabeculectomy

C. Tebbs · M. Batterbury · A. Nelson · A. Floyd · J. Rhodes · I. Grierson

Introduction

A successful trabeculectomy is dependent on the wound-healing response; certain patients are at a higher risk of surgical failure due to excessive scarring. At present, the antifibrotic drugs 5-fluorouracil and mitomycin C are used to modulate healing, although there is risk of serious side effects due to their toxicity. The potential of a lectin from the edible mushroom *Agaricus bisporus* as a less toxic modulator of wound healing has been investigated. It has been previously shown that *Agaricus bisporus* lectin (ABL) inhibits the contraction of collagen gels seeded with human Tenon's-capsule fibroblasts [1]. In order to determine the effects of this lectin on cell proliferation in monolayer culture, a method of directly counting cells using an image-analysis programme has been devised. This was necessary due to the reduced ability of trypsinisation to remove cells from monolayers in order to count cells using a Coulter counter or haemocytometer after treatment with ABL. This paper demonstrates the reproducibility and accuracy of counting cells using image analysis and describes how the method has been used to determine the effects of ABL on the proliferation of human Tenon's-capsule fibroblasts.

Methods

Cell Culture

Fibroblasts were cultured from explants of human Tenon's capsule, taken post mortem or at the time of conjunctival surgery with the approval of the local Ethics Committee. Primary cultures on tissue-culture flasks were maintained in Ham's F10 (Gibco BRL, Paisley, UK) containing 50 U/ml penicillin and 50 μg/ml streptomycin (Sigma, Poole, UK), 2.5 μg/ml fungizone (Gibco BRL), and 7.5 ml of a 7.5 % (weight/volume) sodium bicarbonate buffer solution (BDH, Lutterworth, UK). This was then supplemented with 10–20 % foetal-calf serum (FCS, Harlan Sera-Lab LTD, Crawley-Down, UK). After 2–3 weeks of proliferation and migration, cells were washed with phosphate-buffered saline (PBS, Unipath, Basingstoke, UK) and detached by incubation with trypsin/ethylenediaminetetraacetate (EDTA) (0.05 %/0.02 %; Sigma). After neutralisation with serum-containing culture medium, cells were centrifuged at 1000 rpm for 10 min, then resuspended in F10 medium containing 10 % newborn-calf serum (NCS, Gibco BRL), hereafter referred to as standard medium.

Two-Step Growth Assay

Twenty-four-well tissue culture plates were plated at a density of 20,000 cells/well in 1 ml of standard medium. Cells were washed twice in SF-F10 24 h later before treatment with 1 ml of test media for 3 days.

Cell Counting of Haematoxylin-Stained Cells Using Computer-Assisted Image Analysis

After 3 days, monolayers were fixed with 100 % methanol for 5 min and stained with haematoxylin (Shandon, Runcorn, UK) for 3 min, followed by immersion in running tap water for several minutes until cell nuclei appeared blue. Cell number was counted using Aequitas Image Database and Archiving System (Aequitas IDA; Dynamic Data Links, Cambridge, UK) linked via a video camera to a Nikon Diaphot microscope. Monolayers were counted at 20× magnification. An image of the monolayer was imported into Aequitas IDA. By varying the threshold of the imaging system so that the darkly stained nuclei of individual cells were identified, an automatic cell count could be completed. Five counts per well were made in a cross-like fashion.

Comparison of the Automated Technique with a Manual Reference Standard

Since the automated technique was developed to improve the efficiency of cell counting, comparison with a reference standard was required. First, one operator made a cell count of a stored image by identifying and marking each cell nucleus. Then, the automated technique was performed. The manual count was performed four times, and the automated technique was performed four times for each manual count. The two methods were compared by calculating the difference between the counts obtained. The mean, standard deviation and 95 % confidence limits were computed, and a one-sample *t*-test was performed to detect bias.

Reproducibility of the Automated Technique

Cells were cultured for 3 days in F10 media with or without 10 % NCS. Triplicate cultures were made. An image of each well was imported and stored in Aequitas IDA for later analysis. On three separate occasions, three cell counts of each well were made in random order. Two-way analysis of variance (ANOVA; factors: test condition and repeat count) was performed. Measurement error was derived as the square root of the residual error.

Effect of ABL on Cell Count

For experiments investigating the effects of ABL on proliferation, cells were incubated in F10 media containing 1 % NCS and ABL in PBS (10, 50, or 100 μg/ml) or the appropriate control (SF-F10 or 1 % or 10 % NCS/F10) for 3 days. Test conditions were in triplicate. The experiment was repeated twice. A cell count of each well was made (as described above). Results were analysed using one-way ANOVA, followed by Duncan's multiple-range test to detect non-homogenous groups.

Results

Accuracy of the Automated Technique

Figure 1 shows the results of the comparison of the automated technique with manual counting. The mean difference was 9.2 (SD 7.2, 95 % confidence limits -4.9, 23.38). There is a tendency for the automated technique to underestimate cell number, but this bias is not significant ($p > 0.05$, single sample t-test).

Reproducibility of the Automated Technique

The measurement error was 7.8 (95 % confidence limit 15.35). A significant increase in cell number was observed in the presence of 10 % NCS/F10 when compared with serum-free media (534 ± 89 vs 1319 ± 89.7, $p < 0.01$).

Effect of ABL on Cell Number

Exposure of fibroblasts to ABL resulted in a dose-dependent decrease in cell number (Fig. 2). A significant decrease in cell count was observed in the presence of 50 μg/ml

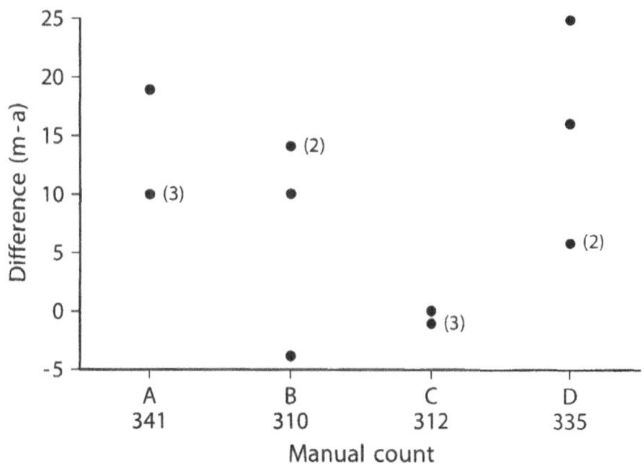

Fig. 1A–D. Comparison of manual and automatic counting. Four repeat counts were made on four stored images (A–D); manual cell counts are shown in *bold*. The difference was calculated between automatic (*a*) and manual (*m*) counts. *Figures in parentheses* represent the number of repeat counts of the same cell number

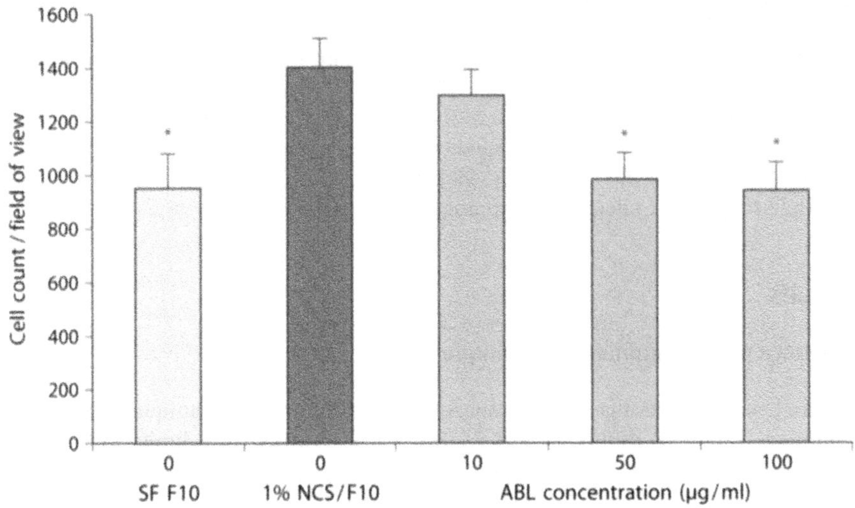

Fig. 2. The effect of *Agaricus bisporus* lectin on the proliferation of human Tenon fibroblasts after 72-h exposure. *SF F10* denotes serum-free F10 medium; *1 % NCS/F10* denotes media containing 1 % newborn-calf serum; * denotes significant difference from 1 % NCS/F10 control at $p < 0.05$

ABL (987.5 ± 102.7) and 100 µg/ml ABL (947.2 ± 110.7) when compared with the 1 % NCS/F10 control (1410.6 ± 106.5). Cell number in the presence of 50 µg/ml and 100 µg/ml ABL was reduced to a level comparable with that observed in SF-F10 (955 ± 133).

Discussion

At present, the drugs 5-fluorouracil and mitomycin C are used to attempt to prevent the failure of trabeculectomy in patients who are at risk of aggressive scarring. However, these drugs are highly toxic and may result in serious side-effects. Preliminary studies using a lectin from *Agaricus bisporus* have demonstrated an antiproliferative effect on human Tenon's-capsule fibroblasts in culture. However, quantification of this effect has been made difficult by the reduced ability of trypsin to detach cells from tissue-culture plastic in order to count by conventional methods such as with a Coulter counter. The present study has demonstrated that a method of cell counting using an image-analysis package is an accurate and reproducible method of quantifying cell number.

Initially, a comparison was made between counts conducted by the computer automatically and those done manually by the operator in order to determine whether counting by image analysis was an accurate method. Results have indicated that there is a tendency for the computer to underestimate cell numbers, which is probably due to the computer not recognising very lightly stained nuclei in its count. This effect can be minimised via careful checking by the operator to ensure that all cell nuclei are marked before counting. However, the error between automated and manual counts is low when compared with the total number of cells counted and was felt to be acceptable.

To determine the reproducibility of the automatic technique, images of cell monolayers were stored, and repeated counts were made. This has demonstrated that automated counting is highly reproducible, as a low measurement error was obtained; a difference between counts of more than 15.35 is unlikely to be due to chance at the 95 % level. This method of counting is therefore also able to demonstrate small differences in cell number between different test conditions; a highly significant difference in cell number between serum-free and serum-containing media was observed.

The present method of counting has been used to determine the effects of ABL on the proliferation of human Tenon's-capsule fibroblasts. This has demonstrated that there is a significant antiproliferative effect in cells exposed to ABL for 3 days. However, the reduction in cell number does not fall below that observed in serum-free conditions, suggesting that ABL may be of low toxicity. This has been verified by trypan-blue dye exclusion and by a live/dead assay (Molecular Probes, Leiden, The Netherlands), both of which indicate that, at the doses of ABL required to inhibit proliferation, cytotoxicity of less than 5 % occurs (data not shown). In addition, it has been previously documented that ABL inhibits the contraction of collagen gels seeded with human Tenon's-capsule fibroblasts in a dose-dependent fashion. At present, the mechanism behind these effects is not clear. However, these preliminary studies demonstrate the need for further investigation into this novel antiproliferative agent with respect to its use in modulating wound healing as an alternative to the toxic drugs 5-fluorouracil and mitomycin C.

References

1. Batterbury M, Grierson I (1996) Investigation of mushroom lectin as a modulator of ocular wound healing. Invest Ophthalmol Vis Sci 37:S117

CHAPTER 35

Non-Penetrating Trabeculectomy with Aspiration of the Inner Wall of Schlemm's Canal and Juxtacanalicular Trabeculum

Alain Béchetoille · H. Bresson-Dumont · N. Urier

Introduction

In the very beginning there was the sky and the earth, then Adam and Eve, and a little bit later, von Graefe and his iridectomy – brilliant, but it does not work in all cases. In addition, at the turn of this century, full-thickness fistulizing procedures were described and popularized by Lagrange, Eliott, Hoylt and, later on, by Sheie. With these procedures, a full-thickness piece of sclera was removed, leaving only the conjunctiva as a barrier to the aqueous humor. Results were excellent, but with a high rate of disturbing complications.

During the most difficult period of the East–West cold war 60 years later, many realized that it was probably possible to do a better job. At that time, Morton Grant was also demonstrating, through perfusion studies, that the main resistance to the aqueous outflow was located within the trabeculum, between the anterior chamber and the Schlemm's canal. With these principles in mind, Harms, from Germany, invented the trabeculotomy, an efficient procedure used in cases of congenital glaucoma; in addition, Cairns invented the trabeculectomy, which, in his mind, was a specific procedure for the resistant trabeculum. It was eventually discovered that trabeculectomy was a fistula, only partly protected from complications by the scleral flap.

Meanwhile, in the scientifically isolated USSR, Krasnov believed that the main resistance to aqueous outflow was located between the Schlemm's canal and the outer sclera. From this assumption, he very logically proposed the sinusotomy, which removes a piece of sclera from between the Schlemm's canal and the subconjunctival space [1]. Russians performed many sinusotomies during this period, with fairly good results, according to Russian physicians. Later, they specified that sinusotomy works in part by lifting the collapsus of Schlemm's canal; they were probably correct on this point. Some years later, they started performing sinusotomies under the protection of a superficial scleral flap, calling it the "new surgery of glaucomas", and this technique was very close to what we perform today.

During this period, no one or almost no one in the Occidental world was interested or even confident in what Russians said. But Arenas, in Colombia, performed this procedure regularly, without speaking about it or publishing it; this was also true of Zimmerman in the United States, especially in aphakic patients, and he published good results [2, 3]. Zimmerman abandoned this technique, not because of the results, which were almost as good as those of the classical trabeculectomy, but because he found it difficult technically, and especially difficult to teach.

Meanwhile, the Russians were not inactive, and Fyodorov, as well as Koslov and Anisimova, pushed their dissection forward to the Descemet membrane and proposed an additional collagen implant as well as the term "deep sclerectomy" [4, 5]. The company, Staar, in contact with them, developed another collagen implant and started to promote the process, especially in Europe, since the implant was not approved at that time by the Food and Drug Administration in the United States. Anisimova, in connection with Staar, came to Demailly's place of work (Hopital Saint Joseph, Paris), where Valtot and Mermoud learned Anisimova's procedure before modifying it a bit and promoting it very strongly.

However, in South Africa, Stegmann quite independently proposed something a bit different, called viscocanalostomy [6]. Stegmann was committed in his country to operate on black patients affected with very severe glaucomas, with very high intraocular pressure (IOP). As the conjunctival-scarring process of black patients is very active, viscocanalostomy was designed to avoid filtration. The procedure starts like deep sclerectomy, but the dissection is pushed forward deliberately to the Descemet membrane, transforming the sclerectomy into a sclerokeratectomy. Then, after deroofing Schlemm's canal, Stegmann injected viscoelastic sideways into the opened canal edges, thus probably making a sort of viscotrabeculotomy. According to Stegmann, the results were good and were obtained without a filtration bleb.

Finally, it is probable that some Russians, especially Fyodorov [4], and certainly Zimmerman in the US and Valtot in France, insisted on the necessity of removing the external trabeculum (where 80 % of the resistance to aqueous outflow is located) in order to get better results; i.e., according to Prof. Bill's group, the 14-μm pieces of tissue adjacent to the canal, including its internal wall and the juxtacanalicular trabeculum (JXCT), is removed [7]. With such a design, the procedure becomes an external trabeculectomy. Valtot and Mermoud removed that tissue using small forceps. We propose to mechanically aspirate the inner wall of the canal and the JXCT matrix.

Purpose

To determine retrospectively the short and mid-term efficiency and safety of non-perforating trabeculectomy, with aspiration of the inner wall of the canal and JXCT [non-penetrating trabeculectomy with aspiration (NPTA)], in decreasing the pressure of primary open-angle glaucoma (POAG) patients.

Method

Of 60 POAG patients (24 male and 36 female, 58 Caucasian, 2 Black, mean age: 55.9 years), 73 eyes with their IOP only partly controlled by means of 1.9 glaucoma medication, and having a significant and progressive alteration of the visual field, were consecutively operated upon using the following protocol. All patients underwent topical anesthesia with tetracaine (1 %), eventually completed with a neuroleptanalgesia procedure. After opening the conjunctiva at the limbus, a superficial (1/4 of the scleral thickness) semicircular scleral flap of 5-mm diameter was created. Then a second, deep homothetic, limbus-based, corneoscleral flap was created just inside the first one and removed, leaving Schlemm's canal either opened or, if not, prepared to be deliberately unroofed. A scleral diathermy was performed just behind Schlemm's canal. At that stage, the aqueous humor was percolating from the trabeculum. A mechanical aspiration of the inner wall of Schlemm's canal and JXCT was then performed, using either an aspirating olive-type probe or a probe originally designed for scratching and aspirating. This action immediately increased the aqueous flow through the remaining trabeculum by severalfold. The second flap, containing the corneoscleral stroma, was then removed down to the Schwalbe's ring using Vannas scissors. No collagen implant was used. The semicircular initial scleral flap was then closed and sutured with two 10–0 nylon sutures. The Tenon's capsule and the conjunctiva were closed with separate 10–0 vicryl sutures. The patients were treated postoperatively with rifamycin (0.1 %) (·2) and tropicamide (0.40 %) (·1) drops for a mean duration of 10 days. Dexamethazone (0.1 %) drops were occasionally used for a short period of time.

Intraoperative episcleral applications of mitomycine were performed in four cases (one second procedure, one allergic conjunctivitis, two black patients) before creating the first scleral flap. Intraoperative episcleral applications of 5-fluorouracil (FU) were also performed in an allergic conjunctivitis eye.

The initial procedure was completed by yttrium-aluminum garnet (YAG)-laser goniosynechodialysis in 2 cases and YAG-laser ab interno trabeculotomies (goniopunctures) in 15 cases. Postoperative use of subconjunctival injections of 5-FU associated with oculo-digital massages were used in 19 cases, 13 of which were the same as the YAG-treated ones. Medical treatment of elevated IOP was ended in all cases before surgery, but eventually reintroduced postoperatively if necessary, especially if the target pressure of the treatment for IOP was not reached.

Results

Mean IOP decreased from 22 ± 4.2 mmHg (mean follow-up 419 days), with 1.9 glaucoma medication, to 11.6 ± 6.7 mmHg (day 1) (0.3), to 14.5 ± 7 mmHg (day 8) (0.3), to 15.6 ± 4.8 mmHg (day 30) (0.2), to 15.7 ± 4.6 mmHg (day 90) (0.1), to 15.9 ± 3.8 mmHg (day 180) (0.2) (range 8–24 mmHg) and to 15.9 ± 3.2 mmHg (day 360) (range 9–21 mmHg) ($p < 0.0001$) (Mann-Whitney rank sum test) (Table 1). Only 11 cases needed additional medical treatment, but with only 1.3 medication instead of 2.2 preoperatively. Finally, additional argon-laser trabeculoplasty was performed in two cases.

Best corrected mean visual acuity was 7.4 ± 2.6 (on a decimal scale for subjective normal visual acuity) at day 360 compared with 8.1 ± 2.7 preoperatively (5.9 ± 2.6 at

Table 1. Effect of non-penetrating trabeculectomy with aspiration (NPTA) on intraocular pressure (IOP) at days 90, 180, and 360 after surgery and units of glaucoma medication eventually used to achieve IOP control

Days	IOP (mmHg)	Medication
0	22±4.2	1.9
90	15.7±4.6*	0.1
180	15.9±3.8*	0.2
360	15.9±3.2*	0.3

* $p < 0.0001$, Mann-Whitney rank sum test.

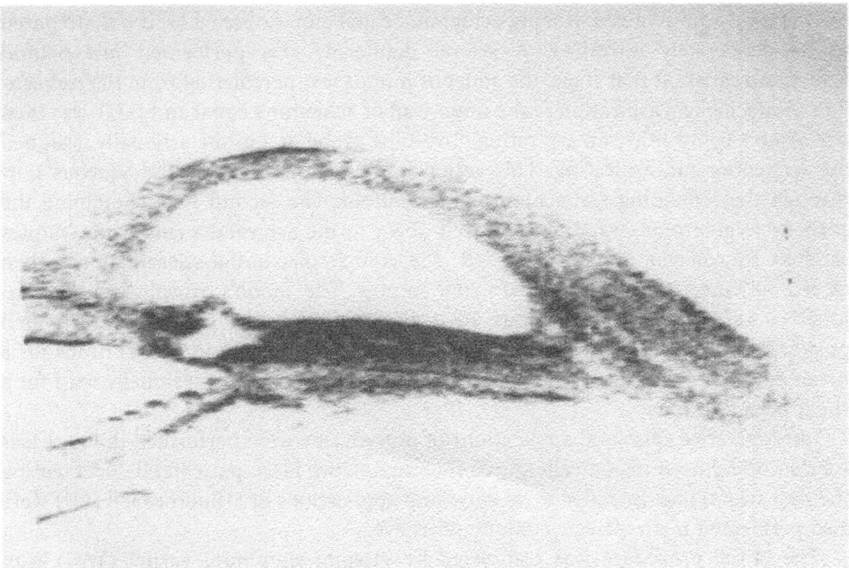

Fig. 1. Ultrasound biomicroscopy of the anterior segment of an eye operated upon 1 year with non-penetrating trabeculectomy. The thin trabecular membrane, which is also a barrier to complications, can be seen between the anterior chamber and an intermediate chamber created by surgery. One can also see, in this case, a large filtering bleb (doc. F Valtot)

day 8). The visual field, assessed by means of a Humphrey Field Analyzer program 30/2, showed a mean deviation of –8.2 ± 6.2 dB and a corrected-pattern standard deviation of 6.2 ± 3.5 dB at day 360, compared with, respectively, –8.4 ± 7.0 dB and 5.1 ± 4.1 dB preoperatively.

Filtration blebs were observed in most cases. On an evaluation scale of 0 (no bleb) to 4 (exuberant), 9 were scored 0, 10 were scored 1, 15 were scored 2, 6 were scored 3 and 4 were scored 4. Information was not available in 33 cases (Fig. 1).

The complication rate was very moderate when compared with standard trabeculectomy. We did not identify any flat or even narrow anterior chambers, any clinically-observed cilio-choroidal detachments [we did not perform ultrasound biomicroscopy (UBM)], or long-standing severe ocular hypotony. We did not observe hyphemas, although a hematic tyndall was noted in one case. Very light anterior-chamber inflammation was noted in four cases, of which one was linked to microperforation. We did not observe any postoperative synechia, but we observed one significant, light opacification of the lens, likely due to a reaction (corneal ulcer) to a subconjunctival injection of 5-FU. Finally, delayed conjunctival scarring was more consistently observed than in standard trabeculectomy (12 cases showed a Seidel sign at day 8), raising the hypothesis of a different scarring process due to a different composition of the filtering aqueous humor.

Discussion

The main advantage of NPSG is that the goal of decreasing IOP is achieved with a very low rate of complication. There is no flat or narrow anterior chamber, no clinically observed cilio-choroidal detachments – although Mermoud identified flat ciliary detachment through UBM examination – and no long-standing severe ocular hypotony. The eye is not opened, with very positive consequences for early outcome on operated subjects, including none or a very light inflammatory reaction, no hyphema, and good postoperative visual acuity. However, one case of malignant glaucoma was reported. The only significant complications are observed when microperforations of the remaining structure happen during surgery. Blebs are observed in most cases. They are ordinarily quite flat and look very nice. Very few of them are cystic or fragile. Mermoud stated that using a collagen implant results in a flatter bleb. Viscocanalostomy surgeons claim that their procedure works without any bleb. Finally, the only significant question is regarding the long-term results of the different procedures.

We like to focus on the value of doing something more than plain deep sclerectomy – we call it external trabeculectomy; Bill's group demonstrated in monkeys that 80 % of aqueous outflow resistance is located within 14 μm of tissue adjacent to the internal side of Schlemm's canal. Mermoud, Valtot and others proposed to peel off, with a small forcep, this strip of tissue, in fact a little bit more, including the inner wall of Schlemm's canal, JXCT and part of the corneoscleral trabeculum, leaving only the remaining permeable trabeculum as a barrier to complications. Our proposition is to mechanically aspirate the 14 μm, including the inner wall of the Schlemm's canal and the matrix of the JXCT. In fact, during surgery, the percolation of the aqueous humor increases severalfold as soon as the mechanical aspiration starts. This increased percolation continues after stopping the aspiration. During the days following surgery, IOP frequently ranges between 8 mmHg and 12 mmHg. It stabilizes within 1 week in the 10–18 mmHg range. At the present time, we have no objective information on the nature of the aspirated tissue or on the scarring process of this tissue.

However, there is some concern about the amount and the duration of IOP lowering provided by this procedure. Trabeculectomy is still standard practice in the surgery of glaucoma.

Conclusion

NPSG is steadily growing in several countries as an alternative to standard trabeculectomy. In addition to deep sclerectomy, with or without collagen implant and viscocanalostomy, NPTA without collagen implant merits further consideration because, so far, it has an interestingly good efficiency in decreasing IOP in chronic open-angle glaucoma patients for at least 6 months. This goal is achieved with a very low rate of significant complications. Aspiration of the inner wall of Schlemm's canal and JXCT might be important in this success. Some surgeons already think that, in terms of glaucoma surgery, one reason for a shift from trabeculectomy to NPSG procedures (NPTA being one of these proposed procedures) might be its improved safety profile. If the initial therapeutic results are confirmed and are long-lasting, the shift would be as important as that from extracapsular cataract extraction to phaco, in terms of cataract surgery.

References

1. Krasnov MM (1969) Méthode de traitement chirurgical et microchirurgical du glaucome sans fistulisation du globe oculaire. Ann Oculist 202:859–873
2. Arenas E (1991) Trabeculectomy ab externo. Highlights Ophthalmol 9:XIX
3. Zimmerman TJ, Kooner KS, Ford VJ, Olander KW, Mandlekorn RM, Rawlings FE, Leader BJ, Koskan AJ (1984) Effectiveness of non-penetrating trabeculectomy in aphakic patients with glaucoma. Ophthalmic Surg 15:44–50
4. Fyodorov SN, Ioffre DI, Ronkina TI (1984) Deep sclerectomy: technique and mechanism of a new glaucomatous procedure. Glaucoma 6:281–283
5. Koslov VI, Bagrov SN, Anisimova SV, Opipov AV, Mogilevtsev VV (1990) Non-penetrating deep sclerectomy with collagen.IRTC, "Eye Micro Surgery". 3. RSFSR Ministry of Public Health, Moscow, pp 44–46
6. Stegmann R (1996) Viscocanalostomy. Binkhorst lecture. European Society of Cataract and Refractive Surgery, Göteborg
7. Maeepa O, Bill A (1992) Pressures in the juxtacanalicular tissue and Sclemm's canal in monkeys. Exp Eye Res 4:879–883

CHAPTER 36

Non-Penetrating Deep Sclerectomy with Collagen Device Versus Trabeculectomy

P. Demailly · M. Berkani · Y. Lachkar

Introduction

Non-penetrating deep sclerectomy (NPDS) is a new antiglaucomatous filtration technique. It was used by Zimmerman et al. (1984), then by Arenas, under the name of trabeculectomy ab externo. It was further developed and extended to the plane of Descemet's membrane by Fyodorov (Koslov et al. 1990).

The principle of non-penetrating deep sclerectomy involves the ablation of a deep triangular or rectangular scleral flap, with a limbal base under a superficial scleral. The procedure involves opening the external wall of Schlemm's canal, flat leaving in place only the plane of the juxta-limbal Descemet's membrane. The anterior chamber is not opened. The aqueous humor filters through the opened Schlemm's canal, the uveal tract and Descemet's membrane.

To improve this aqueous filtration route, Koslov et al. (1990) proposed inserting a collagen implant in the deep scleral bed opposite Schlemm's canal. The collagen implant (2.5 × 1 × 0.5 mm) is biocompatible, made from porcine scleral tissue. This material is known for its high water content (greater than 99 % water), and its failure to elicit systemic immune reactions, as it is destroyed by the body, absorbed and replaced by a porous and low-density meshwork of young collagen fibrils. This implant provides support for the elimination route of aqueous humor and acts like a sponge. It also creates a space between the deep scleral plane and the superficial scleral flap, thus allowing the aqueous humor to flow freely.

The collagen implant has the appearance of a cigarette filter, covered with holes (0.1–1 μm in diameter) along its length. It therefore acts like a drain that carries the liquid by capillary action, pumping the aqueous humor out of the anterior chamber toward the scleral bed. The aqueous humor is then evacuated further, along the same routes as those used in a trabeculectomy – mainly the subconjunctival space. It is therefore a filtration technique.

The collagen implant comes in a sealed packet and is sterilized by irradiation. Full guarantee against viral contamination is provided.

This technique aims to eliminate or minimize the complications of classical trabeculectomy. The purpose of this study was to compare this technique with a trabeculectomy in primary open-angle glaucoma (POAG).

Table 1. Populations: non-penetrating deep sclerectomy (NPDS) and trabeculectomy (TLY)

	NPDS	TLY
Patients (*n*)	25	25
Eyes (*n*)	25	25
Average age (years)	63.4±10.37 (41–82)	61.46±11.12 (41–79)
Average follow-up (months)	18 (7–9)	16.56 (10–26)
Preoperative medications	2.2	2.37
Preoperative therapeutic Duration (months)	107.88 (10–228)	108.96 (2–360)

Materials and Methods

Of 50 patients with uncontrolled open-angle glaucoma, 50 eyes were prospectively assigned to have either NPDS or a trabeculectomy by the same surgeon (Ph.D). Age, mean follow-up, preoperative medications and preoperative therapeutic duration were similar in both groups (Table 1).

The NPDS Technique

A bridle suture (3/0 silk) was placed under the tendon of the superior rectus muscle. A limbus base conjunctival flap was prepared superiorly. One-third to one-half thickness rectangular scleral flap (approximately 5 × 6-mm long) was then dissected to the clear cornea. A triangular deep scleral flap with a limbal base was dissected. This cautious dissection must leave in its posterior section only a thin layer of sclera, opposite the ciliary body.

In the anterior section, the dissection was performed using a diamond knife. The external wall of Schlemm's canal was opened, leaving in front of it only the Descemet plane; the internal wall is removed with a forapes care must be taken to avoid perforating it. At this stage, the aqueous humor must rise from the anterior chamber along all the trabeculo-descemetic surface. The anterior section of the collagen implant must rest on Schlemm's canal and not on Descemet's membrane. The implant should be secured in place by a deep stitch with nylon 10/0.

The scleral flap was sutured using two 10–0 nylon sutures. The conjunctiva was closed with a single running vicryl suture. Post-operative care is simple, with the instillation of local corticosteroids or non-steroidal anti-inflammatory medication for 3–4 weeks. No eye-pad is required.

Post-operative follow-up is done on an ambulatory basis on days 3, 6, 14, 30, 60, 90 and 180. In addition to a standard examination, follow-up will require a gonioscopy for early detection of possible goniosynechiae opposite the filtration site, especially during the first 15 days after the operation. The filtration bleb is slightly inflated, translucent, avascular, and not very different from a trabeculectomy bleb.

Trabeculectomy Technique

The trabeculectomy technique was similar to the NPDS technique except, of course, for the resection of an anterior trabecular block (approximately 1 × 3 mm) and a basal iridectomy. The scleral flap was sutured with three 10–0 nylons. No releasable suture or anti-metabolites were used in these eyes. In the early postoperative period, a topical cycloplegic (atropine, 1 % every day) and corticosteroid (dexamethasone, three times daily) were prescribed routinely for 2 weeks and then slowly tapered off.

Results

Tonometric Results

Tonometric results are presented in Table 2.

Complications

Complications are listed in Table 3. The most frequent postoperative care in the NPDS group was an early rise in the intraocular pressure (IOP) caused by one of two factors:

1. An internal obstruction due to insufficient filtration through the trabeculo-descemetic plane or iris prolapse against the filtration site. It must be quickly

Table 2. Non-penetrating deep sclerectomy (NPDS) versus trabeculectomy (TLY): tonometric results. Rates of success (Kaplan-Meier method): IOP<20 mmHg

	NPDS (%)	TLY (%)
Without treatment[a]		
6 months	100	100
12 months	96	100
18 months	85	84
With medical treatment (monotherapy)		
6 months	100	100
12 months	100	100
18 months	100	91

[a] $n = 16$ eyes for NPDS without treatment. In all other cases, $n = 12$ eyes. All differences established between NPDS and TLY are statistically insignificant.

Table 3. Complications: non-penetrating deep sclerectomy (NPDS) versus trabeculectomy (TLY)

	NPDS Eyes (n)	TLY Eyes (n)
Hyphema	0	1
Shallow AC	0	2
Post. synechiae	0	1
Lens opacities	0	9
Choroidal detachment	0	2
Endophthalmitis	0	0

NPDS, non-penetrating deep sclerectomy; TLY, trabeculectomy.

treated with Nd-yttrium/aluminum garnet (Nd:YAG)-laser bursts (3–4 laser bursts, 6 mJ or 7 mJ for the opening of Descemet's membrane).
2. An external obstruction at the filtration bleb due to conjunctival fibrosis. It can be treated with injections of 5-fluorouracil (5-FU) into the bleb.

Discussion

In this new type of surgery, both negative and positive aspects can be observed. Some questions still remain.

The Positive Aspects

From a tonometric point of view, this procedure is effective; more than 80 % of eyes are well controlled after 18 months. The second positive aspect is the absence of the postoperative complications usually encountered in the course of trabeculectomy, in particular the absence of inflammatory reactions and the absence of any reaction to the collagen drain.

The patient retains pre-operative visual acuity and does not require a dressing on the eye, with an excellent post-operative quality of life. The filtration bleb has the same appearance as that observed after trabeculectomy.

The Negative Aspects

The success rate for NPDS appears to be slightly lower than that for trabeculectomy reported in the literature over the same follow-up period (70–85 %), and was 100 % for Migdal, although the latter was a prospective study. The difficulty of the technique constitutes a second negative aspect. It requires a fairly long training period and very-high-performance diamond knives.

The recurrence of hypertonia is variable both during the first few days and after a few months. It is unpredictable and requires close and regular monitoring. The recurrence of hypertonia may be linked to an internal obstacle. It is the result of two mechanisms:

1. Insufficient filtration through the trabeculo-descemetic plane; it may be caused by a technical error if the sclerectomy was not deep enough. It may also be the result of a poor-quality filtration membrane.
2. Contact between the iris and the filtration site. This phenomenon occurs when filtration is active and the iridocorneal angle is narrow. This is why closed-angle glaucoma, goniosynechia and, in general, narrow-angles, are a contraindication to the method unless iridoplasty can be conducted before surgery and miotic agents can be instilled after surgery for three or four weeks.

An external obstacle is the second cause of failure. NPDS is filtering surgery, in which the filtration bleb may be subject to fibroblast infiltration. Needling with injection of 5-FU into the bleb may reduce fibroblast infiltration.

Questions That Still Remain

The actual mechanism of filtration through the trabeculo-descemetic plane is, in fact, still unknown. Collapse of Schlemm's canal may be involved. It is worth noting that when the wall is stripped, the aqueous humor rises. This spurting of the aqueous humor may, however, come from the opened lateral extremities of the canal. The cribriform trabeculum and the internal wall of Schlemm's canal may also be included in the dissection.

The value of filtration through Descemet's membrane is, a priori, arguable, due to its role as a physiological barrier. Histological studies are necessary. In any event, thinning of the juxta-limbic cornea up to the descemetic plane enables goniopuncture to be conducted at this level using a Nd-YAG laser.

The same problem is posed regarding the role of the uveal trabeculum, to which the Russian authors attach great importance. In any event, a further problem is the determination of whether the collagen implant is really of use in the filtration of aqueous humor. A retrospective study, comparing the results of NPDS with or without collagen drain, does not demonstrate any significant difference. In any event, long-term results are vital.

Conclusion

NPDS with or without a collagen implant is a filtering technique which is subject to the same risk of fibroblast infiltration. It has the enormous advantage of giving rise to practically no complications. It is technically difficult to conduct and requires a wide angle. The level of IOP obtained was slightly higher than that obtained via a trabeculectomy.

References

Demailly P, Jeanteur-Lunel MN, Berkani M, Nouri-Madhavi K, Ecoffet M, Kopel J, Kretz G, Lavat P, Valtot F (1995) Sclérectomie profonde non perforante associée à la pose d'un implant de collagène dans le glaucome primitif à angle ouvert. Résultats rétrospectifs à court terme. Ophtalmologie 9:666–670

Demailly P, Jeanteur-Lunel MN, Berkani M, Ecoffet M, Kopel J, Kretz G, Lavat P (1996) La sclérectomie profonde non perforante associée à la pose d'un implant de collagène dans le glaucome primitif à angle ouvert. Résultats rétrospectifs à moyen terme. J Fr Ophtalmol 19:659–666

Demailly P, Lavat P, Kretz G, Jeanteur-Lunel MN (1997) Non-penetrating deep sclerectomy (NPDS) with or without collagen device (CD) in primary open-angle glaucoma. Middle-term retrospective study. Int Ophthalmol 20:131–140

Kozlov VI, Bagrov SN, Anisimova SY, Osipov AV, Mogilevtsev VV (1990) Non penetrating deep sclerectomy with collagen, IRTC "Eye Microsurgery" 3. RSFSR Ministry of Public Health, Moscow, pp 44–46

Zimmerman TJ, Kooner KS, Ford VJ, Olander KW, Mandlekorn RM, Rawlings EF, Leader BJ, Koskan AJ (1984) Trabeculectomy vs. non penetrating trabeculectomy. A retrospective study of two procedures in phakic patients with glaucoma. Ophthalmic Surg 15:734–740

Surgery III

A Retrospective Analysis of the Incidence of Endophthalmitis in Eyes with Chronic Bleb Leaks

A. Gemperli · G. Nelson · J. T. Wilensky

Introduction

Bleb leaks are a known risk factor for late, bleb-related endophthalmitis [1]. The route of infection is thought to involve migration of organisms through the bleb wall. The risk of this occurring increases when a leak is present, affording a focal transconjunctival passage. Many techniques have been developed to repair bleb leaks, including use of bandage contact lenses, autologous blood injection, fibrin tissue glue, and surgical bleb revision [2]. Some leaks, however, may persist in spite of several attempts at repair. Furthermore, some patients may refuse further intervention. For these reasons, some eyes may have bleb leaks that persist for months or years.

There is an extensive literature on bleb leaks and their association with endophthalmitis. Various investigators have explored the most common offending organisms, predisposing factors for endophthalmitis, and visual outcomes [1, 3–6]. Much attention has been given to different methods of repairing leaks. However, no one has reported the actual incidence of endophthalmitis in patients with chronic bleb leaks or whether chronic antibiotic administration is effective in protecting eyes from infection. This study investigates the incidence of endophthalmitis in a group of patients with long-term chronic bleb leaks.

Methods

We identified 21 patients being treated at the University of Illinois Eye and Ear Infirmary who had chronic bleb leaks in 22 eyes. Their records were reviewed, and the following information was obtained: type of filtering surgery, whether antimetabolites were used as an adjunct to surgery, methods used to treat the bleb leak and whether they were successful, duration of the bleb leak, whether topical antibiotics were used and, if so, which ones, whether the eye became infected, and visual outcome.

Results

Eight of the patients were female and 13 were male. None of the patients had shallow anterior chambers, choroidal effusions, or maculopathy resulting from the leaks. Three filtering procedures were repeat trabeculectomies, 13 were primary trabeculectomies, and 6 were full-thickness procedures. Mitomycin C was used in three of the

Table 1. Prophylactic topical antibiotics used by patients

Topical antibiotic	No. of eyes
Polytrim	4
Ciloxan	8
Ocuflox	5
Tobrex	2
Sulfa	1
Gentamicin	1

primary trabeculectomies, while 5-fluorouracil (5-FU) was used in two of the primary trabeculectomies, the three repeat trabeculectomies, and one of the full-thickness procedures. Eleven of the bleb leaks were successfully treated or stopped spontaneously, while the other 11 have continued to leak. Twenty-one eyes were placed on prophylactic antibiotics. The antibiotics initially used are listed in Table 1, although in many eyes the antibiotic was changed or rotated periodically. The methods used in an attempt to control the bleb leaks are listed in Table 2. The bleb leaks in all eyes were present for an average of 37.4 months.

Four of 22 (18 %) eyes with chronic bleb leaks developed endophthalmitis. Prophylactic topical antibiotics were being used in all four cases when the infection occurred. Endophthalmitis developed an average of 20 months after the bleb leak was discovered. Visual results in the infected eyes were poor. One patient maintained his preoperative 20/40 level of vision. The second patient's vision dropped from 20/40 to count fingers (CF) at 4 feet. The third and fourth patients' acuities fell from 20/40 and 20/70, respectively, to no light perception. Culture results were available on two of the infected eyes. One grew α-hemolytic *Streptococcus* from a vitreous culture, while a second eye grew *Hemophilus* influenza.

We compared the average intraocular pressure (IOP) during the time of the bleb leak for eyes that developed endophthalmitis with the IOP for those that did not. The average IOP in the group that developed endophthalmitis was 10.3 mmHg; the average IOP in the group that did not develop endophthalmitis was 9.3 mmHg.

Discussion

Of the eyes with chronic bleb leaks in our series, 18 % developed endophthalmitis. As a result of this complication, two of these patients completely lost vision in what had been their better eye, while a third eye dropped to CF vision. The import of such infections is clearly major.

When confronted with a bleb leak, most physicians will start treatment with prophylactic antibiotics to hopefully protect against endophthalmitis, although previous reports have indicated that prophylactic antibiotics cannot always prevent infection. In a study evaluating initial filtering surgery, Lamping and coworkers noted that, of four eyes that developed bleb infections, all but one were on chronic topical antibiotics [7]. Also, in the endophthalmitis vitrectomy study, topical povidone-iodine had been administered before cataract surgery in 40.3 % of the study patients (who all developed endophthalmitis), and antibiotics had been administered in the cataract-infusion fluid in 11.5 % of these patients [8]. All four eyes that developed endophthal-

Table 2. Clinical course of patients

Patient	Filter	Antime-tabolite	Date leak noted	Date leak stopped	Intervention	Antibiotic	Endophthal-mitis?	Vision
R.D.	Trab (1989)	No	July 1991	July 1994	Patching, glue, collagen shield, Simmons shell	Tobrex	No	20/100
C.B.	Trab (1985)	No	February, 1990	January 1992	Krupin implant after vitrectomy stopped leak	Sulfa	Yes (1/92)	20/40
S.G.	Trab (1992)	MMC	June 1996, still leaking		Needled 94	Gentamicin	Yes (7/97)	NLP
A.K.	FTF (1986)	No	February, 1991	May 1994	Patch, bleb revised (successful)	Polytrim	No	20/400
P.P.	FTF (1992)	No	January 1993, still leaking		Bandage lens	Ciloxan	No	20/30
M.L.	Trab (1987)	5-FU	November 1987, still leaking		Needled	Ocuflox	No	10/160
W.A.	FTF (1990)	No	October 1991	February 1992	Revised (successful)	Polytrim	No	20/30
L.W. (OS)	PPA FTF (1992)	No	March 1993, still leaking		Patch, glue × 2	Ocuflox	No	20/50
S.J.	Inferior FTF (1988)	5-FU	March 1989, still leaking		Argon laser conjunctival flap	Ciloxan	No	20/400
J.P.	Trab (1994)	Unknown	January 1995, still leaking		Conjunctival flap × 2, autologous blood injection × 2	Ciloxan	No	20/30
M.R.	Trab (1992)	5-FU	September, 1993	April 1994	Patched, Simmons shell	Citoxan	No	
J.J.	Trab (1993)	5-FU	November, 1993	June 1996	Needled (successful)	Ciloxan	No	CF 5 feet
V.C.	Trab (1993)	5-FU	February 1997, still leaking		Needled, comp. suture	Ocuflox	No	20/140
D.K.	Trab (1985)	No	November 1991, still leaking		Patching	None	No	NLP
M.D.	FTF (1990)	No	April 1990	October 1991	Patching, lubricants	Tobrex	No	20/25
L.B.	Trab (1988)	No	August–October 1991; 1997, still leaking-int.		Patching, lubricants, comp. suture	Ocuflox	No	
S.K.	Trab (1993)	?	1994	1995	Contact lens, bleb revision (successful)	Polytrim	No	
W.T.	Trab (1988)	No	August 1996	February 1997	Autologous blood injection (initially successful)	Polytrim	Yes (2/97)	NLP
D.W.	Trab (1992)	5-FU	February 1993	October 1995	Fibrin glue, conjunctival flap	Cifoxan	Yes (10/95)	CF 4 feet
L.W. (OD)	Trab (1989)	No	January 1996, still leaking-int.		None	Ocuflox	No	
J.B.	Trab (1991)	MMC	January 1993	June 1997	Revised (successful)	Cifoxan	No	CF
M.C.	Trab (1991)	MMC	October 1996, still leaking-int.		Patch	Ciloxan	No	20/25

OS, left eye; OD, right eye; PPA, pars planar approach; Trab, trabeculectomy; FTF, full-thickness filter; 5-FU, 5-fluorouracil; MMC, mitomycin C; NLP, no light perception; CF, count fingers.

mitis in this study did so while on topical antibiotics. Whether the rate of endophthalmitis would be higher without the use of prophylactic antibiotics is unknown, as this has not been studied. Our results reinforce the position that one cannot rely on prophylactic topical antibiotics to protect eyes with chronic bleb leaks against the occurrence of bacterial endophthalmitis.

One might hypothesize that more significant leaks would lead to a greater risk of bleb infection. Assuming that larger leaks would correlate with a lower IOP, the quantity of leakage did not affect the risk of endophthalmitis in this group. The average IOP during the time of the bleb leak for the endophthalmitis group (10.3 mmHg) was slightly higher than that for the group that did not develop endophthalmitis (9.3 mmHg). This indicates that the eyes that developed endophthalmitis did not have larger leaks than the other eyes in the study.

Some studies have indicated that antimetabolite use leads to a higher rate of late bleb leaks [9]. Similarly, studies investigating the rate of endophthalmitis in various filtering procedures have indicated that there is a higher rate when antimetabolites [1, 5] are used. The incidence of endophthalmitis for trabeculectomy without an antimetabolite has been reported as 0.1–1.5 %. Wolner et. al. [1] reported bleb-related endophthalmitis in 3.0 % of eyes following superiorly placed trabeculectomies with 5-FU. In other studies, the incidence of endophthalmitis following superior filters with mitomycin C was reported as 1.1–1.6 %. Inferiorly located trabeculectomies with antimetabolites have a greater incidence of endophthalmitis: 9.4 % when 5-FU was used and 7.8–8 % with mitomycin C [5, 6]. Antimetabolites did not appear to significantly increase the risk of developing endophthalmitis in our group. An antimetabolite has been used in 9 of the 22 (41 %) eyes that later developed leaking blebs. In the four eyes that did develop endophthalmitis, half had received an antimetabolite; mitomycin C was used in one case and 5-FU was used in the other.

In summary, 4 of 22 eyes with chronic bleb leaks eventually developed endophthalmitis. Three of the four patients became legally blind following the bout of endophthalmitis. All four patients were on chronic topical antibiotic therapy at the time they developed the infection. This study indicates that chronic bleb leaks are an important risk factor for endophthalmitis and visual loss. Even if the leak is small and there are no complications from hypotony, bleb repair should be attempted promptly. When initial attempts fail, other methods should be used to try to stop the leak. Administration of topical antibiotics cannot prevent the occurrence of endophthalmitis in this population.

Acknowledgement. Supported in part by an unrestricted grant from Research to Prevent Blindness, Inc., New York, N.Y. and the Carson Gabriel Fund.

References

1. Wolner B, Liebmann JM, Sassani JW, et al. (1991) Late bleb-related endophthalmitis after trabeculectomy with adjunctive 5-fluorouracil. Ophthalmology 98:1053–1060
2. Asrani SG, Wilensky JT (1996) Management of bleb leaks after glaucoma filtering surgery: use of autologous fibrin tissue glue as an alternative. Ophthalmology 103:294–298
3. Mandelbaum S, Forster RK, Gelend H, et al. (1985) Late onset endophthalmitis associated with filtering blebs. Ophthalmology 92:964–972

4. Ciulla TA, Beck AD, Topping TM, et al. (1997) Blebitis, early endophthalmitis IPO late endophthalmitis after glaucoma-filtering surgery. Ophthalmology 104:986–995
5. Higginbotham EJ, Stevens, RK, Musch DC, et al. (1996) Bleb-related andophthalmitis after trabeculectomy with mitomycin C. Ophthalmology 103:650–656
6. Greenfield DS, Suner IJ, Miller MP, et al. (1996) Endophthalmitis after filtering surgery with mitomycin. Arch Ophthalmol 114:943–949
7. Lamping KA, Bellows AR, Hutchinson BT, et al. (1986) Long term evaluation of initial filtration surgery. Ophthalmology 93:91–101
8. Endophthalmitis Vitrectomy Study Group (1995) Results of the endophthalmitis vitrectomy study: a randomized trial of immediate vitrectomy and of intravenous antibiotics for the treatment of postoperative bacterial endophthalmitis. Arch Ophthalmol 113:1479–1496
9. Parrish R, Minckler D (1996) "Late endophthalmitis" - filtering surgery time bomb? Ophthalmology 103:1167–1168

Retinectomy Lowers Intraocular Pressure in Otherwise Intractable Glaucoma. Long-Term Follow-Up

B. Kirchhof · K.-U. Bartz-Schmidt · G. K. Krieglstein · K. Heimann

Introduction

Treatment of glaucoma that is unresponsive to conventional therapy has, until recently, been singularly disappointing. Treatment options for intractable glaucomas fall into two groups: those reducing aqueous production and those enhancing aqueous outflow. Cyclodestructive procedures have a high rate of serious complications, which include visual loss, phthisis (especially in eyes with neovascular glaucoma), severe pain and inflammation, and transient postoperative intraocular pressure (IOP) elevation that, at times, can be profound. Conventional filtration procedures are disappointing for three reasons: early hypotony often leads to choroidal detachment, continuing proliferation of fibrovascular tissue invariably blocks off the internal opening of the fistula and bleb fibrosis causes similar obstruction to the external opening of the fistula. Antiproliferative drugs are applied to inhibit excessive scarring after filtration surgery.

Preliminary results suggested that eliminating the retinal barrier to facilitate transit of aqueous humor from the vitreous to the choroid may be suitable as a therapeutic tool for decreasing IOP. Experimental evidence for this hypothesis has been shown previously [1, 2]. Since increased IOP is only due to abnormal resistance to drainage, while aqueous flow is largely constant and independent of the current IOP, one size of retinectomy – the size that establishes normal fluid conductance – should normalize different IOPs.

Retinectomy could be advantageous over conventional filtration procedures, since a retinal hole is not at risk of closing by wound healing. This report is concerned with long-term follow-up of retinectomy in patients with refractive glaucoma of manyfold etiologies.

Patients and Methods

Due to their unfavorable prognosis by a conventional treatment regimen, 45 eyes (42 patients) were recruited from the Glaucoma Service of the Department of Ophthalmology, University of Cologne. Patients selected for retinectomy had various forms of glaucoma and had uncontrolled IOP, despite maximum tolerable medical therapy and conventional surgery when applicable (Table 1). Most eyes were painful and their visual acuity was between legal blindness and 20/20 [37 of 45 eyes ranged between 20/200 and no perception of light (NL)]. The goal of retinectomy was to normalize IOP,

Table 1. Patients selected for retinectomy had various forms of glaucoma and had uncontrolled intraocular pressure

Type of glaucoma	No. of eyes	Patient age min/max/ median (years)	Follow-up time min/max/ median	Preoperative topical antiglaucoma medication (% of column 2)	Preoperative systemic medication (carboanhydrase inhibitors) in % of column 2	Postoperative topical antiglaucoma medication (% of column 2)	Postoperative systemic medication (carboanhydrase inhibitors) (% of column 2)
Neovascular (diabetes, CVO)	7	26/80/57	93/1180/796	5/7	6/7	10/7	1/7
Juvenile	3	3/41/4	96/315/144	3/3	1/3	0/3	0/3
Trauma	4	14/86/30	98/1568/661	2/4	1/4	2/4	1/4
Congenital cataract	12	8/31/14	188/1186/708	18/12	5/12	12/12	1/12
Uveitis	8	11/59/29	94/1264/137	11/8	5/8	8/8	3/8
Others	11	27/65/43,5	96/1080/494	15/11	3/11	11/11	3/11
All patients	45	3/86/31	93/1568/530	54/45	21/45	43/45	9/45

to render additional medical therapy unnecessary and to preserve preexisting visual acuity. All patients gave informed consent regarding their treatment, describing retinectomy as a new investigative approach and cyclodestructive therapy, filtering procedures combined with chemotherapy or implants as the traditional approach. Advantages and disadvantages of each procedure were explained, and the patients were allowed to select between the treatments.

Preoperative evaluation included measurement of visual acuity, measurement of IOP, gonioscopy, anterior and posterior slit-lamp biomicroscopy, indirect ophthalmoscopy and ultrasonography when required. Patients were examined daily on days 1–7, thereafter weekly for 2 months, and at least once a month throughout the follow-up. Preoperative medications were discontinued. Topical antiglaucoma drugs as well as carboanhydrase inhibitors were applied for several weeks after surgery when needed.

All patients were operated on under general anesthesia. IOP was lowered to near normal values 30 min preoperatively by 125 ml i.v. mannitol 17 (Osmofundin 15 % N; Braun Melsungen, Melsungen, Germany) to reduce the risk of choroidal effusion following paracentesis. Vitrectomy was performed using the standard three-port technique under the operating-microscope control. Endophacoemulsification of the lens was applied to all eyes. If necessary, panretinal photocoagulation was performed, except on the area of the retina to be excised. The area selected for retinectomy was crescent-shaped and was located in the temporal or nasal-superior quadrant. The peripheral, convex border of the cut-out was delineated by the ora serrata over 2–3 clock hours. The concave border ran half the distance between *ora serrata* and the temporal or nasal vascular arcade.

Retinectomy was performed by first delineating the area to be excised by endodiathermy. The retina was then mobilized and excised by aspiration into the vitrectomy probe. The procedure was concluded by endolaser photocoagulation to the edge of the retinectomy and by either fluid gas or fluid-silicone-oil exchange.

In patients with active rubeosis, the procedure was modified to two steps: (1) vitrectomy and panretinal- and ciliary-body (270°) endolaserphotocoagulation; (2) retinectomy and fluid-gas exchange at the time of silicone-oil removal (when still necessary and only after rubeosis had regressed, usually about 2–3 months later). Recently, we united retinectomy, endolaserphotocoagulation and silicone-oil tamponade into one step.

Results

Preoperative IOP ranged from 20 mmHg to 61 mmHg (median 41 mmHg). Final postoperative IOP ranged from 4 mmHg to 50 mmHg (median 19 mmHg), representing a mean decrease in IOP of 19 ± 13 mmHg and a median decrease in IOP of 23 mmHg. All patients demonstrated a decrease in IOP, the smallest change being 4 mmHg and the largest being 53 mmHg. Immediate postoperative IOP after retinectomy and fluid-gas exchange was normal for 1–3 days, then rose to preoperative levels, sometimes requiring systemic medication for 1–2 weeks, when the IOP tapered off to normal with absorption of the gas tamponade. Immediate postoperative IOP after retinectomy with silicone-oil tamponade was usually normal. Without systemic medication, 64 % of eyes showed an IOP of less then 21 mmHg 1 year post-operation. Phthisis was observed in two patients. Four eyes developed hypotony. No intraoperative complications were observed. On the third postoperative day, one eye was complicated by a rupture (Ehlers-Danlos Syndrome). In one eye, the retina detached, resembling rhegmatogenous retinal detachment. Three eyes developed proliferative vitreoretinopathy (PVR), two with retinal detachment. In eyes complicated by PVR, usually children or juvenile patients, we did not succeed in inducing a posterior vitreous separation. The posterior hyaloid detached spontaneously 4 days to 6 weeks postoperation, often associated with retinal starfolds.

Discussion

The unsurpassed persistence of the pressure-lowering effect of retinectomy is best explained by the fact that a large retinal hole cannot close. Thus, once the retinal barrier to water transfer is irreversibly damaged, the regulation of IOP should be permanent. Hypotony following retinectomy was apparent within 2–3 months postoperation and was a complication of secondary retinal detachment. Otherwise, hypotony was observed in two patients below the age of 17 years. Correspondingly, persistent hypertonia was registered beyond the age of 75 years and after panretinal photocoagulation. These data led us to speculate that "posterior drainage" varies with choroidal perfusion. We therefore recommend a limit on the size of retinectomy in children to two clock hours of peripheral retina. In circumstances signaling poor choroidal perfusion, we suggest removal of four clock hours of peripheral retina. The size of retinectomy should not be adjusted to the preoperative IOP. Since IOP is only determined by resistance to aqueous outflow, and flow is largely the same with normal as with increased IOP, the size of retinectomy that reconstitutes normal fluid conductance regulates all elevated IOPs. We found that a retinectomy including half of one peripheral retinal quadrant reconstitutes normal fluid conductance in the adult.

Following the patients of our first communication for more than a year [3], we found that a retinectomy including two peripheral quadrants is at risk of hypotony. This is also true for eyes with active rubeosis and retinectomy with fluid-gas exchange. The clinical picture, then, was that of massive blood ocular-barrier breakdown and continuous fibro-vascular proliferation also on the ciliary body, leading to aqueous insufficiency and phthisis. To avoid this problem in the current study, retinectomy was only performed when there was either no rubeosis or regressed rubeosis. In eyes with active rubeosis, new-vessel formation was addressed first by retinal photocoagulation and silicone-vitreous tamponade. The silicone filling was performed because we have the impression that rubeosis regresses faster with silicone than without. However, we have no data to support this notion. We speculate that rapid regression of rubeosis is advantageous, because earlier stages of rubeosis may allow reopening of the trabecular meshwork, rendering rectinectomy unnecessary as in 91 % of our patients with neovascular glaucoma. Lately, we noted that retinectomy can be safely performed even with active rubeosis when the eyes are filled with silicone oil. Surprisingly, silicone oil did not reduce the pressure-lowering effect of retinectomy, possibly because the silicone bubble still allows aqueous humor to the retinectomy site even in the superior retinal circumference. Furthermore, silicone-filled eyes with retinectomy omit the transient postoperative pressure rise typical for retinectomy with fluid-gas exchange.

From our data we suggest the following surgical strategy for refractive glaucoma. If there is no rubeosis, then retinectomy and fluid-gas exchange is advised in a one-step procedure. If rubeosis is present, then retinectomy should be combined with a silicone-oil tamponade to prevent complications from blood ocular-barrier damage and also to avoid even a transient pressure rise. The most serious complication of retinectomy is PVR and retinal detachment, which is rare in conventional glaucoma surgery. However, comparing long-term functional results of retinectomy to conventional glaucoma surgery, we note that, despite surgical complications unusual for glaucoma patients, retinectomy is still advantageous. It appears to us that the risk of retinal detachment and PVR in conjunction with retinectomy coincides with inability to detach the posterior hyaloid, especially in children. In the future we hope to be able to reduce the incidence of retinal detachment by enzyme-assisted detachment of the hyaloid.

References

1. Kirchhof B, Ryan SJ (1993) Differential permeance of retina and retinal pigment epithelium to water: implications for retinal adhesion. Int Ophthalmol 17:19–22
2. Rezai KA, Kirchhof B, Heimann K (1995) Posterior drainage of intraocular fluid: an experimental approach on bovine cadaver eyes. Ger J Ophthalmol 4:275–278
3. Kirchhof B (1994) Retinectomy lowers intraocular pressure in otherwise intractable glaucoma: preliminary results. Ophthalmic Surg 25:262–267

5-Methylurapidil, 8-Iso Prostaglandin E_2: New Drugs to Increase Aqueous-Humor Outflow Facility

J. B. Serle · S. M. Podos · R.-F. Wang · T. Mittag · P.-Y. Lee · B. Becker

Abstract. *Purpose:* Although the trabecular meshwork is thought to be the primary site of pathology in open-angle glaucoma, drugs that improve trabecular outflow facility, such as pilocarpine and epinephrine, are increasingly being replaced by agents acting by other mechanisms. We have evaluated an α-adrenergic antagonist, 5-methylurapidil (5-MU), and a prostane analog, 8-iso prostaglandin E_2 (8-iso PGE_2), for their effects on intraocular pressure (IOP) and outflow facility in the monkey eye. *Methods:* Groups of normal monkeys and monkeys with unilateral laser-induced glaucoma ($n = 6$ or 8) were treated topically in one eye with two 25-μl doses of 2 % 5-MU or with a 25-μl dose of 0.1 % 8-iso PGE_2. *Results:* The maximum reduction of IOP in glaucomatous monkey eyes was 7.5 ± 0.8 mmHg (mean ± standard error of the mean) for 5-MU and 6.6 ± 0.8 mmHg for 8-iso PGE_2. For both drugs, the ocular hypotensive response increased over a 5-day period on a regimen of administration of the drug twice daily. Tonographic outflow facility determined in normal monkey eyes increased by 51 % ($p < 0.01$) 2 h after 5-MU and by 48 % ($p < 0.005$) 2 h after 8-iso PGE_2. *Conclusions:* A selective α_{1A}-adrenergic antagonist, 5-MU, and an isoprostane derivative, 8-iso PGE_2, lowered IOP in the normal and glaucomatous primate eye predominantly by increasing traditional outflow facility.

Introduction

Many adrenergic agents, either α- or β-agonists or antagonists, alter aqueous-humor dynamics by a variety of mechanisms; some of these adrenergic agents are clinically effective ocular hypotensive drugs. Pharmacological studies and molecular cloning have shown that there are a variety of adrenergic receptor (AR) subtypes. 5-methylurapidil (5-MU) is an α_{1A}-AR selective antagonist [1], and a potent 5-hydroxytryptamine $(5\text{-HT})_{1A}$ agonist [2]. Preliminary trials indicate that 5-MU lowers intraocular pressure (IOP) in rabbit and monkey eyes [3].

Several prostaglandin $F_{2\alpha}$ (PG) analogues and their prodrugs are potent ocular hypotensive agents. The mechanism by which these drugs lower IOP, primarily by increasing uveoscleral outflow, differentiates them from other agents used to treat glaucoma. PGE_2 is another prostaglandin derivative, which reduces IOP in normotensive human volunteers following topical application [4]. 8-iso prostaglandin E_2 (8-iso PGE_2), an isoprostane derivative, reduces IOP in rabbits and monkeys [5]. The purpose of this paper is to further document the effects of 5-methylurapidil and 8-iso PGE_2 on IOP in glaucomatous monkey eyes and to determine the mechanism by which these drugs reduce IOP in normal monkey eyes.

Materials and Methods

Female cynomolgus monkeys, each weighing 3–5 kg, were used in this study. In eight of the animals, glaucoma had been previously induced unilaterally by repeated argon-laser (65–120 spots; power 1.1–1.5 W; size 50 μm; duration 0.5 s) or diode-laser (60–120 spots; power 1.1–1.2 W; size 75 μm; duration 0.5 s) photocoagulation of the mid-trabecular meshwork for 360°.

The effect of 5-MU or 8-iso PGE_2 on IOP was measured using a calibrated pneumatonometer (Model 30 classic, Mentor, Norwell, Mass.) prior to drug administration (0 h), at 0.5 h, then hourly until 6 h after drug administration. One drop of 0.5 % proparacaine hydrochloride was applied topically 5 min prior to tonometry, and 1–5 mg/kg of ketamine hydrochloride was administered intramuscularly for adequate sedation. Slit-lamp examination was performed in a dark room prior to drug treatment and at 1, 3, and 5 h post-treatment.

5-MU (Research Biochemicals, Inc., Mass.) was freshly prepared as a 2 % (weight/volume) solution by dissolving in 0.1 M hydrochloric acid, followed by adjusting the pH to 7.0 with NaOH. 8-iso PGE_2 (Cayman Chemical Co., Mich.) was freshly prepared by dissolving in dimethylsulfoxide (100 mg/ml). This stock solution was further diluted with 0.9 % NaCl. A multiple-dose study of 5-MU was performed in seven unilaterally glaucomatous monkeys. A multiple-dose study of 8-iso PGE_2 was carried out in eight unilaterally glaucomatous monkeys. Following one baseline day (neither vehicle nor drug were administered) and one vehicle-treated day (50 μl vehicle to the glaucomatous eye at 9:30 a.m. and 3:30 p.m.), 2 % 5-MU or 8-iso PGE_2 was applied to the glaucomatous eye twice daily (at 9:30 a.m. and 3:30 p.m.) for five consecutive days. For statistical analysis, IOP on each of the five drug-treatment days was compared with that on the vehicle-treated day.

Mechanism studies of 2 % 5-MU and 0.1 % 8-iso PGE_2 were performed in normal monkeys. Outflow facility was measured using an electronic indentation tonograph (Alcon EDT-103, Fort Worth, Tex.) 4 h prior to dosing, and repeated at the peak IOP effect of the drugs; 1 h after unilateral dosing with 5-MU and 2 h after unilateral dosing with 8-iso PGE_2. Aqueous-humor flow measurements were performed using a scanning computerized fluorophotometer (Coherent Fluorotron, Coherent, Palo Alto, Calif.). Fluorescein was bilaterally iontophoresed into the corneas of each monkey for 7 min using 10 % fluorescein in 2 % agar gel at 4:00 p.m. on the day prior to aqueous-flow measurements. Baseline aqueous-humor flow rates were measured hourly for 4 h beginning at 9:30 a.m. The following day, flow measurements were performed at the same times as on the baseline day, beginning 1 h after drug administration. The washout period between each test on the same animal was at least 1 week.

The two-tailed paired *t*-test was used for statistical analysis before and after single-dose treatment, and the Bonferroni *t*-test was used for analysis of the multiple-dose study. The Pearson product-moment correlation coefficient was used to analyze the relationship between IOP and outflow facility. All experimental studies complied with the Association for Research in Vision and Ophthalmology Resolution on the Use of Animals in Research and were approved by the Mount Sinai School of Medicine Institutional Animal Care and Utilization Committee.

Results

5-Methylurapidil

5-MU induced maximum reductions in IOP ($p< 0.05$) (drug-treated compared with vehicle-treated values) in glaucomatous monkeys 1 h after application, and, on days 1 and 5, were 6.9 ± 1.3 mmHg and 15.1 ± 2.9 mmHg, respectively. Significant differences in IOP were not observed when comparing the baseline and vehicle-treated days. The ocular hypotensive effect of 5-MU increased with successive dosing (Fig. 1). Mild corneal edema was observed in one of seven drug-treated eyes on day 4, and not noted in any of the eyes on day 5. Mucous discharge was observed throughout the experiment in two animals during the 5-day treatment.

5-MU significantly increased outflow facility measured tonographically by 51 % ($p< 0.01$) in the treated eyes and by 16 % ($p> 0.10$) in the fellow eyes compared with baseline values. IOP was significantly ($p< 0.05$) reduced at 1 h in both eyes when measured tonographically. 5-MU increased aqueous-humor flow rates in eight normal monkeys 11 % ($p< 0.01$) over 4 h in the treated eyes, and 3 % ($p> 0.10$) in the fellow eyes compared with baseline values (Table 1).

8-Iso PGE_2

Enhancement of the magnitude and duration of the ocular hypotensive effect of 8-iso PGE_2 was observed with twice-daily administration for 5 days to eight glaucomatous monkey eyes. IOP was significantly ($p< 0.05$) reduced for 4 h after the first dose, and for 18 h after the sixth dose compared with the vehicle-treated day. The maximum reduction in IOP occurred 2 h after dosing and was 5.0 ± 0.3 mmHg on day 1 and 9.6 ± 0.6 mmHg on day 5, comparing drug-treated and vehicle-treated days (Fig. 2). IOPs on baseline and vehicle-treated days were similar ($p> 0.40$). Mild superficial punctate keratopathy (SPK) appeared in one eye after the fourth dose, and persisted thereafter. Mild conjunctival hyperemia and mucous discharge appeared in two eyes.

Two hours after unilateral application of 8-iso PGE_2 to six normal monkeys, tonographic outflow facility was increased ($p< 0.05$) by 48 % in the treated eyes compared with the contralateral vehicle-treated control eyes, and by 43 % compared with baseline measurements. IOP was reduced ($p< 0.05$) at 2 h in the drug-treated eyes when

Table 1. Effect of 2 % 5-methylurapidil on aqueous-humor dynamics in eight normal monkeys. Adapted from [3]

	Mean intraocular pressure (mmHg±SEM)	Mean outflow facility (μl/min/mmHg±SEM)	Mean aqueous-humor flow (μl/min±SEM)
Treated eyes	13.0±0.6*	0.68±0.10*	1.88±0.21
Baseline	16.0±0.7	0.45±0.04	1.89±0.13
Fellow eyes	12.8±0.6*	0.59±0.06	2.01±0.13
Baseline	14.9±0.5	0.51±0.06	1.94±0.16

* Significantly different compared with baseline measurement (two-tailed paired t-test, $p< 0.05$).

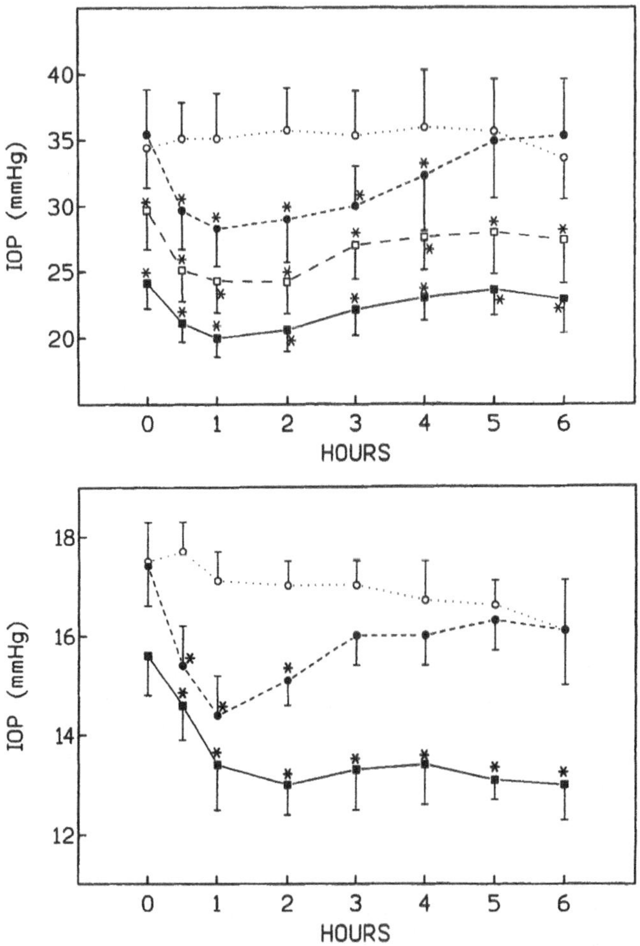

Fig. 1. a Effects on intraocular pressure (IOP) of administration of 2% 5-methylurapidil (5-MU) to eyes with glaucoma twice-daily for 5 days in seven unilaterally glaucomatous monkeys. Points represent means of the IOP on vehicle-treated day (*open circles*), or on days 1 (*closed circles*), 3 (*open squares*), and 5 (*closed squares*) of treatment. *Bars* indicate ± standard error of the mean (SEM). *Asterisks* indicate statistically significant reduction in IOP compared with vehicle-treated values (two-tailed Bonferroni *t*-test, $p < 0.05$). **b** Effects on IOP of the contralateral non-glaucomatous eyes of twice daily administration of 2% 5-MU for five successive days to the eyes with glaucoma in seven unilateral glaucomatous monkeys. Points represent means of the IOP on vehicle-treated day (*open circles*), or on days 1 (*closed circles*) or 5 (*closed squares*) of treatment. *Bars* indicate ± SEM. *Asterisks* indicate statistically significant reduction in IOP compared with vehicle-treated values (two-tailed Bonferroni *t*-test, $p < 0.05$)

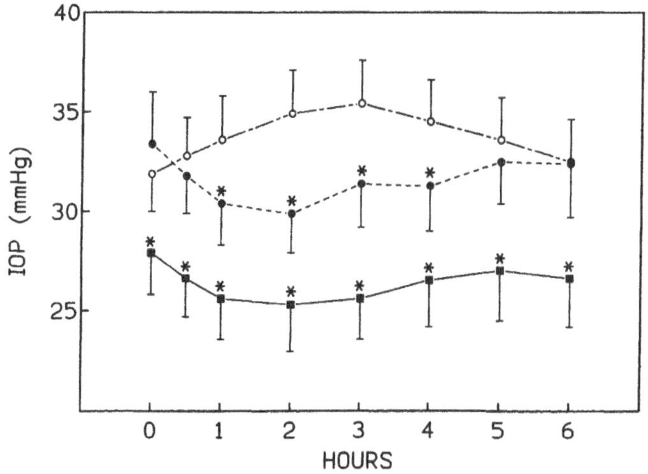

Fig. 2. Effects on intraocular pressure (IOP) of administration of 0.1 % 8-iso prostaglandin E_2 twice-daily to eight unilaterally glaucomatous monkeys for 5 days. Points represent means of the IOP on vehicle-treated day (*open circles*) or on days 1 (*closed circles*) or 5 (*closed squares*) of treatment. The *bars* indicate ± standard error of the mean. *Asterisk* indicates statistically significant reduction in IOP of treated eye with glaucoma compared with vehicle-treated control-day values (two-tailed Bonferroni *t*-test, $p < 0.05$)

Table 2. Effect of 0.1 % 8-iso prostaglandin E2 (PGE_2) on aqueous-humor dynamics in six normal monkeys. Adapted from [5]

	Mean intraocular pressure (mmHg±SEM)	Mean outflow facility (µl/min/mmHg±SEM)	Mean aqueous-humor flow (µl/min±SEM)
Treated eyes	13.0±0.7*	0.83±0.10*	1.88±0.21
Baseline	16.3±1.1	0.58±0.03	1.69±0.29
Fellow eyes	15.7±0.5	0.56±0.06	1.78±0.22
Baseline	15.7±0.6	0.51±0.04	2.01±0.21

* Significantly different compared with either baseline values or contralateral vehicle-treated control eyes (two-tailed paired *t*-test, $p < 0.05$).

measured tonographically (Table 2). A significant correlation was found between the IOP reduction and the increase of outflow facility ($R = 0.81$, $p < 0.05$). The coefficient of determination ($R^2 = 0.66$) indicated that the increase in outflow facility accounted for the majority of the IOP reduction in these normal monkey eyes. Aqueous-humor flow rates were unchanged ($p > 0.10$) for 4 h following single application of 8-iso PGE_2 to the treated eyes of six normal monkeys, compared with baseline values or contralateral control vehicle-treated eyes (Table 2).

Discussion

5-MU is an α_{1A}-adrenergic receptor antagonist and 5-HT_{1A}-receptor agonist. In normal monkeys, the selective 5-HT_{1A} receptor antagonist, 4-(methoxyphenyl)-1-[2'-(*n*-2"-pyridinyl)-*p*-iodobenzamido]-ethyl-piperazine hydrochloride, does not alter the IOP-reducing effects of 5-MU [6]. This suggests that the α_{1A}-adrenergic receptor antagonism of 5-MU is responsible for the effects of this drug on aqueous-humor dynamics. 5-MU has effects on aqueous humor dynamics that are quite different from those of previously studied α-receptor blockers. By increasing trabecular outflow facility, 5-MU reduces IOP. Thymoxamine, prazosin and corynanthine are three other α_1-adrenergic antagonists that do not alter outflow facility. Repetitive dosing with 5-MU produces enhancement of the ocular hypotensive effect in monkey eyes. Repetitive dosing with corynanthine produces tachyphylaxis [7]. In this study, 5-MU induces mild ocular side effects. Further studies on this type of drug are warranted, as they are potential anti-glaucoma agents.

Single-dose administration of PGE_2 to rabbits and normotensive volunteers causes ocular hypertension followed by reductions in IOP [4]. In contrast, ocular hypertension is not observed in monkeys treated with 8-iso PGE_2. Repetitive dosing with 8-iso PGE_2 for 5 days produces enhancement of the ocular hypotensive effect. The mechanism by which 8-iso PGE_2 reduces IOP differentiates it from $PGF_{2\alpha}$ and its derivatives. 8-iso PGE_2 increases tonographic outflow facility by 48 % in monkeys. Laboratory and clinical trials demonstrate only small increases in tonographically measured outflow facility following topical administration of $PGF_{2\alpha}$-isopropyl ester [7] and PhXA34. In isolated human anterior-segment preparations, in which only trabecular outflow facility is measured, PGE_2 [8] – but not $PGF_{2\alpha}$ [9] – increases outflow facility. Mild ocular side effects are noted in some monkey eyes following application of 8-iso PGE_2. Changes in the formulation may reduce or eliminate these adverse effects. The isoprostanes have great potential as ocular hypotensive agents.

Acknowledgements. Supported in part by a grant, EY01867, from the National Institutes of Health, Bethesda, MD, and an unrestricted grant (SMP) from Research to Prevent Blindness, Inc., New York, NY.

References

1. Gross G, Hanft G,Rugevics C (1989) 5-methylurapidil discriminates between subtypes of the α_{1A}-adrenoceptor. Eur J Pharmacol 151:333–335
2. Hoyer D, Clarke DE, Fozard JR, Hartig PR, Martin GR, Mylechrane EJ, Saxena PR, Humphrey PPA (1984) International union of pharmacology classification of receptors for 5-hydroxytryptamine (serotonin). VII. Pharmacol Rev 46:157–203
3. Wang RF, Lee PY, Mittag TW, Podos SM, Serle JB (1997) Effect of 5-methylurapidil, an α_{1A}-adrenergic antagonist and 5-hydroxytryptamine$_{1A}$ agonist, on aqueous humor dynamics in monkeys and rabbits. Curr Eye Res 16:769–775
4. Flach AJ, Eliason JA (1988) Topical prostaglandin E_2 on normal human intraocular pressure. J Ocul Pharmacol 4:13–18
5. Wang RF, Lee PY, Mittag TW, Podos SM, Serle JB, Becker B (1999) Effect of 8-iso prostaglandin E_2 on aqueous humor dynamics in monkeys. Arch Ophthalmol 116:1213–1216
6. Wang RF, Mittag T, Podos SM, Serle JB (1998) Effect of p-MPPI hydrochloride (p-MPPI) applied before 5-methylurapidil (5-MU) on intraocular pressure (IOP) in normal monkeys. Invest Ophthalmol 39[Suppl 488]:2236

7. Serle JB, Podos SM, Lustgarten JS, Teitlebaum C, Severin CH (1985) The effect of corynanthine on intraocular pressure in clinical trials. Ophthalmology 92:977–980
8. Toris CB, Camras CB, Yablonski ME, Brubaker RF (1997) Effects of exogenous prostaglandins on aqueous humor dynamics and blood aqueous barrier function. Surv Ophthalmol 41 [Suppl 2]:S69–S75
9. Gabelt BT, Kaufman PL (1990) The effect of prostaglandin on trabecular outflow facility in cynomologus monkeys. Exp Eye Res 51:87–91

Aqueous Shunting Procedures Versus Trabeculectomy with Antimetabolites for Surgical Control of Glaucoma: An (International?) Clinical Trial

R. K. Parrish II · S. J. Gedde · D. K. Heuer

Introduction

Glaucoma filtering surgery has changed over the past few decades. Trabeculectomy replaced full-thickness procedures when it became clear that a similar success rate could be achieved with a lower rate of complications. Antimetabolites, like as 5-fluorouracil and mitomycin C, were subsequently introduced and improved the success of trabeculectomy [1]. Clinical practice, as determined in a written survey of members of the American Glaucoma Society by Chen et al. in 1997, identified a preference of 77 % for use of an antimetabolite in patients undergoing first-time trabeculectomy [2]. A growing consensus has developed within the North American ophthalmic community that, although antimetabolite trabeculectomies have increased the likelihood of intraocular pressure control, the intermediate- and long-term complications associated with the resultant perilimbal filtering blebs warrant consideration of alternatives. Favorable results have been observed with aqueous shunting procedures (ASP) in the treatment of refractory glaucomas [3, 4]. Comparable complication rates have been reported for ASP and trabeculectomy with antimetabolites [5]. The efficacy and safety of ASP suggests that they may be an appropriate alternative to antimetabolite trabeculectomy. We propose a randomized prospective clinical trial comparing the long-term safety and efficacy of ASP and trabeculectomy with antimetabolites for surgical control of glaucoma.

Proposed Methodology

Patient inclusion and exclusion criteria for the study are listed in Table 1. All patients on tolerated medical therapy with uncontrolled glaucoma and intraocular pressure greater than 21 mmHg would be invited to participate in the study, as long as none of the exclusion criteria were met. Patients with two eligible eyes would undergo randomly determined treatment in the first eye and assignment to the other surgical procedure in the fellow eye.

Patients less than 18 years old or greater than 80 years old would be excluded. Those unwilling or unable to give consent, to accept randomization, or to return for protocol visits would be excluded. Patients unwilling to discontinue contact-lens use permanently after surgery would be excluded. Eyes unable to perceive light, as well as eyes with iris neovascularization, the iridocorneal endothelial syndrome, aphakia (without pseudophakia), or uveitis would be excluded. Eyes that had undergone a

Table 1. Inclusion and exclusion criteria

Inclusion criteria
Uncontrolled glaucoma
Intraocular pressure > 21 mmHg on tolerated medical therapy
Exclusion criteria
Age < 18 years or > 80 years
Unwilling or unable to give consent, unwilling to accept randomization, or unable to return for protocol visits
Unwilling to discontinue contact lens use after surgery
No light perception
Iris neovascularization
Iridocorneal endothelial syndrome
Aphakia (without pseudophakia)
Uveitis
Previous scleral buckling procedure or cyclodestructive procedure
Limbal conjunctival scarring precluding trabeculectomy
Filtering surgery combined with other ocular procedures

scleral buckling procedure or cyclodestructive procedure, or with limbal conjunctival scarring precluding trabeculectomy would be excluded. Patients with eyes undergoing glaucoma filtering surgery alone would be offered to enroll in the study, whereas those undergoing filtering surgery combined with other ocular procedures (such as cataract extraction, penetrating keratoplasty, or retinal surgery) would be excluded.

All participating clinical centers would require local Institutional Review Board approval prior to patient recruitment. After obtaining informed consent, patients would be randomized to undergo trabeculectomy with either antimetabolite or ASP. A trabeculectomy would be performed in a superior quadrant in all patients, using a limbal-based conjunctival flap when possible. The choice of antimetabolite (5-fluorouracil or mitomycin C), duration of antimetabolite exposure, dimensions of the scleral flap, size of the inner block, number of scleral flap sutures, and suture tension would be determined by means of the surgeon's usual practice. Shunt equatorial explants would be placed in the superotemporal quadrant, except in the case of double-plate Molteno implants, which would use both superior quadrants. The method of tube occlusion with non-valved implants would be left to the discretion of the surgeon.

Baseline characteristics of the study population would be tabulated for each treatment group, including age, gender, race, type of glaucoma, number of previous incisional surgeries, and number of ocular medications. Outcome variables to be investigated are shown in Table 2. Outcome discrimination between the two groups would include typical measures of visual function (visual acuity and visual field), intraocular pressure control, glaucoma reoperations, and quality-of-life determination using standardized instruments. Emphasis would also be placed on complication rates, such as bleb leaks determined by Seidel testing, hypotony, bleb dysesthesia, endophthalmitis, cataract, corneal edema, diplopia, and shunt erosion. Sample size calculations would be determined based on predicted rates of successful visual-function outcomes, as well as on complication rates.

Table 2. Outcome variables

Visual acuity
Visual field
Intraocular pressure control
Glaucoma reoperations
Quality of life
Complications (bleb leaks, hypotony, bleb dysesthesia, endophthalmitis, cataract, corneal edema, diplopia, shunt erosion)

Comments

The proposed clinical trial was discussed in the closed meeting of the Glaucoma Society of the International Congress of Ophthalmology held in Edinburgh, Scotland, 18 June 1998. Dr. George L. Spaeth, Philadelphia, USA, commented that the rate of change of both filtering surgery and ASP was too rapid to determine a specific operation that would likely be the procedure of choice at the completion of the clinical trial. It was pointed out that presentations by French investigators regarding deep sclerectomy, with or without collagen implants, challenge the traditional notion of corneoscleral limbal filtration with conjunctival filtering blebs. If this operation, in which the intraocular-pressure-lowering effect does not depend on bleb formation, were to supplant trabeculectomy, then the amount of concern about late-onset wound-leak and bleb infection would be much lower.

Professor Yoshiaki Kitazawa of Gifu, Japan, described the inaccessibility of drainage implants in Japan and the fact that the importation of the devices did not currently enjoy a defined legal status. The unavailability of commercial drainage implants would effectively preclude participation in the proposed clinical trial in Japan.

Dr. Ivan Goldberg of Sydney, Australia, voiced concern over the relative importance of the scientific question posed. The widespread use of antimetabolites in initial filtering surgery, 77 % as demonstrated in a survey of the members of the American Glaucoma Society in 1997 by Chen et al. [2], did not reflect the past or current practice pattern in Australia. Use of mitomycin C is reserved for filtering surgery in patients with poor prognoses, and 5-FU has been employed as an intraoperative adjunct treatment of those patients with somewhat less than the usual good prognosis. Currently, no large-scale patient populations at risk to develop late-onset wound leaks or endophthalmitis exist in Australia.

The concluding remarks suggested that the scientific question regarding late-onset complications may be important and relevant to a highly specific group of patients who largely reside in the United States. Although the consensus of the group strongly favored clinical-trial methodology to define the risks and benefits of new treatments for glaucoma, the general opinion was expressed that this question should be studied in the United States and possibly Canada, where the information is most relevant.

References

1. The Fluorouracil Filtering Surgery Study Group (1996) Five-year follow-up of the Fluorouracil Filtering Surgery Study. Am J Ophthalmol 121:349–366
2. Chen PP, Yamamoto T, Sawada A, et al. (1997) Use of antifibrosis agents and glaucoma drainage devices in the American and Japanese Glaucoma Societies. J Glaucoma 6:192–196
3. Lieberman MF, Ewing RH (1990) Drainage implant surgery for refractory glaucoma. Int Ophthalmol Clin 30:198–208
4. Smith MF, Doyle JW, Sherwood MB (1995) Comparison of the Baerveldt glaucoma implant with the double-plate Molteno drainage implant. Arch Ophthalmol 113:444–447
5. Nguyen QH, Budenz DL, Parrish RK (1998) Complications of Baerveldt glaucoma drainage implants. Arch Ophthalmol 116:571–575

CHAPTER 41

Can Our Patients Afford Our Skepticism?

H. D. Hoskins

Introduction

In every country, the cost of health care continues to be of paramount importance. As populations increase in number and age, competition for the resources available for disease management will intensify. Health policy makers are demanding evidence of the *value* of therapies in terms of reducing human suffering and improving productivity and quality of life. There is increasing effort to compare the value of different disease-management protocols and to compare the value to society of management of various diseases.

With glaucoma, we lack generally accepted screening mechanisms, management protocols, and even definitions of the disease. Thus, it is difficult to use our literature to support investment by countries in early recognition and treatment of glaucoma, as shown by the following quote from the *Journal of Medical Screening*: "National screening programs probably cannot be justified at present given difficulties with test validity, manpower, and some doubts about the natural history of the disease. The situation could change with an improved test with greater validity for primary screening" [1].

Cost effectiveness of screening for primary open angle glaucoma. Boivin JF; McGregor M; Archer C

Canadian Task Force on Periodic Health Evaluation

Benefits = reduction in prevalence of blindness

Assumptions: 75 % Screened and compliant; Rx 50 % effective

Scenario 1: 40-79 yaers, IOP & ON q3y & VF PRN
Scenario 2: 65-79 years, Same; finds 81 % of 1
Scenario 3: 65-79 years, IOP only; finds 59 % of 1

Initial screen T & ON = $25
Confirmation Exam = $45
Treatment = $270 per person per year

J Med Screen, 3(3): 154-63 1996

Fig. 1. Cost effectiveness of screening for primary open angle glaucoma, I. (From [1])

Cost effectiveness of screening for primary open angle glaucoma. Boivin JF; McGregor M; Archer C

Cost per year of blindness prevented:

Scenario 1: $75,000
Scenario 2: $31,000
Scenario 3: $27,000

Heart transplant per year of life prolonged = $10,500
Breast CA Screen per year of life saved = $3,400

"Cost effectiveness ... not competitive"

This study is based on Canadian costs stated in US Dollars.
Costs vary considerably by country

J Med Screen, 3(3): 154-63 1996

Fig. 2. Cost effectiveness of screening for primary open angle glaucoma, II. (This study is based on Canadian costs stated in US dollars. Costs vary considerably by country.) (From [1])

Studies using assumptions derived from the ophthalmic literature imply that the cost of detecting and treating glaucoma is more per year of vision saved than the cost per year of life saved by heart transplants or breast-cancer screening (Figs. 1, 2) [2]. Whether or not we believe these estimates to be accurate, they are likely to influence health policy makers. As clinicians, we are increasingly required to justify the value of what we do and to show that what we do for our patients will reduce suffering and improve their quality of life and productivity; we are also being asked to compare the value (cost/benefit) of what we do to other methods of managing the same disease, and the value to society of managing different diseases.

Lack of general agreement on the definition of glaucoma, the choice of screening methods and effective therapies causes confusion in our literature and in the minds of clinicians. Projections indicate future rapid growth of populations in less-developed countries and aging of populations in developed countries. Both situations will stress the resources available for health care. The World Health Organization estimates that there are 5.2 million people blind from glaucoma today and projects that disability from blindness will double in the next 20–25 years [3].

As advocates for our glaucoma patients and the most knowledgeable physicians dealing with this problem, it is incumbent upon us to resolve these problems by addressing them directly and quickly. As ophthalmologists of the world, we have several challenges facing us. First, we must agree on common definitions and staging of this disease. Second, we must identify a cost-effective screening method to identify treatable cases. Third, we must agree on cost-effective ways to manage this disease.

As scientists, we are required to be skeptical. It is important that we continue to question, to never be satisfied with partial answers, to insist on confirmation and to rigorously debate each and every new concept. As scientists, we seek "proof". Proof may vary by definition or need and can often be elusive [4]. Sometimes we must rely on what we "know", which may be a weaker degree of "proof" arrived at by a consensus of knowledgeable observers.

As clinicians acting on behalf of our patients, we must use what we "know" today to come to a consensus on clinical definitions and management of glaucoma so that our patients will not be denied treatments we "know" to be effective for most of them. As scientists, we should continue our skepticism and collaborate in the design and implementation of studies so that we can "know" more.

References

1. Boivin JF, McGregor M, Archer C (1996) Cost effectiveness of screening for primary open angle glaucoma. Med Screen 3:154–163
2. Wormald RP, Rauf A (1995) Glaucoma screening. Glaxo Department of Ophthalmic Epidemiology, Institute of Ophthalmology, London. J Med Screen 2:109–114
3. World Health Organization (1997) State of the World Health
4. Hoskins HD Jr (1988) Proof: an elusive ideal. Ophthalmic Surg 19:313–314

The manufacturer's authorised representative in the EU is Springer Nature Customer Service Centre GmbH, Europaplatz 3, 69115 Heidelberg, Germany. If you have any concerns regarding our products, please contact ProductSafety@springernature.com

Printed and bound by CPI Group (UK) Ltd, Croydon, CR0 4YY
29/07/2026
02180634-0005